INNOVATIONS IN CLINICAL PRACTICE: A SOURCE BOOK

Volume 2

Edited by
PETER A. KELLER, Ph.D.
LAWRENCE G. RITT, Ph.D.

PROFESSIONAL RESOURCE EXCHANGE, INC.
P.O. Box 15560
Sarasota, Florida 34277-1560

Looseleaf Edition ISBN: 0-943158-02-8
Hardbound Edition ISBN: 0-943158-03-6
Library of Congress Catalog No. 82-7614
ISSN 0737-125x

Printed in the United States of America

PREFACE

We would like to welcome you to the second volume in our **INNOVATIONS IN CLINICAL PRACTICE: A SOURCE BOOK** series. Two years ago, the idea for this series existed only in our imaginations. Therefore, it is difficult for us to believe that we have already completed the second volume and have numerous authors preparing contributions for the third volume.

The series grew out of our feeling that much of what is being currently published for clinicians has little immediate application in professional practice. Consequently, we have attempted to collect and organize the types of materials which address the practitioner's need for useful, "hands-on" information with a format designed to encourage frequent use of these materials. **INNOVATIONS** is an ongoing series of practical source books packed with information which can be copied, shared, and used in the day-to-day conduct of a professional mental health practice. Each book in the series represents the dedicated efforts of our editorial and production staff who have the challenging task of organizing the work of thirty-five to forty prominent contributors into the unified whole you see here.

We have been delighted with the reception given to Volume I during its first year of publication. Feedback from purchasers has been consistently positive and encouraging. Many clinicians apparently share our feelings about the need for such a volume, and many others have found that the volume contains useful materials for training in educational settings.

Recognizing that the volume has the potential to be an effective medium for continuing education training of clinicians, we are preparing examination modules which will allow qualified readers to obtain formal continuing education credits for home study of selected contributions. These modules will be available in a few months and interested readers are referred to the last page in this volume for purchasing information. The Professional Resource Exchange has been approved as an American Psychological Association continuing education sponsor. We are very pleased with this development and hope our readers find the prospect of formal continuing education training and credits of interest.

As with the first volume, there are a number of individuals whose efforts deserve special recognition: Denny Murray, Joel Grace, and Hal Smith for their helpful reviews and critiques; Judy Warinner and Debbie Worthington for their many hours of copy editing, proofreading, and problem-solving. We would especially like to thank our wives, Rhonda Keller and Judy Ritt, for their advice, patience, good humor, and general willingness to put up with us in spite of ourselves.

AN INVITATION TO SUBMIT A CONTRIBUTION

We are currently soliciting contributions for future volumes in the **INNOVATIONS** series as well as seeking ideas for other publications and ways to share information among practitioners. If you are doing something innovative in your work, let us hear from you. Specific guidelines for contributors are included at the end of this volume. Please feel free to contact us if you would like more detailed information.

COPYRIGHT POLICY

Most of the material in this volume may be duplicated. You may photocopy materials (such as office forms and instruments) or reproduce them for use in your practice or share contributions with your students in the classroom. For materials on which the Professional Resource Exchange holds the copyright, no further permission is required for noncommercial professional or educational use. However, unauthorized duplication or publication for resale or large scale distribution of any material in this volume is expressly forbidden.

Any material which you duplicate from this volume (with the exception mentioned below) must be acknowledged as having been reprinted from this volume and must note that copyright is held by the Professional Resource Exchange, Inc. The format and exact wording required in that acknowledgment are shown on the copyright page of this volume. The only exception to this policy is that clinical and office forms (not instruments) for use with clients may be reprinted without including the acknowledgment mentioned above.

There are exceptions to our liberal copyright policy. We do not hold copyright on some of the materials included in this volume and, therefore, cannot grant permission to freely duplicate those materials. When copyright is held by another publisher or author, such copyright is noted on the appropriate page of the contribution. Unless otherwise noted in the credit and copyright citation, any reproduction or duplication of these materials is strictly and expressly forbidden without the consent of the copyright holder.

Peter A. Keller
Lawrence G. Ritt

Professional Resource Exchange, Inc.
Post Office Box 15560
Sarasota, Florida 34277-1560

TABLE OF CONTENTS

SECTION II: PRACTICE MANAGEMENT AND PROFESSIONAL DEVELOPMENT

SECTION III: ASSESSMENT INSTRUMENTS AND OFFICE FORMS

SECTION IV: COMMUNITY INTERVENTIONS

SECTION V: SELECTED TOPICS

INTRODUCTION TO THE VOLUME

This is the second volume in the **INNOVATIONS IN CLINICAL PRACTICE** series and the organization is essentially the same as Volume I. Materials are grouped into five basic sections which reflect the diversity of material contained in the volume and allow for rapid access to the desired contributions.

The first section, ISSUES AND APPLICATIONS, deals broadly with therapeutic concerns. The various contributions are designed, however, to go beyond traditional therapeutic approaches and also address major issues in assessment and treatment with families and individuals suffering from certain behavioral disorders.

The second section addresses PRACTICE MANAGEMENT and includes several basic articles which will be of interest primarily to the clinician or consultant in private practice. We have included this material because of our perception that a growing number of clinicians work independently and need a source of current information on practice management and related professional issues. Many of the articles will also be of interest to students and those who practice in organizational or agency settings.

The third section includes ASSESSMENT INSTRUMENTS AND OFFICE FORMS. The assessment instruments are, for the most part, informal and designed to assist the clinician in the collection of information about clients. Our intention has been to publish screening instruments and forms to assist in the organization of data, rather than more formal psychological tests. There are some exceptions to this rule in the section, but we felt the publication of these instruments would be of use to readers, with minimal potential for misuse by the professionals who purchase the volume. The office forms included here could in no way be described as instruments but should be of interest to practitioners. We have grouped them here for utilitarian reasons.

The fourth section on COMMUNITY INTERVENTIONS reflects our belief that mental health practitioners have much to offer in the community beyond their clinical services. While preventive interventions which appeal to clinicians have been slow to develop, the community orientation has had an important impact on the mental health field, and we would like to encourage this. We hope this section may be of some assistance to those who wish to become more involved in the community.

The fifth section on SELECTED TOPICS includes various contributions we felt were important to include in the **INNOVATIONS** volume but which did not fit clearly into one of the other four sections. The contents range from several useful informational handouts for clients to a valuable collection of structured group exercises. We plan to retain this section in future volumes to accommodate contributions which do not fit neatly into one of the other categories but which we believe would be of value to our readers.

At the end of the volume, we have included information on submitting a contribution to the **INNOVATIONS** series and information with an order blank for the purchase of our Continuing Education modules.

INTRODUCTION TO SECTION I: CLINICAL ISSUES AND APPLICATIONS

The ISSUES AND APPLICATIONS section includes contributions which primarily relate to treatment. There is no other unifying theme intended, and the range of topics is quite broad. We view this section as a means for the experienced practitioner to keep up to date with newer techniques.

Several of the articles address family-oriented interventions. These range from Kaslow's discussion of divorce therapy to the structured, skill-oriented approaches for marital therapy outlined by Bernard Guerney and the innovative use of parents as therapists addressed by Louise Guerney. Levy's contribution presents a practical, eclectic orientation to family therapy which should interest the reader or student who is not yet an experienced family practitioner.

In recent years there has been a developing technology for dealing with many behavioral problems. We have included here articles which address sleep disorders, enuresis, and several problems which have proven amenable to treatment with biofeedback. Each of the articles provides practical suggestions for, or examples of, effective treatment strategies. For instance, in the area of sleep disorders, Hauri and Proeger have presented information on the major disorders about which all therapists should have at least basic knowledge, since certain disorders can be life threatening.

In grouping these articles here, we are not suggesting that every clinician should be competent to administer the various assessment procedures or the techniques of treatment indicated. It is, however, important for practitioners to be knowledgeable about these issues so they can more effectively define the boundaries of their practice and make appropriate referrals that are in the interest of their clients.

STAGES AND TECHNIQUES OF DIVORCE THERAPY

Florence W. Kaslow

All statistics in the last decade and a half have shown divorce to be a rapidly spiraling phenomenon. Whether work is cited that sets the figures at 33% or at 50% (both rates are bandied about), clearly the magnitude of the situation is great. Despite the fact that in many social circles the stigma of divorce has diminished as divorce laws have been liberalized and the frequency of marital dissolution has escalated, the traumatic impact of divorce does not seem to be lessened on the individuals who experience it. Also, a ripple effect occurs, profoundly affecting all members of the nuclear family and at least some of the family of origin of the separating spouses (Kaslow & Hyatt, 1981; Spanier & Hanson, 1981).

Although marital counseling began in a formalized way in the late 1930's and writings about family therapy began to appear in the professional literature in the early 1950's (Kaslow, 1980), the concept of divorce therapy as a substantive aspect of marital and family therapy did not begin to be discussed in the literature until about the mid-1970's. Some of the attention riveted on the impact of divorce upon children (Gardner, 1976; Hetherington, Cox, & Cox, 1977; Kessler & Bostwick, 1977) and some on the adult's readjustment and re-entry into the singles' world (e.g., Froiland & Hozman, 1977; Hyatt, 1977; Kessler, 1975; Krantzler, 1974). Recognition of the special plight of couples who divorce, the impact on their children and their families of origin, and correspondingly, recognition that many mental health professionals did not have a conceptual framework for understanding the dynamics and trauma of the divorce process nor training in effective intervention strategies, led Esther Fisher, a New York based therapist-educator also trained in law, to found the JOURNAL OF DIVORCE, first published in 1977. The advent of this journal and the growing number of articles, chapters, and full books on divorce related topics published since 1977 (e.g., Fisher, 1981; Kaslow, 1979/80; Kaslow & Steinberg, 1982; Stuart & Abt, 1981; Wallerstein & Kelly, 1979, 1980) are indicative of the fact that mental health and social service professionals have finally acknowledged the divorced individuals' needs for attention and assistance and begun to concentrate their knowledge and skill on dealing with those affected by the divorce process.

Given the fact that a rising percentage of patients seen in public and private clinical practice are members of divorcing, divorced, or remarriage families, I was asked to focus this contribution on the practical aspects of divorce therapy. I will do this within the "diaclectic" conceptual framework which I have been evolving since 1977.

THE DIACLECTIC MODEL OF DIVORCE THERAPY

The term diaclectic was first coined to convey the fact that this paradigm draws **eclectically** from a variety of sources on behavior dynamics and stage theory, and seeks a dynamic, **dialectic** synthesis of what is known of the emotions experienced, actions exhibited, and tasks to be accomplished during the divorce process if reasonably successful resolution is to be achieved (Kaslow, 1979/80). Eclectic and dialectic were merged into diaclectic as a confabulated, yet simplified labeling word (Kaslow, 1981a, 1981b).

What type of intervention is selected as the keystone of the treatment is contingent upon a clear understanding of where the patient(s) is in the divorce process sequence. Thus, a brief summation of two of the main stage theories of the divorce process, interwoven with some personal comments, will be given as a backdrop against which to view therapeutic strategies. Those interventions which have proven most effective in my clinical practice and which other clinicians elaborate as valuable in their writings, will be discussed in relation to each stage - what is transpiring when, and what will help reduce the pain and chaos and maximize each involved person's capacity for fruitful living. My own current philosophical orientation is a blend of psychodynamic object-relations and humanistic-existential theory; clinically the therapeutic approach utilizes analytic, gestalt, structural, strategic, family of origin, contextual, and behavioral techniques, depending on the presenting problem, personality dynamics, ego strength, and stage in the life cycle and divorce process (Kaslow, 1981a). In many ways, it is closely akin to Lazarus' multimodal approach (Lazarus, 1981). All of this will be later integrated and incorporated in Table 1.

Bohannon (1973) clearly articulates a six "station" process. He emphasizes that, on both the individual and societal levels, the usual way of coping with devastating traumas such as divorce is to first try denial and hope the terrible problem will disappear. When this does not occur, the reality of the situation is slowly allowed into consciousness where it can gradually be accommodated. The stations do not occur as an invariant sequence, nor is the intensity the same at each phase or for all people. Inevitably, each stage must be experienced and its tasks mastered before a new equilibrium is established.

Emotional divorce is, in Bohannon's schema, the first station. During this period, the pair become increasingly aware of their disenchantment and dissatisfaction with one another, sense that their relationship is deteriorating, and may begin to distrust each other. One or both become disillusioned about the marriage being viable and worth keeping; they become critical and harp on the negative features of the spouse and the marriage.

The seeds of this dissatisfaction can be deeply sown. It can occur as an outgrowth of a long-standing and cherished childhood fantasy, nourished by fairy tales and motion pictures, that one will grow up, meet Prince Charming or Beautiful Princess, fall in love, be awakened sexually by the lover's kiss, and get married and ride off into the beautiful distance to "live happily ever after." Or, coming from an unhappy, abusive, or depriving household, one may enter marriage yearning for a second chance to be cared for and nurtured, craving parenting more than the reciprocal give and take of a healthy adult peer relationship. If either of these scenarios predate the marriage and the unrealistic dreams remain present during the early years of marriage, disappointment and anger are the inevitable consequences when the needs continue to be unmet and the spouse feels cheated and unloved. When the deficiency needs are tremendous (Maslow, 1962, 1968), clinging-pouting or more demanding spouses may be expecting their mates to be not only parents but also best friends, lovers, confidantes, helpmates, playmates, limit setters, and protectors all rolled into one, and capable of discerning which role to assume to harmonize with their mood of the hour. Such inordinate demands leave the caretaker spouse depleted and frustrated. In therapy they often say, and quite accurately, "Nothing I do is enough. It seems like a bottomless pit." The helplessness and dependency, originally great attractions, turn into infuriating deficits. The grandiosity and authoritative manner which was exciting or engendered feelings of security deteriorates into a pompous and repetitious litany of promises never delivered.

Sometimes the early years go quite well, and conflict does not evolve until much later. Since, at any given period of time, people choose exactly the kind of person they most need, consciously and unconsciously, a relationship capable of surviving is most likely one with a solid balance between symmetrical and complementary elements (Pollock, Kaslow, & Harvey, 1982), and in which the partners agree that they should communicate openly, conveying clearly how they think and feel and what they want, and listening attentively and responsively to each other. In addition, some agreement to negotiate important differences and accept each one's right to privacy and being his or her own person as well as part of a couple is probably essential (Sager, 1976). Where these ingredients are not threads of the marital tapestry, the changes which inevitably occur as individuals grow in their life experiences are likely to disrupt the homeostatic balance, particularly if one grows while the other seems to stagnate, or if each grows but in incompatible directions. Problems related to the external environment, like job loss or job relocation, financial difficulties, death of a parent or child, sexual dysfunction or disinterest, a severe injury, or other major life crises can place the couple under extreme stress for which they may blame each other, causing the relationship to become intolerable. Any one or a combination of the above factors can lead to sufficient disenchantment and unhappiness, and ultimately to the emotional divorce. Kessler (1975), who presents a seven stage model, labels Stages I and II disillusionment and erosion, respectively. These are both inherent in the emotional divorce.

It is during this period that the partner who does not want the divorce, the one who is very discontent but ambivalent about the idea of divorce and all of its implications, may seek therapy. At this point, marital therapy should be seriously considered. Research indicates that couples who enter marital therapy are more likely to repair and improve their marriage (since the emphasis is on what is good for the couple as a unit as well as for each partner) than those in which one or both go into individual therapy (Whitaker & Miller, 1969).

PREDIVORCE STAGES IN THERAPY

In marital therapy, each of the member's complaints, criticism, and disappointments should be heard first. Such ventilation provides some relief, at least temporarily, and gives them a chance to put the sources of conflict out in the open in order to begin assessing and seeking solutions.

Meanwhile, the therapist can evaluate the couple and each individual (their strengths and weaknesses, quality of relationship, willingness to change, wellsprings of anger, whether the relationship is triangulated and, if so, with whom, sexual expression of the difficulty, personality integration). Asking partners to recount how they met, the basis of their attraction, and what positives still remain may enable them to break through the excessive negativism and realize that, despite the shattered dreams, they still care about one another and want to work at building or rebuilding a more solid relationship. Alternately, one or both may have feelings of being trapped and really be requesting help in extricating from the no longer wanted marriage. The therapist gets caught in a dilemma when one wants to save the marriage (and may even threaten suicide if the other leaves) and the other wants to dissolve the union. It is ultimately the client's decision; however, the therapist can help them explore the consequences of both choices, can suggest temporary alternatives like a trial separation, and help them move toward feeling each has a part in the decision making. If one is determined to leave, then the therapist's role may shift to helping the partner who feels spurned and victimized take charge of planning his or her own future and enabling both of them to make divorcing as constructive an experience as possible.

Couples Groups. Short term couples group therapy is another efficacious approach at this point. Because of space limitations here, just a brief highlighting of this modality must suffice. (The interested reader is referred to Kaslow, 1981c, and Kaslow and Lieberman, 1981, for greater explication of this approach.) I prefer working with a group of five couples, all of whom are experiencing marital turmoil and none of whom have a member who diagnostically falls into either the severe psychotic or personality disorder categories (APA, 1980). Each couple is first seen separately, and we jointly determine whether single couple or couples group therapy is likely to constitute the treatment of choice for them. If they find the idea of group therapy intriguing and I think they are good candidates, a contract is signed in which they both agree to attend 12 weekly sessions. Fulfilling the contract and terminating on time are crucial aspects, since most participants have not experienced others keeping their word or holding them accountable for commitments. Because dependence-independence is customarily the main theme that emerges in this psychoanalytically oriented, closed end, short-term group, the couple rapidly focuses on the need for connectedness with and separateness from each other, their children, siblings, and parents. Through the group process, members become mirrors for one another, reflecting back what they see, and to confront each other's blind spots and rationalizations (Kaslow, 1982). Healthy attachment, closeness, and individuation are supported; however, group members point out and challenge symbiotic clinging and retreating into silence as a defense against intimacy.

Since the usual pattern is to have a heterosexual cotherapy pair as leaders, they also: (a) can structure their interventions to serve as role models for male-female interaction and constructive problem resolution; (b) function as parent substitutes from whom members can derive some nurturing, reducing the demands on the spouse and coming to the realization that no one person can or should be expected to provide for all of their caretaking and gratification; (c) serve as parent surrogates against whom participants can ventilate some of their anger and distress, deflecting the stress from the marriage and enabling them to have a breathing space in which to enjoy each other; (d) convey their belief that some of the problems predate the marriage and need to be worked through with each spouse's family of origin; and (e) communicate their belief that the couple is capable of deciding whether they prefer to stay together and improve their marriage, with each taking responsibility for his or her own change process, or whether they will ultimately fare better if they agree to separate, planning to do so in a way that will increase their self-esteem and respect rather than be demeaning. The preset time frame provides a useful structure for the group; since they have a limited time to work on the problems which propelled them into group therapy, they become more focused and learn techniques for problem resolution and decision making.

Couples group therapy is a lively, interesting modality that patients report finding extremely enlightening. It helps free up bound energy as they stop clinging to past hurts and quarrels and making excessive demands on each other and, instead, begin to create a larger resource network for fulfillment and enjoyment. It is also interesting and fun for the therapists!

Those couples who recognize and resolve the difficulties during Stage I, either with or without therapy, tend not to move on to the next phase. The prognosis is fairly good for their marriage at this point, and divorce therapy per se is not required.

Just as Kessler calls her Stage II erosion, I see a second phase of the predivorce period as a time of despair when the realization hits that the marriage is in severe jeopardy. It is a time of extreme ambivalence, wavering between denial, a pretense that everything is fine, and attempting to win back the spouse's affection. Feelings of dread, chaos, confusion, inadequacy, and failure are prominent. Often one or the other may turn to family, friends, or clergy to entreat or pressure the spouse who wants to leave into staying. If they have been in marital therapy, one partner may no longer be willing to be seen in tandem. Individual therapy might well be in order here to help one deal with feelings of rejection and failure and the other with guilt over breaking up the marriage and hurting the spouse (or even for feeling relief that the nightmare may soon be ended).

THERAPY DURING DIVORCE

This period merges into Bohannon's second and third stations, the legal and economic divorce, when one or both parties seek legal counsel. Today, with the advent of divorce mediation (Coogler, 1978; Haynes, 1981), individuals who want to maximize their own input into the final agreement regarding custody and property distribution, and who dislike the prospect of litigation, are turning to this alternative form of dispute resolution. If they can decide to cooperate and seek a solution that attempts to embody what is likely to be in the "best interest" of everyone involved, then this period may be one in which they feel empowered to make their own choices and feel increasing self-respect as they exercise their own judgment and take responsibility for refashioning their own lives.

If adversarial proceedings are the route pursued, then the litigants are more likely to feel helpless, pessimistic, detached, and depressed since the negotiating is largely in the hands of the attorneys and the decisions regarding custody, parental responsibility, and partitioning of the assets rests with the judge. There is a great deal of anxiety emanating from uncertainty. From the admixture of confusion, loneliness, sadness, and grief over all the losses entailed in the break up of the marriage and family, vindictiveness may well become a factor. The distribution of valued possessions, purchased or inherited as part of their dream of a fine life together, is a painful experience. Prolonged quarreling may represent unwillingness to let go of the last remnants of the union. Kessler (1975) designates Stage III as detachment, Stage IV as physical separation, and Stage V as mourning. On the master chart which appears in Table 1, these are interwoven with Bohannon's Station 2 and 3 and my discussion of feelings and tasks.

Invariably, I work from a theoretical stance of a family systems perspective, although often I will see subsystems or individual members of the system-in-flux, and I believe this is the most comprehensive and illuminating perspective for the divorce therapist (Isaacs, 1981). In this context, when the decision to separate has been made, it is often advisable to work with the couple around how they have been handling feelings and developments with the children, and what needs to be done now. The therapist can help them understand the powerful impact of their actions on the children and indicate that the nature of their adjustment will correlate with the children's adjustment (Wallerstein & Kelly, 1980). The children's needs to have access to both parents, to feel both parents continue to love them and be actively interested in them, to remain loyal to both and not be torn between them, and their right not to hear either parent denigrate the other (Bodin, 1982) should be highlighted. If the couple cannot be in conjoint sessions, and with dissolution of marriage their goal, it may be more valid to have separate sessions at this stage. The words "may be" are critical since, in some instances, this is a time for family sessions, including the children, so that feelings and wishes can be aired openly in the therapist's safe sanctuary, and all can have a say in shaping the evolving two single parent families. Sometimes, if the couples' parents are unduly pressuring them to make or alter a decision and they cannot contend with it alone, this is an appropriate occasion for a multigenerational, family of origin session with each of their respective parents and siblings. In addition, since the children may well need total attention and empathy and caring from a therapist, individual child therapy may well be in order (with play therapy an important modality so they can act out the turmoil, hostility, and longings). Art therapy integrated into verbal psychotherapy also enables children and adolescents to draw out their internal conflicts, some of which they have great difficulty articulating. This can also provide the therapist with a better diagnostic understanding, an additional avenue through which to establish a therapeutic alliance, and a multipronged way of treating.

For Bohannon, the fourth station is entitled "coparental divorce and the problems of custody." In my paradigm, this is included in the "during divorce" stage and is closely intertwined with the legal and economic divorce since often what is labeled a custody battle revolves around financial considerations. It is important for divorce therapists to be cognizant of the laws in their state regarding divorce (whether it is fault or no fault, the accrual of time for the required waiting period and when that begins to be calculated, how likely a temporary agreement is to become permanent) and child custody (whether there is a preference for joint custody, joint parental custody, or a sole noncustodial arrangement), and what kind of guidance clients may be receiving from their mediator or attorney. It may be important for the therapist using any reality oriented, here and now approach, to make clear his or her own value stance (Abroms, 1978) regarding a "best interest of the child" position and emotional considerations that are at least as important and long lasting as financial ones. Children often seem neglected in the "during divorce" stage when their parents are so tense, hurt, and volatile, and energies are being directed toward physically and financially separating, quarreling over provisos of the agreement, or perhaps taking on additional jobs to handle the economic drain. There may be little time or energy left for the children and little sensitivity to their bewilderment and pain. Conversely, some parents become overly possessive, protective, and intrusive, trying to shield their children from additional anguish or feelings of desertion, or trying to make them an ally against the other parent. For children at this time, group therapy with other children of divorce is a valuable approach. The therapist can create an environment where they can ventilate their sorrow, explore their feelings, gain understanding of the crises, derive support from each other through being with a sympathetic group of peers and a gentle, caring adult, and consider options for handling the difficult situations they are likely to confront. Kessler and Bostwick (1977) vividly describe the "how to" for children's groups. This may also be valuable in the post-divorce stage for children who still have many unresolved issues to deal with but do not wish to do so when parents are present.

POST-DIVORCE ISSUES

As the legal divorce is nearing completion, the kind of support system the individual has is a critical factor. Do they have family to help them with their concerns and to fill the lonely void? What about friends? Are they accessible or does the divorce impinge on friends' religious convictions or threaten their own marriages. Bohannon labels his fifth station "community divorce and the problem of loneliness." Bach (1974) suggests that some kind of divorce ceremony helps facilitate closure. For the most part (except for Orthodox Judaism which has traditionally performed a religious divorce ceremony using a tribunal of three Rabbis to convey sanction of the marital dissolution), there has until very recently been a deficit of ceremonies or rituals to help mark and ease the divorce transition. For patients who need something specific and are religiously oriented, therapists can encourage them to talk to their clergyman about creating a special service (Kaslow, 1981b). Because of the dearth of community support, support groups like Parents Without Partners arose. Later, social agencies and churches began running groups for divorced adults, and the combined social-educational and support emphasis is appealing to many. It offers an alternative to the bar scene as a way of meeting people and serves as one of the passageways in the post-divorce period.

Once the divorce is finalized, the two new family units begin to function. Visitation should slowly smooth out, new identities begin to be forged, and the adults re-enter the larger world. The rhythm which characterizes "letting go" of the past marriage and becoming involved anew or differently in work, recreation, and social activities, is a very individual matter. The therapist must respect the person's individual tempo. It may be slow paced, as when the person is allowing the grieving process to be completed and getting the family and home reordered before entering into new relationships; or fast paced, as when he or she plunges into the social whirl to find excitement, prove sexual appeal and prowess, or as an antidote to loneliness. There is no one right way during the aftermath. If he or she is still extremely emotional, the therapist can help the person cognitively reframe and restructure perceptions and his or her new life. Conversely, if the individual is utilizing intellectualization as the main defensive mechanism against allowing his or

TABLE 1: DIACLECTIC MODEL OF STAGES IN THE DIVORCE PROCESS

Divorce Stage	Station	Stage	Feelings	Actions and Tasks	Therapeutic Interventions
Predivorce A time of deliberation and despair	1. Emotional Divorce	I	Disillusionment Dissatisfaction Alienation Anxiety Disbelief	Avoiding the issue Sulking and/or crying Confronting partner Quarreling	Marital therapy (one couple) Couples group therapy
		II	Despair Dread Anguish Ambivalence Shock Emptiness Anger Chaos Inadequacy Low self-esteem Loss	Denial Withdrawal (physical and emotional) Pretending all is okay Attempting to win back affection Asking friends, family, clergy for advice	Marital therapy (one couple) Divorce therapy Couples group therapy
During Divorce A time of legal involvement	2. Legal Divorce	III	Depressed Detached Angry Hopelessness Self-pity Helplessness	Bargaining Screaming Threatening Attempting suicide Consulting an attorney or mediator	Family therapy Individual adult therapy Child therapy
	3. Economic Divorce	IV	Confusion Fury Sadness	Separating physically Filing for legal divorce Considering economic arrangements Considering custody arrangements	Children of divorce group therapy Child therapy Adult therapy

TABLE 1: DIACLECTIC MODEL OF STAGES IN THE DIVORCE PROCESS (CONT.)

Divorce Stage	Station	Stage	Feelings	Actions and Tasks	Therapeutic Interventions
During Divorce (Cont.)	4. Coparental Divorce and the Problems of Custody	V	Loneliness Relief Vindictiveness	Grieving and mourning Telling relatives and friends Re-entering work world (unemployed woman) Feeling empowered to make choices	Children of divorce group therapy Child therapy Adult therapy
	5. Community Divorce and the Problems of Loneliness	VI	Indecisiveness Optimism Resignation Excitement Curiosity Regret Sadness	Finalizing divorce Begin reaching out to new friends Undertaking new activities Stabilizing new life style and daily routine for children Exploring new interests and possibly taking new job	Adults individual therapy singles group therapy Children child play therapy childrens' group therapy
Post-divorce A time of exploration and re-equilibrium	6. Psychic Divorce	VII	Acceptance Self-confidence Energetic Self-worth Wholeness Exhilaration Independence Autonomy	Resynthesis of identity Completing psychic divorce Seeking new love object and making a commitment to some permanency Becoming comfortable with new life style and friends Helping children accept finality of parents' divorce and their continuing relationship with both parents	Parent-child therapy Family therapy Group therapies Childrens' activity group therapy

her feelings into consciousness, the therapist probably should help the person get in touch with the various emotions buried within. As some balance is achieved between the affective and cognitive states, the individual can make sounder decisions about what actions to take.

For many, the immediate post-divorce period is one of exploration of the inner world as well as the outer environment (trying out new activities, pursuing interests that have been dormant or which have arisen as appealing, returning to school, re-entering or changing jobs, and building new social relationships or changing existing ones). It is exciting, liberating, and stimulating. Individual or group therapy of divorced, single-again individuals can provide the "permission" to enjoy the pleasures of this heady new world and help them evolve the values and structure that will channel their pursuits. It can also assist them in learning to juggle the myriad aspects of their life (parent, friend, lover, worker, student, child's chauffeur and helper with homework, homemaker) and mobilize their energy and optimism to utilize the opportunities inherent in their complex life.

For others it continues as a prolonged period of reactive depression, a time of unabated anger, desire for revenge, and a sense of hopelessness and helplessness. Those in this category are the ones most likely to malign their former mates, try to influence their children against their former spouses, indulge in self-pity, and become "stuck" around the divorce as the most critical event in their lives. For them, individual therapy to work through the anger, to accept their own contribution to the marital discord and its eventual dissolution, to alleviate the depression and to extricate the children from unhealthy bonding or becoming parentified, might well be in order. Only then can they, like the former group, complete what Bohannon calls the sixth station or "psychic divorce."

Kessler indicates that most divorcees pass through a second adolescence, which equates with what I have talked about as the time of exploration. Given their life experience, and often the fact of their parenthood and maturity, I do not find that everyone who re-enters the single world "regresses" into an adolescent way of relating. Some are healthy adults whose ability to be creative and playful is reawakened (Maslow, 1968) as they attempt to "make up for lost time" (Hyatt, 1977). Hard work (Kessler, 1975) is essential as the person continues to resolve the psychic trauma and then re-equilibrates into a wholesome new integration that expresses his or her new identity and values in decisions and behaviors and takes full responsibility for the direction of his or her life (Kaslow, 1981b). Only after this occurs are most people ready to and capable of entering into a long term committed relationship or able to decide that they prefer being single and alone for the foreseeable future.

Table 1 on the preceding pages summarizes the above in a chart form to recapitulate and interrelate.

SUMMARY

This article has been written from a combined family systems and stage theory of development perspective. It suggests that the choice of what kind of therapy is likely to be most efficient and most efficacious in any given situation should be determined by assessing in which stage in the divorce process clients are when they seek treatment, their ego strength, cognitive functioning, and resources. It is predicated on an assumption of flexibility in the therapist's own style and philosophic orientation to either encompass modalities that are valid in the different stages (rather than rigid adherence to one purist truth) or to refer patients to someone else who is likely to be more skilled. It recommends a dynamic, diaclectic paradigm of divorce theory and therapy, culled from various theoretical schools as clinicians of different disciplines and orientations pool their hypotheses, hunches, experiences, observations, and research findings to assist people in the community at large and in their patient populations to navigate through the divorce process.

Florence W. Kaslow, Ph.D., is currently in private practice as a clinical and forensic psychologist and is Director of the Florida Couples and Family Institute in West Palm Beach, Florida. She is also a (Visiting) Adjunct Professor of Family Studies at Duke University Department of Psychiatry, Durham, North Carolina. She has published a number of books and articles on divorce and family therapy. Dr. Kaslow may be reached at Northwood Medical Center, 2617 North Flagler Drive, West Palm Beach, FL 33407.

RESOURCES

Abroms, G. The place of values in psychotherapy. JOURNAL OF MARRIAGE AND FAMILY COUNSELING, 1978, **4**(4), 3-18.

American Psychiatric Association. DIAGNOSTIC AND STATISTICAL MANUAL OF MENTAL DISORDERS (DSM III). Washington, DC: APA, 1980.

Bach, G. R. Creative exits: Fight therapy for divorcees. In V. Frank & V. Burtle (Eds.), WOMEN IN THERAPY: NEW PSYCHOTHERAPIES FOR A CHANGING SOCIETY. New York: Brunner/Mazel, 1974.

Bodin, A. M. Explaining divorce to children. In P. A. Keller & L. G. Ritt (Eds.), INNOVATIONS IN CLINICAL PRACTICE: A SOURCE BOOK (Vol. 1). Sarasota, FL: Professional Resource Exchange, 1982.

Bohannon, P. The six stations of divorce. In M. E. Lasswell & T. E. Laswell (Eds.), LOVE, MARRIAGE AND FAMILY: A DEVELOPMENTAL APPROACH. Glenview, IL: Scott, Foresman and Company, 1973.

Coogler, O. J. STRUCTURED MEDIATION IN DIVORCE SETTLEMENT. Lexington, MA: Lexington Books, 1978.

Fisher, B. REBUILDING WHEN YOUR RELATIONSHIP ENDS. San Luis Obispo, CA: Impact, 1981.

Froiland, D. J. & Hozman, T. L. Counseling for constructive divorce. PERSONNEL AND GUIDANCE JOURNAL, 1977, **55**, 525-529.

Gardner, R. PSYCHOTHERAPY WITH CHILDREN OF DIVORCE. New York: Jason Aronson, 1976.

Haynes, J. DIVORCE MEDIATION. New York: Springer, 1981.

Hetherington, E. M., Cox, M., & Cox, R. The aftermath of divorce. In J. H. Stevens, Jr. & M. Mathews (Eds.), MOTHER-CHILD, FATHER-CHILD RELATIONS. Washington, DC: NAEYC, 1977.

Hyatt, I. R. BEFORE YOU MARRY AGAIN. New York: Random House, 1977.

Isaacs, M. Treatment for families of divorce: A systems model perspective. In I. R. Stuart & L. E. Abt (Eds.), CHILDREN OF SEPARATION AND DIVORCE. New York: Van Nostrand Reinhold, 1981.

Kaslow, F. W. A diaclectic approach to family therapy and practice: Selectivity and synthesis. JOURNAL OF MARITAL AND FAMILY THERAPY, 1981, **6**(3), 345-351. (a) (Reprinted in FOCUS PA FAMILIEN in Norwegian, 1982, **10**(2), 60-66.)

Kaslow, F. W. Divorce and divorce therapy. In A. S. Gurman & D. P. Kniskern (Eds.), HANDBOOK OF FAMILY THERAPY. New York: Brunner/Mazel, 1981. (b)

Kaslow, F. W. Group therapy with couples in conflict. AUSTRALIAN JOURNAL OF FAMILY THERAPY, July 1982, **3**(4), 199-204.

Kaslow, F. W. Group therapy with couples in conflict: Is more better? PSYCHOTHERAPY: THEORY, RESEARCH AND PRACTICE, 1981, **18**(4), 516-524. (c)

Kaslow, F. W. History of family therapy in the United States: A kaleidoscopic overview. MARRIAGE AND FAMILY REVIEW. Spring/Summer 1980, **3**(1/2), 77-111.

Kaslow, F. W. Stages of divorce: A psychological perspective. VILLANOVA LAW REVIEW, 1979/80, **25**(4/5), 7/8-751.

Kaslow, F. W. & Hyatt, R. Divorce: A potential growth experience for the extended family. JOURNAL OF DIVORCE, (special issue "Impact of Divorce on the Extended Family"), 1981, **5**(1/2), 115-126.

Kaslow, F. W. & Lieberman, E. J. Couples group therapy: Rationale, dynamics and process. In P. Sholevar (Ed.), HANDBOOK OF MARRIAGE AND MARITAL THERAPY. New York: SP Medical and Scientific Books, 1981.

Kaslow, F. W. & Steinberg, J. L. Ethical divorce therapy and divorce proceedings. In L. L'Abate (Ed.), VALUES, ETHICS, LEGALITIES AND THE FAMILY THERAPIST. Rockville, MD: Aspen Publications, 1982.

Kessler, S. THE AMERICAN WAY OF DIVORCE: PRESCRIPTION FOR CHANGE. Chicago: Nelson Hall, 1975.

Kessler, S. & Bostwick, S. Beyond divorce: Coping skills for children. JOURNAL OF CLINICAL CHILD PSYCHOLOGY, 1977, **6**, 38-41.

Krantzler, M. CREATIVE DIVORCE. New York: M. Evans, 1974.

Lazarus, A. THE PRACTICE OF MULTI-MODAL THERAPY. New York: McGraw Hill, 1981.

Maslow, A. TOWARD A PSYCHOLOGY OF BEING. New York: Van Nostrand, 1962, 1968.

Pollack, S., Kaslow, N. J., & Harvey, D. Symmetry, complementary and depression: The evolution of an hypothesis. In F. W. Kaslow (Ed.), THE INTERNATIONAL BOOK OF FAMILY THERAPY. New York: Brunner/Mazel, 1982.

Sager, C. J. MARRIAGE CONTRACTS AND COUPLE THERAPY: HIDDEN FORCES IN INTIMATE RELATIONSHIPS. New York: Brunner/Mazel, 1976.

Spanier, G. B. & Hanson, S. The role of extended kin in the adjustment to marital separation. JOURNAL OF DIVORCE, 1981, **5**(1/2), 33-48.

Stuart, I. R. & Abt, L. E. CHILDREN OF SEPARATION AND DIVORCE: MANAGEMENT AND TREATMENT. New York: Van Nostrand Reinhold, 1981.

Wallerstein, J. S. & Kelly, J. B. Divorce and children. In J. D. Noshpitz (Ed.), HANDBOOK OF CHILD PSYCHIATRY IV. New York: Basic Books, 1979.

Wallerstein, J. S. & Kelly, J. B. SURVIVING THE BREAKUP: HOW CHILDREN AND PARENTS COPE WITH DIVORCE. New York: Basic Books, 1980.

Whitaker, C. A. & Miller, M. H. A re-evaluation of "psychiatric help" when divorce impends. AMERICAN JOURNAL OF PSYCHIATRY, 1969, **126**, 57-64.

NEUROPSYCHOLOGICAL SCREENING

Susan B. Filskov

Neuropsychological screening is needed to evaluate large numbers of psychiatric and general medical patient referrals in a cost-effective manner. Typically, patients are referred for neuropsychological testing when the evaluator, through the past history, present behavior, or soft neurological signs, suspects that central nervous system processing difficulties may be contributing to difficulties in psychological and daily functioning. With so many patients in psychiatric settings where these questions are raised, an entire six-hour evaluation cannot be given to everyone. However, a neuropsychological screening may be conducted for intact persons in about an hour by an examiner with general clinical skills. The findings then dictate whether further evaluation is warranted. This contribution will cover some of the underlying issues that need to be addressed while conducting such screening procedures and outline a basic screening battery which covers the primary areas of cognitive functioning.

The battery should be able to provide information about general questions of diagnosis, deterioration, patients' strengths and weaknesses, and a data base for additional long-term comparisons. Such a battery should be comprehensive in the sense that a variety of cognitive functions are measured. A range of tasks from very simple sensory-motor skills to more complex abilities in problem solving and new learning are covered. The testing should include tasks that are generally affected by nonspecific dysfunction as well as items that can give some information regarding lateralization. For the most effective interpretation, a battery incorporates multiple methods of inference. The general level of performance, differences among tests (scatter), differences in the performance of one side of the body compared with the other side and pathognomic signs are inspected (Reitan & Davison, 1974). Testing procedures should also be validated and standardized for group comparisons. As the reader can quickly discern from the above criteria, there is usually no five minute answer to the complex question of brain dysfunction.

Some patient history should be taken. Specifically, questions about the onset of difficulties, premorbid level of functioning (e.g., education, occupation), and concurrent psychiatric problems are important in order to interpret the data and to make better predictions regarding rehabilitation efforts for that patient. The reader is referred to Filskov and Leli (1981), which gives a more comprehensive review of the history-taking procedure.

Clinical observations, so called "qualitative" aspects of performance, are also important in the overall context of a neuropsychological screening examination. Strub and Black's (1977) text, THE MENTAL STATUS EXAMINATION IN NEUROLOGY, is an excellent source of information regarding behavioral observations. In general, any perseverative behavior, recent memory difficulties, motor awkwardness, and language or comprehension difficulties should be noted.

Additionally, it is important to have specific information regarding important group characteristics of patients traditionally evaluated with neuropsychological instruments. Such patient populations as chronic schizophrenics (Golden, MacInnes, Ariel, Ruedich, Chu, Coffman, Graber, & Bloch, 1982; Heaton & Crowley, 1981; Malec, 1978), the elderly (Botwinick, 1981; Wells, 1979), and alcoholics (Parsons & Farr, 1981) all have somewhat characteristic patterns of performance which are important in understanding the complex interactions between neuropsychological difficulties, psychological problems, and day-to-day problems in living. Interpretations about an individual's performance must be made within the parameters of what is known about the group of which he or she is a member when membership is known to have an impact upon test data. For example, subtests on the Wechsler Adult Intelligence Scale (WAIS) involving psychomotor speed are corrected for age. Likewise, the level of performance of alcoholics on motor, memory, and new learning tasks is related to the length of time since detoxification.

Many screening batteries have been devised recently (Barrett, Wheatley, & LePlant, 1982; Erickson, Calysn, & Sheupbach, 1978; Golden, 1976; Kaplan, 1981; Mezzich & Moses, 1980) to name a few. There has also been a fair amount of work using the Trail Making Test exclusively (Gordon, 1978; Mezzich & Moses, 1980) and with specific populations (Goldstein & Neuringer, 1966). Although Trails B has been demonstrated to have strong predictive validity for general organicity, the use of a single test is not recommended because it gives very little specific information. The screening batteries which are validated assess a broad variety of cognitive functions including language and related skills, memory, problem solving, general intellectual ability, sensory perceptual functions, visual-motor skills, and practic functions. Many of the tests that are specified combine parts of established, well validated batteries which have been shortened to fit the needs of time limitations. Most of these tests have specific information regarding the effects of age and education on the scores which are obtained. For instance, the Reitan-Indiana Aphasia Screening Test, specific subtests from the WAIS, and memory items from the Wechsler Memory Scale are frequently used in battery composition.

THE ASSESSMENT PROCESS

Based on the patient's ability to perform in a test situation, a hierarchical sequence of test procedures can be implemented. Certainly an initial determination of the patient's capability can be made through a brief mental status examination (10 item orientation questions; Kahn, Pollock, & Goldfarb, 1961; Pfeifer, 1975) with these initial findings then dictating the type of battery that is given. For the severely disabled patient, beginning with some testing of auditory and visual acuity is important. Information gained from the Aphasia Screening Test and Sensory-Perceptual Examination can usually establish basic visual and auditory receptive abilities. Further formal testing may be warranted from these findings. We have found that, particularly in an elderly population, part of some patients' difficulty is an inability to hear. Simpler and less time consuming parts of the examination are completed first and a determination is made whether to continue with more difficult procedures. Obviously, the more intact person is started with the higher level tasks; testing proceeds very quickly with such persons and can usually be finished within an hour. In general, the examiner looks at the test data using several methods of inference. Initially, nonspecific or generalized indicators of dysfunction are interpreted (e.g., impaired cutoff scores) at the same time that signs indicating decrements in level of performance and pathognomic signs related to lateralization or localization are ascertained. Diffuse cerebral dysfunction usually manifests itself in many areas of functioning with generally lowered levels of performance and evidence of deficits on more complex tasks which require attention or simulate new learning. Information regarding lateralization is obtained from differences among the tests and by noting pathognomic signs.

A comprehensive screening examination includes the five basic areas of cognitive functioning: intellectual functioning, new learning and problem solving, language and related skills, visual-spatial abilities, and sensory-perceptual functions. Each of these areas will be discussed briefly.

INTELLECTUAL FUNCTIONING

Changes in intellectual functioning, especially using the WAIS, are probably most well documented in the literature (Matarrazo, 1972). In fact, poor performance on a Wechsler Intelligence measure frequently identifies difficulties which lead to more specific neuropsychological testing. The current level of intellectual functioning is compared with premorbid estimates of intelligence based on education and occupation (Leli & Filskov, 1979). Subtests most resistant to brain damage (Information and Vocabulary) can also be compared to those that appear to be most sensitive to impairment (Digit Symbol and Block Design). A deficient performance on Digit Span when compared to other better performances should also be noted. If an entire WAIS has been given, significant Verbal-Performance differences must be explained. Certainly alternative hypotheses for decrements (e.g., low academic background, depression, thought disorder) should be considered along with questions of brain impairment. A significantly lower Performance IQ can be associated with diffuse or right hemisphere difficulties. A comparatively lower Verbal IQ can indicate left hemisphere dysfunction. A pattern analysis inspecting new versus old learning differences (similar to the old Deterioration Index) or severe decrements on one specific scale are specific patterns that are observed in brain damaged individuals. Certainly any pathognomic sign which is encountered (e.g., rotations on Block Design, word finding difficulties, extreme concreteness on Similarities) should be further investigated.

NEW LEARNING AND PROBLEM SOLVING

Frequently, some of the more nonspecific signs which are associated with all types of brain impairment are those involved in the acquisition of new learning or novel tasks. Although perhaps not technically included here, problems in abstract reasoning and shifting set could be seen as problems under this general category. There are many tests which are available to assess this area. Some tasks on the WAIS can be measures of new learning ability (e.g., Digit Symbol, Block Design, Similarities, Arithmetic). The Category Test, the Wisconsin Card Sorting Test, the Stroop Color Test, and the

Trail Making Test could also be seen as fairly quick measures of new learning ability. As noted above, the Trail Making Test (particularly Trails B) has well documented validity and is the shortest of all these measures to give. Certainly, among severely impaired persons where these decrements are obvious, it would be unnecessary to put them through the agony of repeated failures. Well-validated screening batteries use the Stroop Color Test or the Wisconsin Card Sorting Test (Pendleton & Heaton, 1982) along with the Trail Making Test.

LANGUAGE AND RELATED SKILLS

Direct clinical observations and administration of verbal subtests from the WAIS serve as a screening for language impaired patients. Additionally, however, the Aphasia Screening Test is used in most batteries to cover word finding difficulties, articulation problems, comprehension difficulties, and other language related skills such as reading and writing. Although persons with diffuse cerebral impairment can demonstrate aphasic symptoms, patients with left hemisphere difficulties usually show some language disorder.

VISUAL-SPATIAL ABILITIES

Drawing tasks are usually used to reveal difficulties in visual-spatial functions. The Bender-Gestalt Test is probably the most widely used. Good performances on the Memory-For-Designs Test, on the Benton Visual Retention Test, or a Visual Reproductions from the Wechsler Memory Scale would preclude the necessity for an extended evaluation of constructional ability. Simple figures from the Aphasia Screening Test which include a Greek cross, a square, a triangle, and a key have been used successfully in a number of screening batteries. Severe difficulties with copying most usually occur in patients with right hemisphere damage. However, patients with diffuse and right hemisphere damage also demonstrate copying difficulty at times.

SENSORY-PERCEPTUAL FUNCTIONS

Difficulties with primary sensory input (i.e., tactile, auditory, visual) may be associated with lesions in the posterior cortex. A brief sensory-perceptual examination (Reitan & Davison, 1974) also is included in screening batteries. This particular brief examination tests for tactile, auditory, and visual perception under conditions of bilateral simultaneous stimulation. A low level of performance or apparent differences in performance, comparing one side of the body to the other, can be lateralizing signs of impairment. However, certainly among normal elderly patients, the ability to perceive fingertip number writing (a very refined tactile perception) may be somewhat diminished.

SUGGESTED SCREENING TESTS

The following tests or subtests cover the areas of functioning mentioned above. There are several more complete treatments of these tests available, including Matarrazo (1972), Lezak (1976), and Filskov and Leli (1981). Most of the interpretation on these familiar tests is already known to the trained clinician. A clear presentation of the relationship between different types of cerebral impairment and testing for various cognitive functions is covered in a chapter by Goodglass and Kaplan (1979).

The time required for well functioning individuals to complete the tests is given in parentheses. Good initial tests that are most sensitive to cognitive decrements are starred (*). If a patient completes more difficult items, simpler items of the same type can be eliminated.

1. WAIS (Full test - 45 min.):
   Information (4 min.)   Block Design (8 min.)
   Vocabulary (4 min.)   Digit Span (3 min.)*
   Digit Symbol (3 min.)*

2. TRAIL MAKING TEST (3 min.):
   Trails B (90 sec.)*

3. WECHSLER MEMORY SCALE (Entire scale - 20 min.):
   Orientation (1 min.)
   Logical Memory (3 min.)
   Visual Reproductions (3 min.) } Delayed Recall (Russell, 1975)
   Paired Associates (5 min.)*

4. APHASIA SCREENING TEST AND ASSOCIATED EXAMINATION FOR SENSORY-PERCEPTUAL DISTURBANCES (entire test - 15 min.)

5. CATEGORY TEST (Booklet Form - 8 min.)*

6. WISCONSIN CARD SORTING (5 min.)*

CASE ILLUSTRATIONS

CASE #1 - MS. H

Ms. H, a 66-year old woman, was referred by a psychiatrist who had been seeing her for problems concerning her family and difficulties with a recent retirement. She had been a high school history teacher who had earned a Master's degree on a Fullbright Scholarship. She was an extremely articulate woman who was angry about being referred and was quite disparaging to the examiner. Results of the screening battery are presented below.

Ms. H's Neuropsychological Screening

WAIS: Vocabulary - (16)*   Block Design - (7)
      Information - (15)   Digit Symbol - (6)
      Digit Span - (9)

WMS: Logical Memory - (8)
     Visual Reproduction - (5) } 50% delayed recall

Trails B - 155 sec.

Aphasia Screening Test and Associated Examination for Sensory-Perceptual Disorders - normal except for slight bilateral fingertip number writing difficulties

Category Test - 105 errors

*Age corrected scaled scores

Vocabulary and Information scores, which are the most resistant to brain damage, show this woman had a superior premorbid level of functioning which is consistent with her education and occupational history. In contrast, the score on Digit Symbol, even with the age correction, was below average functioning. Digit Span, a short-term auditory memory test, although below her highest score, was in the average range. Memory testing indicated below average performance on logical memory, visual reproductions, and paired associate learning. The delayed recall indicated that this woman could only recall 50% of her original performance. The Aphasia Screening Test and Associated Examination for Sensory-Perceptual Disturbances showed slight bilateral fingertip number writing difficulties but was otherwise within normal limits for a woman of her age. Her copied drawings from this examination, although somewhat shaky, were also seen as within normal limits for her age group. Ms. H became extremely agitated during the administration of the Category Test (Booklet Form). Her performance was prorated with 105 errors. On the basis of this screening, it was felt that this woman was having significant difficulties with recent memory, problem solving, and new learning in contrast to her premorbid level of functioning. This type of pattern is frequently encountered with the onset of dementia in the elderly. Intact verbal and social skills, in contrast to severe difficulties with recent memory and learning tests, are quite common. Additional neuropsychological evaluation and Cat Scans corroborated the above initial findings. It was also felt that, on the basis of interaction with this woman and personality findings, a significant depression also existed. Again, this is quite common among persons who are showing initial signs of loss of cognitive functioning. It was suggested that some supportive measures be implemented immediately for this woman to aid in her adjustment to the above difficulties.

CASE #2 - MR. R

A 54-year old architect with his own firm was referred by a gerontological specialist with complaints of memory difficulties. Mr. R had stated that he had always had some problems concentrating but that he found his difficulties were recently exacerbated. The results of his initial screening are shown below.

Mr. R's Neuropsychological Screening Results

WAIS: Vocabulary - (15)*   Block Design - (14)
      Information - (13)   Digit Span - (10)
      Digit Symbol - (16)

WMS: Logical Memory - (15)
      Visual Reproductions - (16)   } 90% delayed recall
      Paired Associate Learning - (15)

Trails B - 50 sec.

Aphasia Screening Test and Associated Sensory Perceptual Examination - within normal limits

Category Test - 33 errors

*Age corrected scaled scores

The brief intellectual evaluation did not show the same differences in scores as were apparent with the previous examination. This patient exhibited scores appropriate for his level of education and occupation. An age correction on performance tasks placed him within the expected level for his intellectual ability. The Aphasia Screening Test and associated sensory-perceptual examination, copying tasks, and tests involving new learning and problem solving were all within expected levels for his age. Mr. R's performance on the Wechsler Memory Scale subtest was also within expected limits with delayed recall at a half hour being over 90% for logical memory and visual reproductions. Some difficulty was seen on Digit Span where he earned an average scaled score. He was able to improve his score on this particular test at a later time during the examination, although it still fell within the average range. Based on the fact that Mr. R did not show decrements in more complex tasks with delayed recall (which are usually deficient in persons beginning to experience memory difficulties), it was felt that many of Mr. R's complaints could be accounted for by anxiety and depression. Personality testing corroborated the above finding. It was reported that symptoms significantly improved as he was seen in psychotherapy and identifiable problems were brought to light.

These cases are typical illustrations from our files of screening evaluations. As can be noted in the above cases, the ruling out of brain impairment versus psychological difficulties often coexist rather than some simple dichotomy between the two. This has been a brief presentation and has certainly not thoroughly covered many aspects of brain-behavior relationships, but rather sought to outline basic screening procedures. The interested reader is encouraged to explore this topic further, using the list of recommended resources given here.

Susan B. Filskov, Ph.D., is currently Associate Professor of Psychology, Psychology Department, at the University of South Florida and also holds a clinical appointment in the Department of Psychiatry at USF School of Medicine. She received her doctorate in clinical psychology in 1975 from the University of Vermont. In addition to her research and teaching activities, she consults with various mental health agencies in the Tampa Bay area and has co-edited the HANDBOOK OF CLINICAL NEUROPSYCHOLOGY and numerous other articles. Dr. Filskov can be reached at the Department of Psychology, University of South Florida, Tampa, FL 33620.

RESOURCES

TEST RESOURCES

APHASIA SCREENING TEST

Halstead, W. C. & Wepman, J. M. The Halstead Wepman Aphasia Screening Test. JOURNAL OF SPEECH AND HEARING DISORDERS, 1959, **14**, 9-15. (Reitan's modification of the above battery)

Boll, T. J. Diagnosing brain impairment. In B. B. Wolman (Ed.), CLINICAL DIAGNOSIS OF MENTAL DISORDERS. New York: Plenum, 1978. (Contains Reitan's modification of the above battery)

Russell, E. W., Nevringer, C., & Goldstein, G. ASSESSMENT OF BRAIN DAMAGE. New York: Wiley, 1970. (Appendix B) (Contains another form of the test)

BENDER VISUAL MOTOR GESTALT TEST

This test is available through Western Psychological Services and Psychological Corporation.

BENTON VISUAL RETENTION TEST

This test is available through Psychological Corporation.

BOOKLET CATEGORY TEST

DeFilippis, N. A. & McCampbell, E. Available from Psychological Assessment Resources, Inc., P. O. Box 98, Odessa, FL 33556. This is a booklet version of the widely utilized Halstead Category Test. The test is portable and easily administered. It is sold with a manual and scoring forms.

MEMORY-FOR-DESIGNS TEST

This test is available through Psychological Test Specialists, Box 1441, Missoula, MT 59801.

STROOP COLOR AND WORD TEST

Stroop, J. R. Studies of interference in serial verbal reactions. JOURNAL OF EXPERIMENTAL PSYCHOLOGY, 1935, 18, 643-662.

Golden, C. J. Identification of brain disorders by the Stroop Color and Word Test. JOURNAL OF CLINICAL PSYCHOLOGY, 1976, 32, 621.

TRAIL MAKING TEST

Reitan, R. M. Testing brochure is available through the author, Department of Psychology, University of Arizona, Tuscon, AZ 85721.

WECHSLER MEMORY SCALE

Wechsler, D. & Stone, C. P. Available from Psychological Corporation, 757 Third Avenue, New York, NY 10017, and regional offices. A brief standardized scale which yields a Memory Quotient. It is available in two forms. The delayed recall is described in Russell, 1975.

WISCONSIN CARD SORTING TEST

Grant, D. A. & Berg, E. A. Psychological Assessment Resources, Inc., P. O. Box 98, Odessa, FL 33556. This test is used primarily to assess perseveration and abstract thinking. Two decks of cards for the test, response and scoring forms by R. K. Heaton, and two manuals are available from the publisher.

PUBLICATIONS

Barrett, E. T., Wheatley, R. D., & LaPlant, R. J. A brief clinical neuropsychologic screening battery: Statistical classification trials. JOURNAL OF CLINICAL PSYCHOLOGY, 1982, 38, 375-377.

Botwinick, J. Neuropsychology of aging. In S. B. Filskov & T. J. Boll (Eds.), HANDBOOK OF CLINICAL NEUROPSYCHOLOGY. New York: John Wiley and Sons, Inc., 1981.

Erickson, R. C., Calysn, D. A., & Sheupbach, C. S. Abbreviating the Halstead-Reitan neuropsychological test battery. JOURNAL OF CLINICAL PSYCHOLOGY, 1978, 34, 922-926.

Filskov, S. B. & Leli, D. A. Assessment of the individual in neuropsychological practice. In S. B. Filskov & T. J. Boll (Eds.), HANDBOOK OF CLINICAL NEUROPSYCHOLOGY. New York: John Wiley and Sons, Inc., 1981.

Golden, C. J. The identification of brain damage by an abbreviated form of the Halstead-Reitan neuropsychological battery. JOURNAL OF CLINICAL PSYCHOLOGY, 1976, 32, 821-826.

Golden, C. J., MacInnes, W. D., Ariel, R. N., Ruedich, S. L., Chu, C., Coffman, J. A., Graber, B., Bloch, S. Cross-validation of the ability of the Juria-Nebraska neuropsychological battery to differentiate chronic schizophrenics with and without ventricular enlargement. JOURNAL OF CONSULTING AND CLINICAL PSYCHOLOGY, 1982, **50**, 87-95.

Goldstein, G. & Neuringer, C. Schizophrenic and organic signs on the Trail Making Test. PERCEPTUAL MOTOR SKILLS, 1966, **22**, 347.

Goodglass, H. & Kaplan, E. Assessment of cognitive deficit in the brain-injured patient. In M. Gazmaniga (Ed.), HANDBOOK OF BEHAVIORAL NEUROBIOLOGY. New York: Plenum Press, 1979.

Gordon, N. G. Diagnostic efficiency of the Trail Making Test as a function of cutoff score, diagnosis and age. PERCEPTUAL MOTOR SKILLS, 1978, **47**, 191-195.

Heaton, R. K. & Crowley, T. J. Effects of psychiatric disorders and their somatic treatments on neuropsychological test results. In S. B. Filskov & T. J. Boll (Eds.), HANDBOOK OF CLINICAL NEUROPSYCHOLOGY. New York: John Wiley and Sons, Inc., 1981.

Heaton, S. K. & Heaton, R. K. Testing of the impaired patient. In S. B. Filskov & T. J. Boll (Eds.), HANDBOOK OF CLINICAL NEUROPSYCHOLOGY. New York: John Wiley and Sons, Inc., 1981.

Kahn, R. L., Pollock, M., & Goldfarb, A. I. Factors related to individual differences in mental status of institutionalized aged. In P. H. Hoch & J. Lubin (Eds.), PSYCHOPATHOLOGY OF AGING. New York: Grune & Stratton, 1961.

Kaplan, E. Neuropsychological screening battery. Unpublished test. Boston VA Hospital, 1981.

Leli, D. A. & Filskov, S. B. Relationship of intelligence to education and occupation as signs of intellectual deterioration. JOURNAL OF CONSULTING AND CLINICAL PSYCHOLOGY, 1979, **47**, 702-707.

Lezak, M. D. NEUROPSYCHOLOGICAL ASSESSMENT. New York: Oxford University Press, 1976.

Malec, J. Neuropsychological assessment of schizophrenia versus brain damage: A review. JOURNAL OF NERVOUS AND MENTAL DISEASE, 1978, **166**, 507-516.

Matarazzo, J. D. WECHSLER'S MEASUREMENT AND APPRAISAL OF ADULT INTELLIGENCE (5th ed.). Baltimore: Williams & Wilkins, 1972.

Mezzich, J. E. & Moses, J. A. Efficient screening for brain dysfunction. BIOLOGICAL PSYCHIATRY, 1980, **15**, 333-337.

Parsons, O. A. & Farr, S. P. The neuropsychology of alcohol and drug use. In S. B. Filskov & T. J. Boll (Eds.), HANDBOOK OF CLINICAL NEUROPSYCHOLOGY. New York: John Wiley and Sons, Inc., 1981.

Pendleton, M. G. & Heaton, R. K. A comparison of the Wisconsin Card Sorting Test and the Category Test. JOURNAL OF CLINICAL PSYCHOLOGY, 1982, **38**, 392-396.

Pfeiffer, E. A short portable mental status questionnaire for the assessment of organic brain deficit in elderly patients. JOURNAL OF THE AMERICAN GERIATRIC SOCIETY, 1975, **23**, 433.

Reitan, R. M. & Davison, L. A. (Eds.). CLINICAL NEUROPSYCHOLOGY: CURRENT STATUS AND APPLICATIONS. Washington: Winston, 1974.

Russell, E. W. A multiple scoring method for assessment of complex memory functions. JOURNAL OF CONSULTING AND CLINICAL PSYCHOLOGY, 1975, **43**, 800-809.

Russell, E. W., Neuringer, C., & Goldstein, G. ASSESSMENT OF BRAIN DAMAGE: A NEUROPSYCHOLOGICAL KEY APPROACH. New York: John Wiley and Sons, Inc., 1970.

Strub, R. L. & Black, F. W. THE MENTAL STATUS EXAMINATION IN NEUROLOGY. Philadelphia: F. A. Davis Company, 1977.

Wells, C. E. Pseudoementia. AMERICAN JOURNAL OF PSYCHIATRY, 1979, **136**, 7.

INTRODUCTION TO FILIAL THERAPY: TRAINING PARENTS AS THERAPISTS

Louise F. Guerney

Filial Therapy is a behavioral intervention for children under twelve years of age using parents as the primary therapists. Parents are trained and supervised by professionals to provide child-centered (client-centered or nondirective) play therapy sessions to their emotionally or behaviorally disordered children. Hence the name Filial, which literally means "pertaining to a son or daughter." Filial Therapy is more formally known as Filial Relationship Enhancement Therapy because the first of its four major goals is the enhancement of the filial relationship. The other goals are the reduction of child symptoms, increasing child competence and confidence, and improvement of the quality of the parents' child-rearing skills.

Filial Therapy (FT) was conceived by Dr. Bernard Guerney, Jr., then Director of the Rutgers University Psychological Clinic, in an effort to address several problems which he perceived in the method of psychological service delivery to families. Guerney contended that (a) the exclusion of parents from children in the typical "child guidance" model tended to develop defensiveness and resistance on the part of parents to therapeutic measures taken on behalf of the children; (b) parents are in the position of having a uniquely powerful impact on children which should be utilized in treating their troubled children; (c) the role of parents in treatment ought to be that of active ally instead of passive observer, co-client, or even antagonist; and (d) the limited number of professional therapists available to provide the much under served child population could be better utilized if they were to act as supervisors and consultants to primary therapists, such as parents and others indigenous to the environments of children (Guerney, 1964). Working with a group of colleagues in clinical psychology (Dr. Lillian Stover, Dr. Michael Andronico, and this author), Guerney slowly and carefully researched the method since it was such a departure from traditional therapies. It was, in fact, the first systematic, programmatic effort to utilize parents as therapists. Since then, of course, behavioral therapy has made wide use of parents as primary change agents (e.g., Hargis & Blechman, 1979).

The first parents to be utilized as filial therapists were placed in groups, composed of parents unrelated to each other, which were conducted by one of the experienced psychologists named above. By 1970, successful experience with the method allowed the training of graduate students to utilize the methods with related and unrelated parents, single parents, and foster parents in one parent, couples, or group formats. No parents are excluded except those who are clinically depressed or otherwise severely disturbed.

Originally, children with the slightest suspicion of even minimal organicity were excluded from the treatment since it was conceived as one for behaviorally and emotionally based problems. However, with increased experience, it was recognized that secondary problems of children with primary organicity were appropriately responsive to the filial approach. Currently, the author and colleagues exclude only autistic and schizophrenic children. A modified version of FT is used, however, with autistic children by a group at the University of Texas at Galveston (Hornsby & Applebaum, 1978).

A considerable amount of research has been done to demonstrate that parents can learn to conduct the play sessions in a satisfactory way and that training to do so makes a significant difference in the way mothers behave in relation to their children in an observed behavioral interaction (Stover & Guerney, 1967); that parents and children participating in the program make significant improvements in four months of treatment while no changes take place during a four month wait period (Sywulak, 1977); that changes continue to increase at six months and are maintained for at least three years, the latter demonstrated in an extensive follow-up study (Sensué, 1981).

Before proceeding to more detailed descriptions of the method, it would seem important to lay out for the reader the advantages to this approach when working with families with children identified as emotionally or behaviorally disordered.

WHY THE ROLE OF CHILD-CENTERED PLAY THERAPIST FOR PARENTS?

As is commonly known by therapists working with children, the therapist enjoys a very special place in the life of the child, a place so special it is sometimes a threat to parents. Nonetheless, it is a very circumscribed place, limited to the relatively short period of therapy both in place and time. On the other hand, the parent spends more time with the child and will be present in some capacity at least throughout the child's young life in the great majority of instances. Even when the parent-child relationship is problematic, it is an ongoing relationship in all but the rarest of circumstances with affective and instrumental components of profound significance for both parent and child. Engaging the parent as therapist then builds on this existing powerful relationship. The method permits parents to function in that relationship at the "highest and best way" possible for the development of the child and the strengthening of the relationship itself.

The behaviors of a play therapist represent some of the most facilitative behaviors as yet identified as important in helping children learn and relate effectively and develop self-confidence. The work of Baumrind (1971) with young children indicates that a parent who is warm and understanding of children, yet at the same time communicates an expectation for appropriately mature behavior, encourages the greatest social competence in those children. The play therapist does just that in that the play therapist is warm and empathic and very understanding of the child's needs, but at the same time places responsibility on the child for management of his or her behavior: to initiate activities and to stay within the limits of the play session. The therapist is permissive only to a point but is authoritative in demeanor beyond that. However, the play therapist is never authoritarian. The child-centered play therapist is accepting, nonjudgmental, warm and encouraging, but leaves it to the child to accept the responsibility for his or her own direction.

Of course, proponents of FT do not mistake the play session for real life or the play therapist for the parent as the latter must function outside of the playroom. However, it is impressive how similar the characteristics of the authoritative parent of Baumrind (1971) and Coopersmith (1967) who studied parents of older children, resembles the child-centered play therapist. Except for the teaching and socializing specifics of parent behavior outside the playroom, most of the important components of successful parenting can be acquired in the context of learning play therapy. At the same time, the parent is providing the child with a powerful treatment and enhancing the parent-child relationship. The play session serves as a learning laboratory, bringing into focus in the context of the child's play and in the parent's responses to the child, the salient issues in the respective dynamics of the parent and the child and in their relationship. Parents who are very submissive to children in real life have trouble setting limits. Parents who are not sensitive and understanding of their children's needs demonstrate problems in mastering the empathic and accepting elements of the therapist role. Instruction and concern from the therapist for the parents' positions helps them overcome these problems, at first in the playroom, and, in due time, in the real world as well.

While groups of six to eight are the most common format for training parents, a single parent or single couple may be seen. The child with problems (i.e, the target child) is played with by the participating parents in their own home with supervision by the professional therapist through detailed reports from the parents. However, the other children of the family whose age permits (i.e., those approximately 3-10 years) are also provided with play sessions by the parents. Older children may be given Special Times, to be described later. Thus, it is frequent that all of the children and both parents will be engaged in the therapy program.

The Filial Therapy Program can be divided into five periods or phases: the teaching of parents to do play sessions; parents' practice sessions; home play sessions; a generalization phase; and an evaluation and planning phase.

PHASE 1:   THE TEACHING OF PLAY SESSIONS

In this initial phase, therapists teach parents the rationale of the child-centered play session, the process and the special nature of the adult-child relationship in the play session, typical child behaviors in play sessions, stages of play therapy, empathic understanding and expression, structuring and limit setting for the playroom, and recognition of one's own feelings. Expression of adult feelings is not taught in this phase, since the play session is intended to be limited as nearly as possible to facilitation of child expressions.

In this phase, short lectures laced with many examples are presented. Therapists demonstrate play sessions using all the age-appropriate children of the participating families. Parents observe these demonstrations through one-way vision or screen arrangements. If these cannot be obtained, a barrier of any sort over which parents can watch the session (e.g., a bookcase or table) can be used to create the illusion of isolation of child and therapist from the parent observers.

Parents will be intensely interested in how their own children behave in the session as well as observant of the behavior of the therapist. Therefore, a number of sessions are required to provide complete instruction. Discussions of what happened in the play sessions follow the demonstrations, with ample opportunity for parents to ask questions about the child's and therapist's behaviors. During this phase, the therapist is primarily instructional about therapeutic techniques except for dealing with the parents' feelings about their children's observed behaviors and their concerns about their own future performances as therapists. Such concerns are handled empathically, with a limited amount of instruction on realistic expectations of children at their respective developmental levels.

Skills practice on empathic understanding and responding are conducted as well as practice in limit setting. Role-played play sessions with the therapist as the child are carried out before parents try to play with their children.

Before describing the next phases of FT, it would seem appropriate to explain a bit more fully the nature of the child-centered play session as utilized in FT.

The Play Session. The child-centered play session has been described by Axline (1969) in her book, **PLAY THERAPY**. Essentially, these play sessions are based on the developmental and therapeutic principles of Axline's mentor, Carl Rogers (1951). Axline stresses the great value of acceptance and of permitting self-direction with only the limitations "that are necessary to anchor the therapy to the world of reality and to make the child aware of his responsibility in the relationship" (Axline, 1969, p. 76). Limits are not spelled out in a list at the beginning but introduced as required. Adult efforts are directed toward dealing with the child empathically and labeling his or her feelings and actions in a way that communicates acceptance. The therapist is warm, friendly, and ready to participate as requested by the child in games, role playing, or conversation.

While most children quickly enjoy the opportunity to direct themselves and the therapist, some children are at first confused about the lack of adult direction. In such instances, the therapist empathizes with the child and provides more explicit structure (e.g., "You're wondering why I don't tell you some things to do. In this playtime, it is what you want to do that is important. You may play with any of these toys that you like." Or, "You're worried about whether I'll want to play with you. In here, you may do just as you would wish. I will be here to play with you if you would like that sometimes.").

Children really are free to choose from the toys provided and are not guided toward any that the adult might prefer or think important to the child's problems. The opening statement that we rehearse parents to use is, "This is your special time to do just about anything you would like." Parents also tell the children that they will be there and let the child know if there is something that the child should not do. Some children are worried that the adult has a hidden game plan and this last statement reassures them.

We use the toys recommended by Axline (1969) with only a few modifications. The toys are heavily loaded with those which encourage the expression of the typically most troublesome feelings, dependence and aggression, as well as those which permit age-appropriate play and social interaction with the therapist if desired by the child. Included are a soft rubber knife, a gun of some sort, miniature soldiers and military vehicles, a puppet family including a baby, a ferocious puppet (e.g., an alligator or wolf), clay, crayons, pencil, paper, a building set of some sort (e.g., Leggo's), a punching bag doll of a figure who can be safely aggressed against (e.g., Popeye or Superman), and miniature cooking and water play equipment. Paint and sand are omitted from our playrooms since they are too difficult for parents to manage. We make a point of having no play objects in the playroom at the training site which are not suitable for parents to handle in their home play sessions.

PHASE 2: PARENTS' PRACTICE SESSIONS

After the parents have observed a number of demonstrations with their children and practiced the skills in role-play format, they conduct two sessions with their child(ren) to practice what they have learned. These sessions are observed by the filial therapist and other parent participants. Following the sessions which are kept brief (10 minutes at first and then 15 minutes), parents are given extensive feedback on their adherence to the principles, attitudes, and behaviors appropriate to client-centered play therapy. They are also encouraged to express in detail how they felt about the behaviors. Were they comfortable? What impulses did they have to inhibit? Of course, much positive reinforcement is given. Expectations for the first session attempted are merely the omission of unacceptable therapist behaviors (e.g., directing the child, giving their own views). The second session should include some evidence of use of positive behaviors (e.g., empathic statements, appropriate structuring). If a parent fails to meet the expectations, additional sessions can be scheduled as part of the practice phase. Therefore, it is good to keep the time for this phase flexible in outlining the program. In order to prevent parents from practicing the skills outside of the playroom before they are competent, they are asked not to use them until a later phase of the program. This request has the added value of reassuring parents that there is no indirect goal harbored by the therapist that parents should try to employ play session principles in everyday living at this early stage. The intake procedures and first session orientation make this very clear to parents. However, some are so eager for solutions or have such guilt feelings that they again must be cautioned that the play sessions at this point are their only responsibility.

PHASE 3: HOME PLAY SESSIONS

Following evidence of at least minimal mastery (some parents are quite good almost from the start) of the play therapy, parents begin to conduct play sessions at home. This phase is considered the high point of the program. Parents have become proficient enough to operate without immediate supervision, and the children generally appreciate the privilege of being able to have regular home sessions with their parents. Supervision is provided through parent reports. Occasionally audio tapes are made.

A very important session is held before parents begin the play sessions at home. The therapist follows a checklist with each parent participant which contains all of the issues that are known to be relevant in structuring for the success of home sessions. Detailed discussion is held with each parent about the following points in relation to anticipated home play sessions:

When: The time should not conflict with a high priority activity of the child. It should be a low-stress time for the parent.

Where:	The room in the house should be one in which the parent will not be worried about the child's play.
Supports:	Someone needs to be available to keep the other children from disrupting. Even the family dog should be contained. The play session is intended to be a time that focuses entirely on the child, undiluted by others, even beloved pets or friends.
Limits:	The boundaries necessary for facilitating an atmosphere of acceptance will probably differ from those of the treatment site. For example, if the parent has designated the basement as the play session area, will the section with the washer or dryer be out of bounds? The therapist and parent consult on how the parent will react to possible boundary issues and agree on what the limits will be. The therapist also rehearses parents, if it seems appropriate, in the actual statement of the limits. Thus, the problem of parental confusion over strict limit enforcement is eliminated.
Toys:	Parents are issued a kit of toys to be used for the home session, which is paid for as a treatment expense. The final point of structuring for home sessions is a realistic plan for storing toys at home between sessions. The toys are not to be available except for the special play times.

If parents have no satisfactory place to play at home because of limited space, as in the case of a small trailer or apartment, the "home" sessions can be scheduled at the treatment site, either as a part of regular parent meetings or at a separate time. If the latter is the case, the therapist would not necessarily wish to observe all of the sessions. However, it is recommended that the parent be told that the therapist might observe at some point so that the option is open. It is from such passing observations, done on an unscheduled basis, that it has been possible to substantiate at least to some degree the accuracy of parent play session reporting.

Continued parent demonstrations – parent meetings. It is important to include continued observed demonstrations at the treatment site in addition to the home sessions. These observations permit monitoring of the parents' application of the skills and of the children's reactions and progress in the play sessions. The frequency of these demonstrations with the family depends on the number of parents with whom the therapist is working at a given time. If a multi-family group is the format, parents would demonstrate no more than every three to four weeks. If a single family is being worked with, the therapist might wish to have a play session demonstration by the parent(s) each week, which would become a routine part of the meeting with the parent(s). If observed sessions are held on a regular basis, the filial therapist might wish to dispense with home sessions. While the extremely positive advantage of the home sessions in facilitating the generalization process for the parents will be lost in dropping regular home sessions, as long as parents adopt the therapeutic role and are perceived by their children as capable of behaving in these therapeutic ways, the essential purpose of FT will be attained.

The nature of the play in the home sessions follows the known patterns of play sessions which have been analyzed in treatment centers (Finke, 1947; Guerney & Stover, 1971). Children typically follow one of two patterns in relation to home versus observed sessions. Some follow the same themes as in the treatment site demonstrations, making no distinction between the two sets of conditions. Others have a set of themes and styles at home and different themes or styles for the observed sessions. Such differences become the focus for rich discussions between parent and therapist about the dynamic sources of the themes. While no empirical work has been conducted on them, clinical observation indicates that even if different, there is no incompatibility between themes in relation to dynamics. One child, for example, who had suffered neglect from his mother because of circumstances in her life, played out themes requiring great nurturance from her at home, and at the treatment site played out themes that allowed him to develop independence. The entire dependence-independence dimension was the dynamic issue between him and his mother.

PHASE 4: GENERALIZATION PHASE

Typically after parents have conducted four to six home sessions and have been observed two or three times at the treatment site, the sessions cease to offer them technical difficulties. At this point, the emphasis in the parent feedback and discussion sessions falls on the child's reactions to the parents' session behavior and the implications these have for the relationship and for life outside the session in general. However, the therapist does not omit feedback to the parents about their fulfillment of the play session role requirements. At this point, this is more likely to consist of reinforcement on how far the parent has come in handling certain situations than on the actual mechanics of their performance. The level of parent reinforcement is very high. A therapist-parent exchange in this phase might go as follows:

Therapist: Marie was testing the limits very vigorously in relation to the new rule which you had to bring in tonight. But, you didn't back down for a second. You let her know that you accepted her desire to do it but stuck with your position that it would not be all right. How did you feel about that?

Parent: Well, I was a little scared when it came up since she doesn't like rules and since this one was new. Because she'd never tried to shoot at the lights before, I thought she might get nasty like she does at home with rules.

Therapist: It's kind of scary for you when you realize that it's necessary to interfere with Marie's wishes at home and here.

Parent: Oh, yes. You've heard how she can get.

Therapist: However, in the play session you were able to show her that she was not at fault but rather that the behavior she wanted to carry out was not acceptable. Also, you seemed sure of yourself and cool about it. You were really accepting of her feelings but nonetheless firm. Does it ever happen like that in real life? That is, when you're able to accept her desires but be cool and firm about their expression?

Parent: Well, not very often because in real life, I'm not as sure of myself and I'm likely to get mad or upset. I'm not so sure that she'll listen to me unless I come down on her pretty hard.

Therapist: It's more complicated outside of the playroom. You're less confident of your ability to control her. This leads to your getting into emotional high gear.

Parent: Yes. She usually doesn't take any restrictions unless I go all out to make her see I'm serious about it.

Therapist: You've gotten into a pattern where things don't work as needed unless you both get into high gear.

Parent: Right.

Therapist: You have seen that in the playroom when you can feel that you **can** control her with the limits procedures you've learned, and you feel obliged to use them, that you can understand Marie's feelings and yet with calm and conviction you can let her know that all feelings are permitted but that you do not permit her to act them out. She takes you seriously. I believe that it is both these factors - first, you feel like you can control her, and second, this allows you to express your understanding. In the playroom you have broken the pattern of the power struggle. We have found that once a negative pattern has been broken in the play session it is possible to break out of it outside as well. You are different and Marie responds differently to you and you're both on your way into a good cycle. What do you think about that, Mrs. D.?

Parent: Well, I think that is true. Whether I can be as calm at home I'm not sure.

Therapist: It's a little more complicated in real life, isn't it? The play session simplifies it. However, the process is the same. Let's try to think of a recent situation at home where Marie ignored your efforts to stop her or to get her to do something.

Parent: Well, actually come to think of it she has been a lot better that way, lately. Maybe it is the play sessions. But I can think of one I'm sure if I take a minute.

Therapist: Perhaps your ability to assert your authority with Marie while not putting her down in the playroom is beginning to pay off already.

Parent: Yeah, I hadn't actually realized that' til now. But she's not completely changed because the other night...(and so on).

Therapist: Now let's go back and see just what happened there and see if it would be possible to apply the limits system you learned in the playroom to that situation. Okay now you say you were outside...(and so on).

Parent and therapist together share ideas and "image" reactions of Marie and parent in relation to dealing with such situations.

Therapist: You are really becoming a master of this method in the playroom. I am convinced from other parents' experiences that you can do the same thing outside if you follow the sequence as we just rehearsed it. Try it once this week and when we meet again, we'll discuss the way it went. If it worked we'll know why. If it didn't, we'll try to figure out together where it broke down and why.

Using the play session as the starting point, parallels in real life are thus considered. Typically by this time parents are feeling reasonably confident about their abilities to both understand and accept more fully what their children are feeling, and their ability to achieve compliance when necessary. They have learned from the play session the principle of cutting out superfluous demands and reducing psuedo-requests such as, "Why is your shirt always out? All the other boys manage to keep theirs in." (This is simply a complaint with none of the authority of a genuine request for compliance.) They have learned what is actually required in the way of conviction and persistence to achieve compliance and that the number of demands for compliance must be a manageable number for both parents and children. It is a matter of the therapist sensitizing and raising the consciousness of parents to help them identify parallels to real life. It is also necessary for the therapist to set low criterion levels until parents have gotten the transfer to real life principles in place.

Once parents are comfortable in this generalization phase in relation to issues that emerge in the play session, additional generalization tasks are assigned to be carried out systematically by all parents, regardless of their and their children's dynamics. Everyone is assigned the task of carrying out a daily empathic responding session (for 5 to 10 minutes), and the tasks of applying structuring and limit setting principles to two different problematic situations in the home. These are thoroughly planned with the therapist in advance just as the home sessions were.

PHASE 5: EVALUATION AND PLANNING PHASE

The final phase consists of three parts, (a) evaluation of the status of the target child and of the parent-child relationship; (b) planning for fading out play sessions; and (c) introduction of additional skills which take into account the additional responsibilities of parents outside the play session, but at the same time are consistent with the philosophy of the interpersonal atmosphere of the play session.

Preparations for decreasing play sessions and/or substituting Special Times are made with the parents as evidence appears that the children's adjustment is improving and parents' and therapists' goals are being met. Typically this is done by having parents cut play sessions to every other week, then every three weeks, and then not at all, unless requested by the child or parent as a kind of "booster." This fading process generally takes about two months. In addition to fading out play sessions, we try to introduce "Special Times" as a substitute for play sessions. While not considered a part of the generalization phase, we believe that Special Times do have the effect of facilitating transfer of the parents' acquired skills to daily living.

Special Times are periods of time arranged between child and parent that are devoted to an activity chosen by the child to share with the parent. It should be an activity which permits the parent to be accepting of the child's feelings, yet low on the necessity for controls. For example, a session with Dad's power tools would require too much monitoring by the parent if the child were young and inexperienced in their use. Parents are instructed to use the skills of the playroom plus the skills added at this time – parent messages and reinforcement for the Special Times. These skills are basic to relating to children in the real world and are seen as expanding on those learned for the playroom. The sequence in the final phase is described next.

A session is held evaluating progress made in the playroom and outside of the play session by the child. Typically we have parents fill out the same behavior checklists and other parent forms that we have had them fill out when first starting the FT program. Also, the therapist evaluates the child's progress in dealing with expression of troublesome feelings, control of problem behaviors, attitudes toward himself or herself and the parent, and others as they occur in the playroom. We would be looking for a diminishing of aggression compared to its peak early in the play session sequence. We would also look for more independence on the part of the child, greater affiliation with the parent, in terms of including him or her in games on a genuine give and take basis, and more positive statements about the self and others, as well as in relation to the future. An example of the above would be, "Next year when school starts I'm not going to let that J. bug me," in contrast to an earlier statement like, "That J. bugs me all of the time. I can't stop him."

Therapist and parent together decide on the basis of the information assembled from this variety of sources (including, where possible, teacher and day care reports), (a) whether additional play sessions are in order; (b) whether fading out of play sessions should be initiated; or (c) whether progress has been so minimal as to require an additional intervention. The latter generally would be a behavioral program of some sort to be conducted by the parent, teacher, or day care provider aimed specifically at a remaining troublesome target problem behavior. Referrals to non-psychological kinds of treatment agents generally would have been made earlier (e.g., speech therapist, learning disabilities specialist, perceptual-motor trainer). However, these might be initiated at this time if parents had chosen not to pursue them earlier because of limited time or money.

Only 10% of the children require extra-filial treatment. About 25% require additional play sessions beyond those of the standard 10-12 home sessions. Special Times are initiated in most cases with those children for whom play sessions no longer seem necessary. If the children are very young, the parents and therapist may agree that the best Special Times remain the play session. For older children who are into competitive games and skills acquisition activities or other modes of fun (e.g., shopping or short trips to a miniature golf course), the Special Times will take a different form. The Special Time is set up for a specific time as is the play session. A session on how to structure for Special Times is held as it was earlier in relation to home sessions. A follow-up study (Sensué, 1981) indicated that a number of parents still continued Special Times three years after finishing the program (something we did not expect). Of course, their form had changed as the children matured.

ADDITIONAL PARENTING SKILLS

Two or three sessions are held to teach, practice, and carry out homework assignments in relation to the two additional skills of parent messages, similar to "I messages" (Gordon, 1970), and reinforcement. PARENTING: A SKILLS TRAINING MANUAL (Guerney, 1978) is used in conjunction with this training. The last lesson in the manual is entitled, "Putting It Altogether," which teaches parents how to decide which skills are appropriate in complex situations based on their goals, the needs of the child, and the reality demands of the situation.

NONCHILD ISSUES

Having spent approximately five months together, there is adequate comfort for parents and therapist to introduce into this last phase any other issues that seem relevant to the parents' continued success. Interpersonal issues external to the play sessions (e.g., the parents' relationship to each other, to in-laws, relatives, baby sitters, school personnel) would be brought in at this point. Intra-psychic issues such as lack of self-esteem or fears are other common themes. Concerns about lack of assertiveness or lack of control rank very high. Having learned to be more appropriate in relating to their children, parents become sensitized to shortcomings elsewhere in their lives and seek changes for them as well. Many successfully generalize on their own, using the skills they have learned with spouses, employers, teachers, and others. Some require more consultation. Such issues can be worked on in the last few weeks of the program if they are relatively circumscribed. Otherwise, it is recommended that the parents seek out other skills training programs such as assertion training, self-control programs, or Marital Relationship Enhancement Skills (Guerney, 1978), or personal therapy.

CONSIDERATIONS OF THE UNIQUE ROLES OF
PARENT AND THERAPIST IN FT

The use of parents as primary therapists for their children places the professional therapist in the role of instructor, skills trainer, supervisor, and consultant to the parents. Secondarily, the filial therapist will serve as a counselor or psychotherapist for the parents. However, it is critical to understand that FT is not a parents' backdoor to therapy for parenting or intra-psychic issues. Issues arise in the context of parents carrying out their play therapist roles. The successes and failures in the mastery process tend to parallel those in the parents' real life relationships with their children and other significant figures. As these are noted by the therapist and the parents in training, attitudes, feelings, and values will emerge. The therapist deals with these using client-centered counseling skills (Rogers, 1951) or the core helping skills (Carkhuff, 1969) until some resolution in relation to their roles as play therapists is reached. Gratuitously, this generally relates to their other life-roles as well. This process resembles that which occurs when the supervising analyst explores with an analyst the intra-psychic issues of the latter as they relate to his or her patients.

The parents are trained exactly as professional students of play therapy would be trained. The parents are taught the rationale for play sessions, the behaviors of the play therapist, and are shown how these behaviors can impact positively on problems in children. They are taught how to provide supervision for themselves and other parents in their group, while the filial therapist serves as a dynamically oriented consultant to this supervision process. Thus, we speak of FT as both didactic and dynamic (Andronico, Fidler, Guerney, & Guerney, 1967).

An example should help to illustrate these points. In the play session a child violently threw a beanbag at her mother. The parent made no effort to place a limit on this forbidden behavior. When it happened a second time, she said, "You really want me to have that." During the feedback session the therapist and other parent observers asked the mother what feelings at the time of the throwing prompted her to let the behavior go unstopped. The parent disagreed that a limit had been required since the child was simply "giving" the beanbag to her. Group members and the therapist offered a counter observation that the child was showing nonverbal signs of anger. Following some empathic exchanges with the therapist about her feelings, the mother recognized that she failed to see the anger because she could not bear to believe that her adopted daughter could have any negative feelings toward her. Permitting the daughter's feelings to be expressed and labeling them correctly at the next session, paired with the empathic understanding of her own needs, allowed the mother to come to terms with her daughter's feelings as well as her own.

To fully utilize the strength of the model, the roles of parent as therapist and therapist as supervisor and consultant must be followed. Diversion to intra-psychic issues of parents are considered reversions of the filial therapist into his or her usual therapist role and an abandonment of the collaborative model between parent and therapist. For dynamically trained therapists, this constraint can present some dilemmas. If one does not deal directly with parent shortcomings, how then do necessary changes in parent behaviors and attitudes occur?

Two factors operate to promote positive changes in parent attitudes and behaviors. The behavioral factor of being required to replace inappropriate behaviors by more desirable ones in the presence of the instructor, and, in many instances, the presence of other parents, brings into play all of the laws of learning new social behaviors. The promise of being able to help one's child and one's self in the process by learning some new ways to behave in a circumscribed therapeutically oriented period has enormous motivational power for parents. This seems considerably more possible to them than trying to follow vague instructions of a parent counselor or therapist who determines by some (perhaps not too clear) means that the parent has some deficiencies which must be removed through his or her advise. Being told that "you are acting out your anger at your own mother with your child" does not really equip a parent to go home and start to act positively. Being shown how and being required to practice, for example, the setting and enforcement of appropriate limits instead of "blowing up," promotes the development of a positive parental behavior repertoire that in due time can replace an existing inappropriate one.

The second factor is the caring and sensitivity demonstrated toward the parents by the therapist. The parent is given the role of an important and necessary ally and collaborator with the therapist in their mutual goal of helping children. But, more importantly, the parent is also accepted as a person who receives the empathy and support of the therapist. While much of the filial therapist's interest in the parents will center around the parent-child relationship and the parent as therapist, the empathy expressed to them as individuals helps parents recognize that they are valued for themselves. The combination of the therapist's respect and concern seems to create an atmosphere that furthers parental insight and growth in the affective and cognitive domains and in the parent-child relationship.

Louise F. Guerney, Ph.D., is currently an Associate Professor of Human Development at The Pennnsylvania State University and heads the Filial Relationship Enhancement Program at the Individual and Family Consultation Center of the College of Human Development. Trained in clinical psychology, her major interest is in the development and evaluation of psycho-educational programs for employment by individuals, families, and professionals and paraprofessionals. Dr. Guerney may be contacted at the Individual and Family Consultation Center, Catherine Beecher House, Pennsylvania State University, University Park, PA 16802.

RESOURCES

PUBLICATIONS

Andronico, M. P., Fidler, J., Geurney, B. G., Jr., & Guerney, L. The combination of didactic and dynamic elements in filial therapy. INTERNATIONAL JOURNAL OF GROUP PSYCHOTHERAPY, 1967, **17**, 10-17.

Axline, V. PLAY THERAPY (Rev. ed.). New York: Ballantine Books, 1969.

Baumrind, D. Current patterns of parental authority. DEVELOPMENTAL PSYCHOLOGY MONOGRAPHS, 1971, **4**(1, Entire issue).

Carkhuff, R. HELPING AND HUMAN RELATIONSHIPS (Vol. I & II). New York: Holt, Rinehart, & Winston, 1969.

Coopersmith, S. THE ANTECEDENTS OF SELF-ESTEEM. San Francisco: W. H. Freeman, 1967.

Finke, H. Changes in the expression of emotionalized attitudes in six cases of play therapy. Unpublished master's thesis, University of Chicago, 1947.

Gordon, T. PARENT EFFECTIVENESS TRAINING. New York: Peter Wyden, 1970.

Guerney, B. RELATIONSHIP ENHANCEMENT: SKILL TRAINING PROGRAMS FOR THERAPY, PROBLEM PREVENTION, AND ENRICHMENT. San Francisco: Jossey-Bass, 1977.

Guerney, B. G., Jr. Filial therapy: Description and rationale. JOURNAL OF CONSULTING PSYCHOLOGY, 1964, **28**(4), 303-310.

Guerney, B. G., Jr. Filial therapy used as a treatment method for disturbed children. EVALUATION, 1976, **3**, 34-35.

Guerney, B. G., Jr., Coufal, J., & Vogelsong, E. Relationship enhancement versus a traditional approach to therapeutic/preventative/enrichment parent-adolescent programs. JOURNAL OF CONSULTING AND CLINICAL PSYCHOLOGY, 1981, **49**, 927-939.

Guerney, B. G., Jr. & Stover, L. FILIAL THERAPY: FINAL REPORT ON MH 1826401. State College, PA, 1971, p. 156. (Mimeograph)

Guerney, L. Filial therapy program. In D. H. Olson (Ed.), TREATING RELATIONSHIPS. Lake Mills, IA: Graphic Publishing Co., Inc., 1976.

Guerney, L. F. PARENTING: A SKILLS TRAINING MANUAL. State College, PA: Institute for the Development of Emotional and Life Skills, 1978.

Guerney, L. F. Play therapy with learning disabled children. JOURNAL OF CLINICAL CHILD PSYCHOLOGY, Fall 1979, 242-244.

Hargis, K. & Blechman, E. Social class and training of parents as behavior change agents. CHILD BEHAVIOR THERAPY, 1979, **1**, 69-74.

Hornsby, L. & Applebaum, A. Parents as primary therapists: Filial therapy. In E. Arnold (Ed.), HELPING PARENTS HELP THEIR CHILDREN. New York: Brunner & Mazel, 1978.

Rogers, C. CLIENT-CENTERED THERAPY. Boston: Houghton Mifflin Co., 1951.

Sensué, M. B. FILIAL THERAPY FOLLOW-UP STUDY: EFFECTS ON PARENTAL ACCEPTANCE AND CHILD ADJUSTMENT. Unpublished doctoral dissertation, The Pennsylvania State University, 1981.

Stover, L. & Guerney, B. G., Jr. The efficacy of training procedures for mothers in filial therapy. PSYCHOTHERAPY: THEORY, RESEARCH AND PRACTICE, 1967, 4(3), 110-115.

Sywulak, A. E. THE EFFECT OF FILIAL THERAPY ON PARENTAL ACCEPTANCE AND CHILD ADJUSTMENT. Unpublished doctoral dissertation, The Pennsylvania State University, 1977.

ADDITIONAL RESOURCES

Annual Relationship Enhancement Workshops, Spring of each year. Contact: Continuing Education, Keller Building, The Pennsylvania State University, University Park, PA 16802.

Guerney, B., Guerney, L., & Vogelsong, E. FILIAL THERAPY: A VIDEO DEMONSTRATION TAPE (50 minutes). The Pennsylvania State University, 1980. (Video Tape)

The Pennsylvania State University. A Selected Bibliography of Problem Solving, Conflict Resolution, Relationship Enhancement Therapy, and Interpersonal Education Programs of the Individual and Family Consultation Center, March, 1982.

MARITAL AND FAMILY RELATIONSHIP ENHANCEMENT THERAPY

Bernard Guerney, Jr.

For over twenty years, since my colleagues and I developed Filial Therapy (described elsewhere in this volume), we have been researching and developing skill training methods of therapy appropriate for children, adults, couples, and families. We have called our methods Relationship Enhancement (RE). This approach to psychotherapy and family therapy is built on the educational model, and is a radical departure from therapies based on the medical model.

We have dealt elsewhere with the broad array of differences in attitudes and procedures which exist between the two models (Authier, Gustafson, Guerney, & Kasdorf, 1975; Guerney, 1977b, 1979, 1982; Guerney, Guerney, & Stollak, 1971/1972; Guerney, Stollak, & Guerney, 1970, 1971). Here we will touch only briefly on the topic. The medical model carries with it the following paradigm for remediation: illness (or maladjustment) $\longrightarrow$ diagnosis $\longrightarrow$ prescription $\longrightarrow$ therapy $\longrightarrow$ cure. In contrast, the educational paradigm of intervention is: motivation (or ambition) $\longrightarrow$ value/goal choices $\longrightarrow$ instructional-program selection $\longrightarrow$ skill training $\longrightarrow$ goal achievement (satisfaction). Of course, the elimination of negative experiences ("symptom" in medical terminology) can be chosen as a goal within the educational model. However, it has become clear to those working within the educational model that such negative goals can be translated into positive ones. For example, the elimination of a phobia or fear can be stated equally well in terms of the acquisition of courage; or the goal of anxiety reduction can be replaced with the positive goal of attaining levels of tension appropriate to a given circumstance or task.

It is important that the practitioner not confuse the use of an educational model with any particular theoretical orientation. For example, many behavior therapists operate almost entirely within the medical model. It is true that certain theoretical positions fit in more readily with such an orientation than others. However, almost any psychotherapeutic theory probably could, at least in part, be translated into a skill training, therapeutic approach. In addition to many skill training therapies based on Skinnarian theory, the theoretical perspectives of Freud, Adler, and Rogers have all been translated in one way or another into skill training models of intervention. The methods of Ellis always were essentially educational in nature.

A second common misconception to guard against is that the educational skill training model is a form of treatment which takes psychodynamics into account less than other methods. In our view, the opposite is often true.

A third frequent misconception is that skill training therapeutic methods are somehow more watered down, less strong, or less suited to severely disturbed populations than traditional psychotherapy. On the contrary, the skill training methods have been shown to be effective with a very wide range of pathology. Regardless of the degree of pathology involved, we are aware of no studies in which traditional psychotherapeutic methods have proven to be superior to a skill training method. There is, however, a rapidly growing body of literature which indicates that skill training methods are superior to traditional psychotherapeutic approaches.

A fourth misconception is that a skill training approach such as RE is applicable mainly to middle-class, educated clients. Such clients are probably easier to work with in any psychotherapeutic approach, but, relative to traditional approaches, the advantages of a skill training approach with the socioeconomically and educationally disadvantaged seem at least as strong as they are with middle-class clients. Goldstein, in fact, developed his skill training therapy precisely because his studies suggested it was the most appropriate form of therapy for such clients (Goldstein, 1973). We think a small number of clients sometimes need very strong and direct understanding, love, nurturance, support, and advice from a therapist, because no one else could possibly provide it. Except in these cases, we think that direct, systematic training programs to teach clients how to get the people in their natural environment to meet their needs have the edge over traditional modes of therapy in which such teaching, if it goes on at all, seems comparatively haphazard and inefficient. We think the advantages of systematic skill training generally apply to all types of clients in all phases of remediation (getting clients to accept a recommendation for treatment, to remain in therapy, to improve with therapy, and having them maintain the gains they achieve after termination of therapy).

GOALS OF MARITAL AND FAMILY RE THERAPY

Generally, the goals of marital and family RE therapy are the same as those which family members typically set for themselves: achieving an attitude of camaraderie and mutuality in which members are reciprocally accepting, supporting, and caring, honor their agreements and commitments to one another, are open and direct in communicating, encourage one another to express feelings and thoughts, value each other's thoughts and feelings, and generally feel positive, secure, and trusting (Fisher, Giblin, & Hoopes, 1982).

Stated in terms more closely related to theory and measurement construction in the marital and family field, the goals of RE are to increase marital or family cohesion, adaptability (Fisher & Sprenkle, 1978; Olson, Sprenkle, & Russell, 1979), and constructive communication. These terms have been defined by Fisher, Giblin, and Hoopes (1982) as follows: **Cohesion** refers to "emotional attraction, differentiation, mature dependency, supportiveness, loyalty, psychological safety, reliability, family identification, physical caretaking, and pleasurable interaction"; **adaptability** refers to "flexibility, leadership, assertiveness, negotiation, rules, roles, and...feedback"; **constructive communication** includes the ability to "attentively listen, indicate messages are heard, paraphrase, checkout, attend to affect and content, value sender, message and self...speak for self, specify, express thoughts, feelings, and intentions, report completely... show congruence of messages, spontaneity, provide feedback...and encourage others to talk" (p. 273).

RANGE OF APPLICATIONS

It is our belief that some psychoses such as schizophrenia have a large biochemical component. However, even in these true diseases, when psychological intervention of any kind does seem appropriate, clinical experience has shown that marital and family RE therapy can be helpful. Clinical experience has also shown RE therapy to be highly effective in treating other severe dysfunctions (e.g., alcohol and spouse abuse). For the less severe types of problems which bring most couples and families for help, there is not only clinical but experimental evidence that RE is effective, that it is more effective than a traditional approach, and that the superiority is maintained after treatment terminates.

RESEARCH

A bibliography of research on RE therapy and very closely related methods is presented in the Resource section. Here I will briefly summarize this research.

There have been a series of controlled experimental studies on RE. Most of these studies have been conducted in a mental health facility in a university setting. Some, however, have been conducted in settings such as local schools and a community mental health center. RE has been tested in both group and individual formats. RE has been compared to no-treatment control conditions and to a variety of alternate treatments. The experiments have covered both intergenerational and marital relationships. Either in terms of the clients' attitudes toward the treatment process, or in terms of outcome variables assessing communication skills and the general quality of the relationship, RE consistently has been found to be superior to no-treatment and to alternate treatments. These alternate treatments have included a behavioral therapy approach, a gestalt approach, a traditional eclectic group approach, and the therapist's own preferred form of treatment. Excluding Filial Therapy (discussed elsewhere in this volume) in which even longer follow-ups have been conducted, RE has been assessed in follow-up periods ranging from ten weeks to six months. Significant gains were still found in every treatment and follow-up study. Perhaps of special interest to the readers of this particular volume is the study in which dyadic marital RE therapy was compared to the therapist's own preferred methods of therapy (Ross, 1982). This study was conducted with staff therapists in a community mental health center. With five therapists involved, a broad range of preferred traditional treatment orientations were represented, including psychoanalytic, behavioral, and Rogerian therapist orientations. These personal preferences had been developed over an average of six years of experience in marital therapy. The therapists received a three-day training program in RE therapy after which couples coming because of marital problems were assigned to them on a random basis to receive either the therapist's preferred form of marital therapy or the RE therapy they had recently been taught. The design was a pre-post comparison after ten weeks of treatment. Clients treated with RE showed very substantial gains in communication skills, marital adjustment, and the general quality of their relationship. These gains were far greater than the insignificant gains shown by the participants in the therapist's preferred treatment method.

COMPOSITION AND FORMATS

Marital or family RE therapy can be used with an individual, a dyad, or a group. The RE method falls in the category of marital and family therapy even when only a single individual is included. This is so because, when working with one person, RE concentrates on preparing that individual for specific interactions with others in the family (session-rehearsed, role-played interactions are implemented at home, and then closely supervised on the basis of detailed reports). In any of the formats to be described further on in this chapter, RE therapy can be conducted with only one member of a family, with a subgroup from a family, with the entire family attending as a unit, with two or more whole family units, or with groups comprised of subunits or individuals from two or more families.

RE can be conducted in an **intensive** format which refers to marathon sessions, lasting six to eight hours or a whole weekend, or mini-marathon sessions, lasting three or four hours. A typical example of a marathon application would be a group of married couples seen for a weekend or a series of weekends. Marital and family RE therapy can also be conducted in an **extensive** format, by which we mean sessions lasting for an hour or two at the rate of one or two a week over a period of many weeks. A typical example of an extensive format would be a married couple seen for a period of ten or fifteen weeks for fifty minutes each week. In a **combination** format, the two previously mentioned formats are combined. An example would be seeing a family for two three-hour sessions during the first two weeks and following this with weekly sessions lasting a hundred minutes each for ten or more weeks. This combination format is especially useful for clients that are in a crisis situation when first seeking help. This format allows the training stage of RE therapy to be completed quickly so that the clients can proceed rapidly to resolve critical problems. The **time-limited** format runs a predetermined length of time (e.g., ten or fifteen weeks). Such time-limited programs are usually associated with the prevention and enrichment uses of RE or with therapy programs limited because of research requirements or because of funding or administrative constraints.

We have coined the term **"time-designated"** (Guerney, 1977a) to apply to the typical time format for marital or family RE therapy. By time-designated we mean that an informal contract is made in which the clients agree to a minimal time commitment (anywhere from two to twenty sessions). At the end of this time, progress is evaluated with a discussion of whether or not both the therapist and the client(s) agree that the criteria for termination have been met. If it is jointly decided that more time is needed to meet the criteria for termination, another mutually agreeable time is designated for a second evaluation where this procedure will be repeated. It is our belief that the time-designated approach offers the best opportunity to achieve the advantages associated with both the open-ended and the time-limited formats of therapy, and to avoid the problems that accompany each.

THEORY

Like most modern approaches to marital and family therapy, RE is based on the view that the family should be regarded as a system. We mean by this that members of a family develop behavior patterns which take into account the thoughts, attitudes, and feelings of other family members. This occurs because they know the tangible and the psychological rewards and punishments likely to follow a given type of behavior in a given type of situation. Also, concepts of self and of others are based in large measure on the history of family interactions. Significant changes in the behavior patterns of one family member are very likely to affect the other members psychologically and emotionally. To be successful, a therapeutic approach should take these phenomena into account.

RE therapy draws upon and integrates a variety of previous psychotherapeutic theories and practices. In some instances, our debt is almost exclusively to a theory as such, rejecting the therapeutic strategies and techniques previously drawn from that theory because we believe that very different and better therapeutic strategies can be derived from the same theoretical base. In other instances, we draw heavily from the technique and general orientation of a method, but reject the general theory behind it because we believe that other theories better explain why such practices should be employed. It is our hope that the theoretical foundation which we have constructed for RE is internally consistent, and that our practices are appropriately derived from the new theoretical constellation. We have not yet published this theory, and do not have the room to do so here. Therefore, we simply offer the reader a very broad overview of the manner in which RE combines psychodynamic, humanistic, and behavioral theory and principles.

Our greatest theoretical debt is to the interpersonal theories of Sullivan as elaborated by Leary. From this theoretical perspective, we accept the principle that the avoidance of anxiety is a major factor in determining interpersonal behavior while rejecting the notion that it is the only, or root, cause of interpersonal behavior or interpersonal pathology. We draw upon Thorndike and Skinner to add reward or reinforcement as a second major principle determining interpersonal behavior. We reject, however, the idea that one can go as far as is necessary in the understanding and changing of behavior simply by analyzing stimulus-response relationships. We draw from Adler the view that the understanding of a person's present behavior can be greatly facilitated by looking upon the person as primarily a goal-striving, future-anticipating being.

We accept from Freud the notion that making the unconscious conscious is often an important ingredient in producing positive changes. While we reject any sort of deification of the unconscious, we do accept what we regard as the essence of Freud's view of the unconscious: that one is often strongly motivated to keep certain feelings and ideas outside of awareness, and that certain preconditions must be met before some ideas are admitted to oneself, and that still others must be met before those ideas are admitted to others. Continuing on Freud's side here against the behaviorists, we also accept the idea that catharsis can sometimes be a positive force in promoting awareness and positive change.

We reject most of the therapeutic techniques used by Freudian or other psychodynamic therapists, because we believe that probing, interpretation, and the like generally are counterproductive to making the unconscious conscious and to therapeutic gains in general. Instead, we accept Roger's view that the best way to bring the unconscious to awareness and the best route in general toward therapeutic gain is the feeling of strength and safety the client derives from an environment of empathy, warmth, and acceptance. We believe, apparently more strongly than most Freudians, in the almost unlimited power of psychological defenses to circumvent probing, direction, suggestion, advice, and interpretation. We believe that defense mechanisms (such as denial or projection) can best be overcome by the conditions advocated by Rogers.

We reject, however, the Rogerian contention that growth in the environment of acceptance results from some mysterious drive toward self-fulfillment. Rather, we take the view that the increased self-awareness and growth which follow unconditional positive regard and empathy are the result of deconditioning and conditioning processes.

We accept the view that the desire for the expression of repressed thoughts and feelings persists over long periods of time. This is not consistent with behaviorism, but is consistent with the positions of both Freud and Rogers. Our view that the fears associated with such thoughts and feelings can be deconditioned through acceptance is similar to the views of Dollard and Miller (1950) who, in our opinion, long ago achieved a rather successful integration of behavioral and Freudian theory along many dimensions. Other reasons we add Rogers to our picture of how therapy works are that we believe compassion and love are far more powerful shapers of behavior than the variables which learning theorists and social learning theorists usually discuss, and that threats to the self-concept are the most important generators of reality distorting defense mechanisms.

Our techniques in training people to bring about desired changes are a blend of Rogerian, Skinnarian, and Bandurian methods (and age-old teaching methods): demonstration, modeling, encouragement, prompting, task-assignment, and bushels full of contingent and no-so-contingent praise, all in an interpersonal environment of unconditional positive personal regard, warmth, empathy, and genuineness (and strong leadership and competence).

In closing this brief theoretical background to RE, we must return to Sullivan and Leary. We accept their position that personality is best understood in terms of interpersonal relationships. These relationships shape personality which in turn shapes interpersonal relationships. A person's every utterance, and every significant nonverbal sign, causes others to respond to him or her in certain ways. We all train others to treat us in certain ways just as they train us. "Interpersonal reflexes," flashing quickly between persons, operate almost entirely outside of awareness, but in largely predictable ways.

RE is essentially a method for changing personality and interpersonal relationships by **teaching people how to gain conscious control over what had previously been unconscious, reflexive, interpersonal behaviors.** We believe that, by learning which types of interpersonal responses commonly elicit what types of responses from others (see Shannon & Guerney, 1973), people can bring their behavior into the service of their conscious goals. In fact, we believe that such knowledge also helps them to better understand their true goals. Also, in RE we teach clients to become acutely aware that their own needs and goals must be considered in the context of others' needs and goals. We teach them how to achieve coordination between their needs and goals and those of others in a way that mutual satisfactions are maximized and pain and sacrifice are minimized. In these ways, self-understanding, mutual understanding, mutual acceptance, and mutual gratification of needs (that is to say cohesion, adaptability, and good communication) are increased, and the individual and the family are strengthened.

We recognize that the above is merely the roughest sort of sketch as far as theoretical exposition is concerned. We recognize, too, that what was said leaves much to be desired with respect to drawing the links between the theory and the practice of RE. We have presented the sketch because we hope that it will provide the reader with at least a taste of RE's theoretical flavor, thereby permitting a comparison with the reader's own preferences.

SKILLS CLIENTS ARE TAUGHT

The skills taught to clients to help them reach the goals described are outlined below. Although we are not covering nonmarital, nonfamily forms of RE here, we have stated the skills in generic rather than family-related terms to allow the reader to see how the method also can be applied to persons coming for help with nonfamily related social adjustment problems. The reader can simply add "in the family" wherever we use the generic "others" in our description of the skills below. For each of the skills mentioned, the client is given numerous, clearly specified operational guidelines to follow. These guidelines may be found elsewhere (Guerney, 1977a; Preston & Guerney, 1982). Here each skill will be described only in terms of its purpose.

1. **Expressive** skill enables clients to (a) better understand their own emotional/psychological/interpersonal needs, (b) express those needs to others in ways least likely to engender unnecessary defensiveness, anxiety, conflict, and hostility, and most likely to engender sympathetic understanding and cooperation, and (c) face up to conflicts and problems with others more promptly and more positively in terms of their own goals and needs (assertively, if you like) and with less anxiety.

2. **Empathic** skill enables clients to (a) better understand the emotional/psychological/interpersonal needs of others and (b) elicit more prompt, frequent, open, honest, relevant, trusting, and intimate behaviors from others.

3. **Conversive** ("mode-switching") skill enables clients to best preserve a positive emotional climate in working through problems and conflicts, and to avoid unnecessary or deleterious digressions, and to bring discussions expeditiously to the root issues.

4. **Problem/conflict resolution** skill enables clients to devise, and to help others involved to devise, creative solutions to problems; solutions which maximize mutual need-satisfaction and, therefore, are likely to prove workable and durable.

5. **Self-change** skill enables clients to implement changes in their attitudes/feelings/behaviors in order to implement interpersonal agreements and objectives.

6. **Helping-others change** skill enables clients to help others to change their attitudes/feelings/behaviors in order to implement interpersonal agreements and objectives.

7. **Generalization** skill enables individuals to train themselves to use relationship-enhancing skills in daily life.

8. **Teaching** ("facilitative") skill enables clients to train others to use relationship-enhancing skills in daily life (i.e., to train others to treat them in ways most likely to enhance their own self-image, psychological well-being, and interpersonal relations).

9. **Maintenance** skill enables clients to maintain usage of such skills over time.

SOURCES OF THERAPIST'S SATISFACTION

When one is used to conducting other types of therapy, becoming an effective RE therapist obviously involves acquiring some specific new skills. Acquiring such skills will not be nearly so difficult for many therapists as doing something else which sometimes may be required - shifting to the types of personal gratification found in conducting RE therapy as opposed to the types of gratification derived from their present mode of conducting therapy. In RE therapy, therapists must derive their gratification not from directly helping clients to achieve insights and reach solutions to their problems, but rather from helping clients learn the skills and then watching them use the skills on their own to achieve insights and reach solutions to their problems. Similarly, except with the unusual client or with the usual client on relatively infrequent occasions, the therapist also must learn to largely forego gratifications derived from directly providing solutions to problems and giving nurturance to the client. Rather, he or she must learn to derive most satisfaction from helping clients learn the skills which will enable them, on their own, to solve problems and win nurturance from the significant others in their natural interpersonal environments.

In our experience, the difference between the traditional therapist who is successful in making the shift to RE therapy, and the one who is not, does not generally lie in a difference in basic capacity to learn RE-related skills. Nor does the difference lie in a therapist's reasoned analysis of competing theoretical positions or comparative research. The difference most often lies in whether or not the therapist is willing to shift the major source of personal gratifications in his or her daily interactions with clients. The therapist's power or control needs and need to nurture are very important in this regard. In our view, one might summarize the basic differences by what we hope is a value-free analogy between the gratifications one derives from parenting young children (much direct help and nurturance as in traditional therapy), and that derived from parenting older children (less of the above and more teaching and promoting independence as in skill-training therapy).

We do not wish to leave a false impression here. There is nothing formal, cold, or distant about RE therapy either in the way family members relate to each other during the sessions or in the way they relate to the therapist. The discussion of issues between family members very often is highly emotional in nature, and a deeply moving experience for the therapist.

THERAPIST ATTITUDES

Two attitudes are extremely helpful for the RE therapist: first, humility concerning one's own powers of understanding what may be best for others (especially when one has only a limited number of hours of observation outside the family's natural habitat) and second, confidence in the ability of others, once given appropriate means and circumstances to do so, to reach self-knowledge, understanding of others, and to work through their personal and interpersonal conflicts in ways better than any outsider may devise for them (however bright, knowledgeable, and experienced that outsider might be). These two attitudes or beliefs generally facilitate learning how to be an RE therapist.

Conversely, practicing RE therapy also greatly facilitates the development of these attitudes. RE therapists encounter case after case in which things are later revealed which they would have needed to know but could not have known if they had decided early in therapy what made the relationship among clients go, or what made it go wrong. Indeed, the therapist would probably never have learned what was needed if he or she acted on such earlier diagnostic and prescriptive "insights." That type of experience strengthens humility. Similarly, experience as an RE therapist affords many examples of skilled clients resolving their conflicts with creativity, efficiency, and wisdom. It is hardly surprising when one stops to think about it. The clients have had thousands of hours of experience with each other and with their problems, and a great deal of experience with attempted solutions that have failed, whereas the therapist has virtually no experience in either sphere. Nevertheless, continually seeing clients actually proceed to reach creative, durable solutions to problems that have long plagued them, does a lot to build the kind of confidence in clients we mentioned.

There is no single widely accepted, let alone validated, theory of family functioning or of diagnosis or of therapy. From the diversity of views in the literature, it seems probable that if five family therapists were picked at random from five areas of the country and each was allowed to interact alone for a few hours with the same family, they would come up with six different diagnostic descriptions and seven different sets of ideas about how the therapy should proceed. Yet, some marital and family therapists believe that, in a few hours or less, they know all they need to know to decide exactly what to change and how to change it in a family. This type of therapist seems equally confident that therapy really was successful even when someone has left the family in a rage; and if failure of therapy is all too obvious, equally confident that some suddenly discovered deep pathology in one or more family members really made success impossible. Such therapists probably will find it difficult to practice RE therapy techniques long enough to acquire the attitudes necessary to become an RE therapist.

THERAPIST SKILLS

The RE therapist needs most of the skills which are valuable in the majority of psychotherapeutic approaches. Predominantly, these are the interpersonal skills which cause the client to view the therapist as warm, honest, compassionate, and competent. Where a therapist works with more than one client, there is a need for additional skills which make all the clients in the groups regard the therapist as impartial and fair and, again, these would be common to most psychotherapeutic group approaches.

Added to these skills, therapists in RE must know how to change client attitudes and behaviors efficiently and effectively. Therapists must know how to elicit formulations of the most important life goals, especially interpersonal goals. They must know how to motivate and inspire people to acquire the attitudes and skills, including how to positively link the skill to be taught to the individual's own values, goals, and aspirations. They must know how to instill and maintain the learner's confidence in his or her ability to learn and to change. Inspiring and maintaining motivation and confidence means knowing when and how to use verbal and nonverbal praise. It means knowing how to use evidence. It means knowing how to fully elicit client doubts about what is being taught, when it is appropriate to try to remove those doubts through discussion, when and how to turn off discussions in favor of allowing concrete experience to answer the doubts, and how, in either case, to ultimately remove the doubts.

RESPONSE CLASSIFICATION

On a more specific level, being an effective RE therapist means knowing how to classify responses a therapist of any school of thought is likely to make. We classify such responses into seven major categories which are RE-inappropriate. These are: Directive Lead; Interpretation; Suggestion, Explanation, or Advice regarding Problem Content; Encouragement, Approval, Reassurance regarding Problem Content; Personal Criticism; and Failure to Correct a Significant Unskilled Response. We also classify therapist responses into seven major responses which are RE-appropriate. These are: Administrative; Social Reinforcement; Demonstrating; Modeling; Encouraging and Prompting; Doubling; and Troubleshooting. This last response is infrequently used but it allows the therapist, following certain guidelines, to do certain things generally proscribed in RE (e.g., to express his or her own opinions, make suggestions, offer interpretations, discuss his or her own feelings about the clients' problems or the therapeutic process, and to provide direct empathy, nurturance, reassurance, and support to the client).

In addition to being instantly able to classify anything they are about to say into any one of these categories, skilled RE therapists, following various guidelines and employing their clinical knowledge and intuitions about the client's abilities and disabilities, know how to choose the most appropriate response(s) from among all appropriate ones to suit any given therapeutic circumstance.

While it is not too difficult for neophyte marital and family therapists, learning to keep the clients at skill practice and problem-solving with each other rather than engaging the therapist in discussions of their problems is possibly the hardest thing for therapists experienced in other approaches to master.

PARADIGMS

THE TEACHING PARADIGM

In teaching the client any RE skill, the following paradigm is used in approximately this order, though sometimes adjacent categories are intermingled:

1. Explain the rationale underlying the skill.
2. Explain all, or the most essential, guidelines the client is to follow and the rationale for them. (Depending on client attention

span, less critical guidelines can be left for interspersion within practice.)

3. Demonstrate the skill by playing demonstration audio tapes or by role playing with the client or a co-therapist.
4. Provide word by word supervision of the client's practice of the skill in the session.
5. Once a suitable level of skill has been reached, provide assignments in which that skill is to be practiced at home.
6. Closely supervise, via self-report or tapes, the home practice of skills.
7. Provide assignments to bring about the use of skills in the course of regular daily living.
8. Closely supervise, via self-report and log questionnaires, the skill's' usage in daily life.
9. See that the skill is incorporated as part of maintenance-skill practice.

TOPIC SELECTION PARADIGM

To facilitate successful experience in skill practice, the following paradigm is used in selecting topics for conjoint RE marital and family therapy:

1. Strongly felt views and feelings which do **not** involve the other family members (such topics are used only until empathic skill has been mastered with some proficiency)
2. Positive views of significant other(s) physically present
3. Enhancement issues (suggestions for improving the relationship that the significant others are also likely to find agreeable)
4. Mild problems
5. Moderate problems
6. Serious problems
7. Enhancement issues again (once all significant problems are solved)

SESSION PARADIGM

The session paradigm generally followed after the first or second session is:

1. Review and supervise home assignments.
2. Conduct follow-up inquiries regarding problem solutions that are due for evaluation.
3. Share positive attitudes/feelings/behaviors of the others physically present at therapist's option, but frequently if feasible.
4. Review for appropriateness the topics chosen by the clients as most important to their relationship and supervise revision if necessary. (Allow no substitutions of less fundamentally important topics, however salient they may be, unless the substitution clearly arises from a critical or urgent need.)
5. Supervise the use of skills on the current topic.
6. Once problem-solving has been learned, follow each problem through to its solution in the session (or at home) unless discussion of another more appropriate one has taken its place.
7. Help the clients prepare for their home assignments.

Innovations In Clinical Practice: A Source Book

Bernard Guerney, Jr., Ph.D., is currently Professor of Human Development and Head of the Individual and Family Consultation Center at The Pennsylvania State University. He was formerly Professor of Psychology and Director of the Psychological Clinic at Rutgers University. A diplomate in Clinical Psychology and in Behavioral Medicine, he is also an AAMFT approved Marital/Family Therapy Supervisor. He has written several books and professional articles on individual, child, marital, and family therapy and is on the Editorial Boards of the AMERICAN JOURNAL OF FAMILY THERAPY, the INTERNATIONAL JOURNAL OF FAMILY THERAPY, and FAMILY STUDIES REVIEW YEARBOOK. Dr. Guerney may be contacted at Catherine Beecher House, Pennsylvania State University, University Park, PA 16802.

RESOURCES

THERAPIST MATERIALS

All of the materials in this section are available through the Individual and Family Consultation Center, The Pennsylvania State University, Catharine Beecher House, University Park, PA 16802, (814) 865-1751.

CONJUGAL RELATIONSHIP ENHANCEMENT PROGRAM - A 34 minute, 3/4", color video cassette tape available on marital RE methods. It shows how the basic RE skills are taught in one format (group and time-limited to 10 sessions).

RELATIONSHIP ENHANCEMENT PROGRAM FOR FAMILY THERAPY AND ENRICHMENT - A 35 minute, 3/4", color video cassette which illustrates family RE. It shows how the basic RE skills are taught in a variety of formats. Both are available either for rental or purchase.

AUDIO TAPES - A number of these are available for use to illustrate RE skills to clients. Using a variety of family constellations (e.g., cohabiting and married couples, fathers and sons, mothers and daughters), the tapes illustrate discussions of a wide variety of issues and problems. Each tape begins with a brief dialogue between the couple showing how the discussion of a given issue or conflict is likely to proceed without the use of skills. This is then followed by a longer dialogue (about 20 minutes) in which the couple discuss the same issue using RE skills. On some tapes, the discussion proceeds all the way through the problem resolution stage. Descriptions of these tapes are available without charge.

FORMS - Many of the forms used with clients in RE therapy may be seen in the book, RELATIONSHIP ENHANCEMENT (Guerney, 1977), and/or are available from the author.

TRAINING - Training is available through The Pennsylvania State University, where three-day training programs in Marital Relationship Enhancement and Family Relationship Enhancement have been held each spring. The program carries Continuing Education Units, and graduate credits can be arranged. These workshops have been approved by the American Psychological Association and by the AMA for continuing education credits. The program is very skill oriented. An instructor is provided for every four to six participants, permitting role playing and a great deal of individualized constructive feedback.

Workshops can also be held where there are six or more people available for training in a community. Certified trainers will travel anywhere in the country to provide such training. IDEALS (the Institute for the Development of Emotional and Life Skills), a nonprofit educational organization founded in 1972, has the major purpose of training therapists in the skill-training methods of psychotherapy, marital, and family therapy. One-day, three-day, and advanced workshops and supervision, which can lead to certification as an RE therapist and trainer, are available. A description of supervisory and certification procedures is available from IDEALS, P. O. Box 391, State College, PA 16801.

PUBLISHED MATERIALS

Authier, J., Gustafson, K., Guerney, B. G., Jr., & Kasdorf, J. A. The psychological practitioner as a teacher: A theoretical-historical practical review. THE COUNSELING PSYCHOLOGIST, 1975, 5(2), 31-50.

Dollard, J. & Miller, N. E. PERSONALITY AND PSYCHOTHERAPY. New York: McGraw Hill, 1950.

Fisher, B. & Sprenkle, D. Therapists' perceptions of healthy family functioning. INTERNATIONAL JOURNAL OF FAMILY COUNSELING, 1978, **6**, 1-10.

Fisher, B. L., Giblin, P. R., & Hoopes, M. H. Healthy family functioning: What therapists say and what families want. JOURNAL OF MARITAL AND FAMILY THERAPY, 1982, **8**, 273-285.

Goldstein, A. STRUCTURED LEARNING THERAPY: TOWARD A PSYCHOTHERAPY FOR THE POOR. New York: Academic Press, 1973.

Guerney, B. G., Jr. The delivery of mental health services: Spiritual versus medical versus educational models. In T. R. Vallance & R. M. Sabre (Eds.), MENTAL HEALTH SERVICES IN TRANSITION: A POLICY SOURCEBOOK. New York: Human Sciences Press, 1982.

Guerney, B. G., Jr. The great potential of an educational skill-training model in problem prevention. JOURNAL OF CLINICAL CHILD PSYCHOLOGY, 1979, **3**(2), 84-86.

Guerney, B. G., Jr. RELATIONSHIP ENHANCEMENT: SKILL TRAINING PROGRAMS FOR THERAPY, PROBLEM PREVENTION, AND ENRICHMENT. San Francisco: Jossey-Bass, 1977. (a)

Guerney, B. G., Jr. Should teachers treat illiteracy, hypocalligraphy, and dysmathematica? CANADIAN COUNSELLOR, 1977, **12**(1), 9-14. (b)

Guerney, B. G., Jr., Coufal, J., & Vogelsong, E. Relationship enhancement versus a traditional approach to therapeutic/preventative/enrichment parent-adolescent programs. JOURNAL OF CONSULTING AND CLINICAL PSYCHOLOGY, 1981, **49**, 927-939.

Guerney, B. G., Jr., Guerney, L., & Stollak, G. The potential advantages of changing from a medical to an educational model in practicing psychology. INTERPERSONAL DEVELOPMENT, 1971/72, **2**(4), 238-245.

Guerney, B. G., Jr., Stollak, G. E., & Guerney, L. A format for a new mode of psychological practice: Or, how to escape a zombie. THE COUNSELING PSYCHOLOGIST, 1970, **2**(2), 97-104.

Guerney, B. G., Jr., Stollak, G. E., & Guerney, L. The practicing psychologist as educator - An alternative to the medical practitioner model. PROFESSIONAL PSYCHOLOGY, 1971, **2**(3), 276-282.

Jessee, R. & Guerney, B. G., Jr. A comparison of Gestalt and Relationship Enhancement treatments with married couples. THE AMERICAN JOURNAL OF FAMILY THERAPY, 1981, **9**, 31-41.

Olson, D., Sprenkle, D., & Russell, C. Circumplex model of marital and family system I: Cohesion and adaptability dimensions, family types, and clinical applications. FAMILY PROCESS, 1979, **18**, 3-28.

Preston, J. & Guerney, B. G., Jr. RELATIONSHIP ENHANCEMENT SKILL TRAINING. Mimeographed manuscript, 625 pages, 1982. Available at cost from author of this chapter at Individual and Family Consultation Center, Catharine Beecher House, University Park, PA 16802.

Rappaport, A. F. Conjugal relationship enhancement program. In D. H. Olson (Ed.), TREATING RELATIONSHIPS. Lake Mills, IA: Graphic Publishing Company, Inc., 1976.

Ross, E. COMPARATIVE EFFECTIVENESS OF RELATIONSHIP ENHANCEMENT VERSUS THERAPISTS' PREFERRED THERAPY ON MARITAL ADJUSTMENT. (Doctoral dissertation, The Pennsylvania State University, 1982). DISSERTATION ABSTRACTS INTERNATIONAL, 1982, **42**, 4610A.

Shannon, J. & Guerney, B., Jr. Interpersonal effects of interpersonal behavior. JOURNAL OF PERSONALITY AND SOCIAL PSYCHOLOGY, 1973, **26**(1), 142-150.

Vogelsong, E. PREVENTATIVE-THERAPEUTIC PROGRAMS FOR MOTHERS AND ADOLESCENT DAUGHTERS: A FOLLOW-UP OF RE VERSUS DISCUSSION AND BOOSTER VERSUS NO BOOSTER. (Doctoral dissertation, The Pennsylvania State University, 1975). DISSERTATION ABSTRACTS INTERNATIONAL, 1975, **36**, 7677A.

Vogelsong, E. L. & Guerney, B. G., Jr. Working with parents of disturbed adolescents. In R. R. Abidin (Ed.), PARENT EDUCATION AND INTERVENTION HANDBOOK. Springfield, IL: Charles C. Thomas, Publisher, 1980.

Vogelsong, E., Guerney, B. G., Jr., & Guerney, L. F. Relationship enhancement therapy with inpatients and their families. In R. Luber & C. Anderson (Eds.), COMMUNICATION TRAINING APPROACHES TO FAMILY INTERVENTION WITH PSYCHIATRIC PATIENTS. New York: Human Sciences Press, in press.

A SLEEP DISORDERS PRIMER

Peter J. Hauri and Terry S. Proeger

According to an Institute of Medicine Report (1979), approximately 5 million adult Americans are issued prescriptions for sleeping pills in a given year. These 5 million are only a tenth, however, of the 50 million people who report some kind of difficulty sleeping. Although physicians are traditionally consulted for sleep disorders, mental health clinicians can play an important role in the diagnosis and treatment of these problems (Hauri, 1982). This chapter includes a brief review of current scientific knowledge pertaining to sleep and then discusses the diagnosis and treatment of specific sleep disorders.

CHARACTERISTICS OF SLEEP

THE FUNCTION OF SLEEP

Despite the subjective importance of sleep in our lives, scientists do not yet understand why we sleep. Numerous theories about the function of sleep have been proposed, including the idea that sleep allows general bodily and cortical recovery (Hartmann, 1973; Oswald, 1974), that sleep protects the body from tissue damage caused by exhaustion (Claparede, 1905), that sleep is a natural mechanism for conserving energy (Allison & Van Twyver, 1970), and that sleep is an innate, species-specific behavior similar to such phenomena as nest building, migration, or courtship dances (McGinty, 1971).

It is interesting to note that sleep needs seem to be finely tuned to the ecological niche of a given species. Animals with few enemies, such as the large cats, or animals that are well protected, such as small burrowing rodents, sleep a great deal of the time, while animals who are at risk during sleep, such as the large grazing animals, sleep very little.

Webb (1974) observed that sleep length is closely related to the time in which it is best for an animal not to respond. He suggested that the inactivity of sleep may have survival benefits. For example, early humans who slept little and were active at night were no doubt frequent victims of animals better adapted to nocturnal hunting, while their sleeping and motionless relatives were more likely to go unnoticed. Also, since subsistence food gathering probably consumed most of the daylight period, those inclined to sleep during the day would soon find themselves starving to death. Thus, there may well have been a survival advantage for those humans who remained unresponsive during darkness, but were active during the daylight hours.

Many of these sleep theories are compatible and it seems likely that sleep serves many functions (Webb, 1979). It may well be, for example, that a certain minimal amount of sleep is required to restore some bodily processes, and that additional sleep may vary according to ecological requirements or specific needs to conserve energy.

STAGES OF SLEEP

Sleep consists of distinct stages which are traditionally measured and defined by electroencephalogram. There are two basic types of sleep, rapid eye movement (REM) and non-rapid eye movement (NREM), as well as a transition phase between wakefulness and sleep. We will briefly define each stage in the following paragraphs; however, the reader is referred to Rechtschaffen and Kales (1968) for a more detailed description of each stage.

The transition phase between wakefulness and sleep is commonly labeled **stage 1 sleep**. Stage 1 occurs at the beginning of sleep and at varying times during the night, especially after a body movement or noise. Stage 1 sleep is also recorded in many experienced meditators during their meditation (Elson, Hauri, & Cunis, 1977). Decreased reactivity to external stimuli and a change in mentation to a more dreamlike state (Foulkes & Vogel, 1965) serve to differentiate stage 1 sleep from wakefulness. However, a person awakened from Stage 1 sleep usually reports a feeling of having been awake.

NREM sleep is divided into stage 2 (normal) sleep and delta (deep) sleep. Stage 2 is the most abundant of sleep stages and occupies 50% to 70% of adult sleep. When persons are awakened from this stage, they usually report short, mundane, and fragmented thoughts (Foulkes, 1962). Delta sleep is the deepest type of sleep and is commonly believed to be the most restorative. It usually occurs early in the night.

REM sleep, the second major type of sleep, is characterized by rapid eye movements which usually occur in bursts. Although muscle tone, particularly in the chin and neck muscles, is lowest during REM sleep, small twitches occur in many muscle groups. Heart rate and respiratory rate are higher and more variable during REM than NREM sleep. In general, about 80% of awakenings from REM sleep yield reports of vivid dreaming.

THE NORMAL ADULT SLEEP CYCLE

Upon going to bed, a normal sleeper initially enters stage 1 and then passes into stage 2 sleep. After 10 to 30 minutes in stage 2, the sleeper gradually enters delta sleep. Sixty to 90 minutes later the sleeper returns to stage 2 and then enters a REM period which lasts only a few minutes. This first REM period is the least intense of the night, both in terms of the physiological manifestations of REM sleep and of dream intensity.

The second sleep cycle begins when stage 2 reoccurs after the first REM period. Depending on age, the sleeper often re-enters delta sleep, although there is usually less of it in the second cycle than in the first. After about 90 minutes of NREM sleep, the second REM period begins and usually lasts 8 to 10 minutes. For the remainder of the night, stage 2 sleep and REM sleep usually alternate in approximately 90 minute cycles with REM sleep typically occupying 15 to 30 minutes of each cycle. REM sleep becomes more intense, both physiologically and psychologically, towards morning. Delta sleep is rarely seen in these later sleep cycles.

Numerous body movements and 5 to 15 spontaneous awakenings a night are spread throughout REM and NREM sleep. In good sleepers, these awakenings typically last from a few seconds to a few minutes each. Although the sleeper is responsive to environmental stimuli during these shorter arousals, the awakenings are usually forgotten by morning.

DEPTH OF SLEEP

Depth of sleep is typically measured by the amount of noise required to awaken a sleeper. Of NREM sleep, delta sleep is much deeper than stage 2, although stage 2 varies greatly in depth. Stage 2 is lighter just after falling asleep and during the early morning, and deeper when adjoining delta sleep (Bonnet, Johnson, & Webb, 1978). The depth of REM sleep, on the other hand, cannot be as easily classified because it has physiological characteristics of both light and deep sleep. However, in terms of noise needed to awaken a person, REM and stage 2 sleep are similar (Rechtschaffen, Hauri, & Zeitlin, 1966).

AGE AND SLEEP PATTERNS

Sleep patterns change with age. On the average, sleep time drops from approximately 17 hours at birth to about 10 hours at age 4, and 9 hours at age 10. The typical adolescent averages about 8 hours of sleep per night. Sleep time then gradually declines to about 6 hours in old age. Also, both delta and REM sleep decrease as a person ages (e.g., about 50% of sleep at birth is REM; this drops to approximately 20% by old age).

From birth to about age 35, actual sleep time is essentially the same as time spent in bed. It appears, however, that after 35, humans spend more time in bed but less time asleep as a result of an increase in middle of the night and early morning awakenings. The nature of problems with sleep also changes with age. A younger insomniac typically has trouble falling asleep; middle and older aged insomniacs have more difficulties with frequent awakenings.

SLEEP NEEDS

Customary sleep time varies widely, even in good sleepers. Some healthy adults require 3 hours or less sleep per night (Jones & Oswald, 1968; Stuss & Broughton, 1978), while others feel sleep deprived and tired unless they are able to sleep 10 to 12 hours per night. Large individual differences in sleep needs characterize children as well as adults. This wide range in sleep needs makes it difficult to objectively define insomnia.

The best currently available measure of sufficient sleep in children or adults is adequate daytime functioning. An individual who remains alert and energetic during wakefulness is apparently getting enough sleep. More sleep would seem to be indicated if, after several weeks on a given sleep schedule, one becomes excessively tired, irritable, or frequently dozes off. However, should drastically increased amounts of sleep not bring alertness after a few nights, the possibility of pathologically excessive daytime somnolence should be investigated.

CIRCADIAN RHYTHMS

The sleep-wake cycle is one of the body's circadian rhythms. Circadian rhythms include those biological cycles which require about a day to complete. When normal individuals live in environments with no time clues, they usually show a sleep-wake rhythm lasting about 25 hours. There are many biological clocks in our body and they do not all keep the same time (Wever, 1976). Thus, unless internal circadian cycles are regularly synchronized with the earth's rotation, humans not only drift out of phase with their social environment, but also experience desynchronization of their different biological clocks. If circadian rhythms become desynchronized, both sleep and wakefulness are adversely affected, because one internal rhythm may be at a low ebb while another calls for wakefulness. People who have lost a synchronized circadian rhythm often complain of being "always sleepy, but never sleeping well."

It is important to note that the most powerful synchronizing impulse may be a regular wake-up time which is an effective way to push back and, therefore, regulate the sleep cycle. This is also practical because wake-up time is under voluntary control. One can force oneself into wakefulness with alarm clocks, cold showers, and similar techniques. Bedtime, on the other hand, is a less powerful synchronizing impulse because falling asleep is not under voluntary control.

SLEEP DEPRIVATION

The immediate effect of sleep deprivation is a sharply increased need to sleep, an alteration in mood, and a subjective feeling of malaise. Initially, there is no serious impairment in objective behavioral performance. However, if sleep deprivation extends beyond a few nights, "mini-sleeps" with short lapses of attention begin to occur during wakefulness. These "mini-sleep" episodes increase in duration and number with increased sleep deprivation until, within about 10 days, it becomes almost impossible to distinguish, either from the EEG or from the person's behavior, whether the individual is actually awake or asleep. Although mood after sleep deprivation deteriorates drastically, it still follows a circadian rhythm and is generally worse during times when one normally would be sleeping. Increased irritability and aggressiveness, a grim listlessness, and a feeling of depletion are also noted in sleep deprived individuals (Hauri, 1979b). Waking performance gradually decreases after extended sleep deprivation.

Although it is still debated, evidence suggests that deprivation of REM sleep has different effects than deprivation of delta sleep. Mood states seem to be affected more by deprivation of REM sleep (Vogel, 1975). Delta sleep deprivation, on the other hand, seems to result in more somatic symptoms, such as increased pain sensitivity (Moldofsky, Scarisbrick, England, & Smythe, 1975).

THE DIAGNOSIS AND TREATMENT OF SLEEP DISORDERS

ASSESSMENT OF SLEEP DISORDERS

While some clinicians feel that only certified sleep disorders centers are qualified to make diagnoses involving sleep problems, we believe that most sleep disorders can at least be tentatively diagnosed through a sensitive interview, especially if the clinician also talks to the patient's bed partner. The decision to refer to a sleep disorders laboratory is a matter of clinical judgment, depending on the clinician's trust in the diagnosis, the seriousness of the problem, and the success of the prescribed treatment. For example, when presented with a patient complaining of insomnia, the clinician might first want to tentatively rule out medical problems, such as sleep apnea or myoclonus, by carefully interviewing the patient and bed partner. If no medical causes are discovered, psychiatric problems might then be considered and, if present, treated. If the treatment based upon the interview diagnosis is unsuccessful, a referral to a sleep disorders center might then be appropriate. The general rule for insomnia is to try all relevant treatments first and then, if not successful, refer to a sleep disorders center. However, if excessive daytime sleepiness is suspected, a referral to a sleep disorders center should be made because this is a medical problem and may be life threatening. The Association of Sleep Disorders Centers, P. O. Box YY, East Setauket, NY 11733, will supply the locations of sleep disorders centers to anyone wishing the information.

BEHAVIORAL CAUSES OF POOR SLEEP

Most sleep disorders involve interactions between psychological and physiological factors. When a person undergoes serious and prolonged stress, such as a divorce, the arousal system responds with increased activity and, as a result, it will usually become more difficult to sleep. If the stress continues for several weeks, other factors usually interact to cause temporary insomnia. Frequently, a maladaptive habit of "trying too hard to sleep" develops. The more persons are sleep deprived, the harder they try to sleep, which increases arousal and results in less sleep. Such individuals usually fall asleep easily when not trying to sleep, such as when watching TV, but become alert whenever they make a conscious decision to try to sleep.

Lying in bed unable to sleep often results in maladaptive conditioning. When this happens, the bedroom environment (i.e., the feeling of the mattress, the room itself) becomes associated with frustration and arousal, rather than with relaxation and sleep. Similarly, customary bedtime rituals, such as brushing teeth and turning off lights, become stimuli anticipating frustration and tension rather than relaxation. People suffering from conditioned insomnia typically sleep better away from their usual sleep environment, such as in the living room or in a hotel. Also, when people sleep poorly because of stress, they often fall asleep towards morning and then oversleep or frequently take daytime naps "to catch up." This behavior leads to a desynchronization of the different biological clocks and causes further sleep difficulties.

As long as sleep is basically adequate, an occasional poor night usually is tolerated. However, in patients who have labeled themselves "insomniacs," a poor night re-confirms the label, and the fear of insomnia often then becomes a self-fulfilling prophecy.

The behavioral factors discussed here contribute to almost all chronic insomnias, whether the insomnia was originally due to psychological upheaval, to environmental stress, or to medical factors. Behavioral factors, therefore, need to be considered and treated, even if the original cause of the insomnia is clearly non-behavioral. The following references can provide detailed information on the behavioral treatment of insomnia (i.e., stimulus control therapy, relaxation therapy, biofeedback, environmental changes): Bootzin and Nicassio (1978), Borkovec (1979), Hauri (1979a), and Ware (1979).

RULES FOR BETTER SLEEP HABITS

While most of the scientific knowledge about good sleep habits is common sense, it is surprising how often these rules are not followed by persons suffering from serious sleep disorders. The following suggestions may help patients with sleep difficulties.

1. Do not sleep any more than is needed to feel refreshed the next day (Hauri, 1977).

2. Maintain a regular wake-up time because this will help to synchronize circadian rhythms.

3. Attempt a long term regular daily exercise program because it tends to deepen sleep (Baekeland & Lasky, 1966). However, omit any strenuous exercise for 3 hours before bedtime.

4. Try to create a sleep environment devoid of loud noises. It has been discovered that occasional loud noises, such as aircraft overhead, disturb sleep even in individuals who feel that they have adapted to the noise (Globus, Friedmann, Cohen, Pearsons, & Fidell, 1973).

5. Maintain a room temperature of 72 degrees or less. A hot environment causes more awakenings, more body movements, less REM sleep, and less delta sleep than a cool room (Otto, 1973; Schmidt-Kessen & Kendel, 1973).

6. Hunger seems to disturb sleep (Jacobs & McGinty, 1971). Eat a light bedtime snack if hungry (Brezinova & Oswald, 1972), preferably something bland and soothing, such as a milk product.

7. Avoid caffeine, cigarettes, and alcohol before going to bed. Caffeine ingestion and smoking increase arousal and make sleeping more difficult (Karacan, Thornby, Booth, Okawa, Salis, Anch, & Williams, 1975; Myrsten, Elgerot, & Edgren, 1977). Coffee can be consumed in the morning but should not be consumed after lunch. Although alcohol often facilitates relaxation, it typically results in fragmented and poor sleep (Johnson, Burdick, & Smith, 1970).

8. Although daytime naps may, depending on the individual, either help or hinder nighttime sleep, poor sleepers should probably avoid all daytime naps (Evans, Cook, Cohen, Orne, & Orne 1977; Karacan, Williams, Finley, & Hursch, 1970).

9. It is best to associate lying in bed with sleep. For those individuals who go to bed and ruminate about personal or business problems, it is usually better to wait until drowsiness occurs before going to bed and to get out of bed after 15 minutes if sleep has not occurred. At such times, reading or watching a TV program which is rather unstimulating is recommended, with return to bed only after

drowsiness has set in. For those individuals who cannot sleep because they try too hard, reading or watching TV in bed may be helpful. The important rule is not to remain in bed trying to sleep without success.

PHARMACOLOGICAL TREATMENT

Two types of medication are generally taken to facilitate sleep. Nonprescription (over the counter) "sleep aids" cause drowsiness, but do not directly induce sleep. These medications sometimes allow the person who tries too hard for sleep to relax and fall asleep.

Prescription sleeping pills, commonly referred to as hypnotics, constitute the other type of sleep medication. Although over 5 million persons may receive prescriptions for hypnotics in a given year, their use appears to be declining. Benzodiazepines, which were originally marketed to relax muscles and relieve anxiety, have replaced barbiturates as the most frequently prescribed hypnotic because they are believed to be somewhat safer.

While certain medications are useful for treating specific diagnostic conditions, the chronic use of hypnotics for the treatment of insomnia is to be avoided, although occasional use is quite acceptable. Arguments against the use of hypnotics include the fact that hypnotic efficacy decreases over time, most hypnotics distort natural sleep (Hauri, 1977), hypnotics may result in "rebound insomnia" when the medication wears off (Kales, Scharf, & Kales, 1978; Nicholson, 1980), and many hypnotics impair waking performance of such activities as driving (Church & Johnson, 1979; Roth, Kramer, & Lutz, 1977). There is also concern that hypnotics often mask the insomniac's medical, behavioral, or psychological problems, which may delay appropriate treatment. Sleep medications carry the risk of medical complications, including overdose, adverse interaction with other medications, and withdrawal symptoms.

Proponents of hypnotics argue that the detrimental side-effects of hypnotics have to be weighed against the detrimental effects of suffering from insomnia. They note that incidence rates for complications and adverse reactions from hypnotics are exceedingly small. Furthermore, evidence concerning the loss of efficacy with chronic hypnotic use may not be relevant in most cases, since most insomniacs take their hypnotics intermittently (Clift, 1975).

It is currently considered acceptable medical practice to prescribe hypnotics to help an individual get through an acute crisis, as long as the patient is also followed and supported through the drug withdrawal period. A nightly prescription of hypnotics over a long time span (months or years) is rarely indicated, although there are a few patients who seem to benefit from long-term low doses of a hypnotic. Occasional use of hypnotics (once or twice a week) sometimes helps to reduce the insomniac's fear that they may never sleep again and allows some needed rest. The benzodiazepines are now generally preferred over other medications because of their relative safety and lack of interaction with other drugs. However, benzodiazepines should not be taken with alcohol, as some episodes of lethal overdose have occurred. Barbiturates are recommended for those individuals for whom the benzodiazepines do not work. There seems to be little advantage in using any of the other currently available hypnotics such as glutethimide, meprobamate, or methaqualone, (Institute of Medicine, 1979).

CLASSIFICATION AND TREATMENT OF SLEEP DISORDERS

A classification system of sleep and arousal disorders has recently been published by the Association of Sleep Disorders Centers (1979). Basically, the ASDC classification system recognizes four major types of sleep disorders: the Insomnias (Disorders of Initiating and Maintaining Sleep - DIMS), Disorders of Excessive Somnolence (DOES), Disorders of the Sleep-Wake Schedule, and Dysfunctions Associated with Sleep, Sleep Stages, or Partial Arousals (Parasomnias). Diagnoses are made based largely upon the patient's primary sleep complaint. For example, a diagnosis of Disorder of the Sleep-Wake Schedule rather than Disorder of Initiating and Maintaining Sleep is made if the sleep disturbance disappears whenever the patient is allowed to follow his or her internal, biological clock. Similarly, if the main complaint is a pathological tendency to sleep when the patient should be awake, a diagnosis of Disorder of Excessive Somnolence rather than Disorder of Initiating and Maintaining Sleep is most appropriate, even though nighttime sleep may also be disturbed.

INSOMNIAS - DISORDERS OF INITIATING AND MAINTAINING SLEEP - DIMS

Psychophysiological DIMS. This classification constitutes the most common sleep-related disorder. Psychophysiological DIMS can be manifested by difficulty in falling asleep, intermittant awakening during the night, and premature, early awakening.

> **Transient and Situational Psychophysiological DIMS** includes sleep difficulties of less than three weeks duration. There is usually a clear reason for the sleep difficulty, such as acute stress or an unfamiliar sleep environment. This type of insomnia is caused by a wake system that is temporarily too active. Hypnotics are often indicated if transient and situational insomnia persists for more than 2 to 3 nights. Hypnotics not only give the patient some rest, but also help to avoid the faulty conditioning which can result in chronic insomnia. Although relaxation exercises and hypnosis are occasionally used to calm an overly active arousal system, these behavioral methods are usually too slow to relieve acute crises.

> **Persistent Psychophysiological DIMS** is the ASDC term for chronic behavioral insomnia. Insomnia is considered a chronic problem if it lasts for more than 3 weeks. This type of insomnia typically develops when a predisposition towards occasional poor sleep is exacerbated by learned, maladaptive sleep habits (Hauri, 1979a).

Tension, anxiety, and mild depression are usually present, but not to the extent that a purely psychiatric diagnosis would be merited. This diagnosis depends mainly on the diagnostician's judgment as to whether the tension, anxiety, and depression are primary or secondary to the insomnia. Persistent psychophysiological DIMS tends to be stable, while DIMS associated with psychiatric disorders usually waxes and wanes along with the other symptoms of the psychiatric disorder.

Persistent psychophysiological insomnias are most effectively treated with behavioral techniques because they are based, at least in part, on faulty habits and conditioning. If somatized anxiety and tension are predominate factors, various forms of relaxation training can be effective (Borkovec & Weerts, 1976). If conditioned associations between bedroom stimuli and arousal are operating, Bootzin's (1973) stimulus control therapy is often effective. Depending on the degree of chronic anxiety, traditional forms of psychotherapy may also be employed. Hypnotics should be prescribed for occasional use only and are prescribed to avoid the helpless panic that many insomniacs experience.

It should be noted that not all psychophysiological insomniacs suffer from tension. Relaxation training is only effective with those insomniacs who are tense. Those insomniacs who are relaxed and still cannot fall asleep often are suffering from an organic predisposition towards poor sleep, and are usually treated more effectively with sensory-motor rhythm (SMR) biofeedback (Hauri, 1981; Hauri, Percy, Hartmann, & Russ, 1981).

DIMS Associated with Psychiatric Disorders

Symptom and Personality Disorders. This classification includes insomnias associated with anxiety disorders, somatoform disorders, and personality disorders. Standard psychiatric treatment, including psychotherapy, and appropriate medication is generally indicated. Some therapists (Kales, Kales, Bixler, & Martin, 1975) caution against becoming preoccupied in therapy with the symptom of insomnia, and suggest that discussions of insomnia be limited to a small part of the therapeutic hour.

Affective Disorders. One of the most common types of insomnia is secondary to affective disorders. Insomnia related to depression is usually characterized by difficulties with frequent middle of the night and early morning awakenings, but not with difficulty falling asleep (Kupfer & Foster, 1978). The severity of insomnia often, but not always, correlates with the severity of the depression (Hauri & Hawkins, 1973a). Early morning awakenings are more common in older patients, with younger depressed patients often showing hypersomnia rather than insomnia (Hawkins, Taub, Van de Castle, Teja, Greyson, Garland, & Talley, 1977).

In Bipolar Disorders, the manic phase is characterized by shorter sleep duration and difficulties in falling asleep. In contrast to the Major Affective Disorders, the depressive phase of a Bipolar Disorder is often associated with hypersomnia. Hypnotics are rarely indicated in Affective Disorders. However, anti-depressant medication might be given at bedtime in order to make use of its sedative side effects (Karacan, Blackburn, Thornby, Okawa, Salis, & Williams, 1975). Sleep usually normalizes with the waning of depression.

Other Functional Psychoses. Acute psychotic decompensation usually results in severe insomnia with the patient kept awake most of the night because of extreme anxiety, racing thoughts, and preoccupation with delusional and hallucinatory experiences. Such individuals often fall asleep during the early morning hours and sleep until midday or later. Day-night sleep cycle reversals are also common. Treatment should be aimed at relevant psychiatric problems.

DIMS Associated with Use of Drugs and Alcohol. The habit of avoiding emotional discomfort through drug use is common to most patients classified in this group. These patients should generally be treated for drug addiction, rather than for sleep disturbance. Usually, the patient using CNS depressants is first stabilized on a steady dose of the drug and then withdrawn quite gradually in order to avoid seizures, severe insomnia, and other side effects. The sustained use of CNS stimulants, including amphetamines, caffeine, and mood elevating drugs typically results in insomnia. Many commonly used drugs, which are not classified as either CNS depressants or stimulants, may also interfere with sleep. Anti-metabolites, thyroid preparations, dilantin, monaminoxydase inhibitors, contraceptives, and many others may result in insomnia. The clinician must decide whether the beneficial effects of the drug outweigh the detrimental side effects. Poor sleep associated with drug withdrawal is common with major tranquilizers, marijuana, and cocaine (Kay, Blackburn, Buckingham, & Karacan, 1976). Heavy use of alcohol also results in a progressive deterioration of sleep, and withdrawal from alcohol is often associated with severe insomnia.

DIMS Associated with Sleep-Induced Respiratory Impairment. Those sleep apnea patients who complain of insomnia usually suffer from central apneas (Guilleminault & Dement, 1978). We have included a more detailed consideration of sleep apneas within this chapter (see the discussion of Disorders of Excessive Somnolence).

DIMS Associated with Sleep-Related (Nocturnal) Myoclonus and "Restless Legs". "Restless legs" and myoclonus appear to be two separate entities, but often appear in the same individual. Nocturnal myoclonus involves episodes of repetitive, stereotyped leg muscle jerks during sleep, which are spaced about 40 seconds apart for periods of up to an hour and are usually bilateral. The myoclonic kick is often followed by partial or full arousal. Estimates of the incidence of myoclonus in insomniacs vary from 1% to 15%. The occurrence of myoclonus in normal sleepers has also recently been reported (Bixler, Kales, Vela-Bueno, Jacoby, Scarone, & Soldatos, 1982), but it does not apparently affect their sleep. This disorder occurs primarily in middle-aged or older persons.

Sleep-related myoclonus may be presented as either insomnia or a disorder of excessive somnolence. Patients typically complain of frequent awakenings and unrefreshing sleep, but usually have no knowledge of their myoclonic twitches. Therefore, reports of bed partners are crucial to the correct diagnosis of this problem.

Sleep-related myoclonus should be differentiated from sleep-related epileptic seizures, from waking myoclonus, and from the hypnic jerks that occur on occasions in many normals when falling asleep. Clonazepan tends to be effective in treating myoclonus (Coleman, Pollak, Kokkoris, McGregor, & Weitzman, 1979; Zorick, Roth, Salis, Kramer, & Lutz, 1978).

The "restless legs" syndrome consists of extremely uncomfortable, but not actually painful, sensations which usually occur deep inside the calf, but occasionally also in thighs, feet, and arms. These sensations begin during periods of relaxation and disappear with leg exercise. The etiology of the "restless legs" syndrome is unknown, although some cases have been linked to motor neuron disease and others to inadequate circulation (Frankel, Patten, & Gillin, 1974). The syndrome usually becomes more severe with age, is exacerbated by sleep deprivation, and often aggravated during pregnancy.

"Restless legs" should be differentiated from leg cramps, "growing pains" in children, and from the agitation and restlessness of anxiety and emotional upset. Regular leg exercises may help. Oxycodone and carbamazepine tend to be effective in treating this disorder.

DIMS Associated with Other Medical, Toxic, and Environmental Conditions. Medical conditions in this category would include CNS disorders, endocrine and metabolic diseases, renal failure, infections, and arthritis. Toxic conditions would include the effects of such substances as arsenic, mercury, and alcohol. Environmental conditions include noise, excessive heat, humidity, and other physical stimuli that disturb sleep. Because these conditions are often chronic, there is usually a large overlay of behavioral factors that aggravate the sleep disturbance. In addition to the apparent medical and environmental interventions, sleep in these patients is often improved by behavioral treatments, discussion of proper sleep habits, and supportive therapy.

Childhood Onset DIMS. Childhood onset insomnia appears to be more serious than adult onset insomnia (Hauri & Olmstead, 1980). Patients in this group tend to take longer to fall asleep and to sleep less than those who become insomniacs as adults. They also tend to have childhood histories of "soft" neurological impairment including hyperkinesis and dyslexia. Many childhood onset insomniacs are exceedingly sensitive to noise and to stimulants. Such patients are often aided by very low doses of Elavil (10 to 25 mg).

DISORDERS OF EXCESSIVE SOMNOLENCE - DOES

Pathologically excessive daytime somnolence usually has a medical origin. Over 90% of patients with Disorders of Excessive Somnolence (DOES) appear to suffer from medical diseases such as narcolepsy, sleep apnea, and drug related DOES. Psychological/behavioral components are clearly identifiable in less than 10% of these patients, in contrast to over 80% of insomniacs who show psychological/behavioral components. Narcolepsy and sleep induced respiratory impairments make up the bulk of the DOES patients.

Excessive somnolence includes the tendency to fall asleep whenever intense stimulation is absent. Persons suffering from DOES report either chronic, excessive sleepiness throughout the waking hours, or an excessive tendency to nap even after relatively adequate sleep at night. This excessive somnolence should be differentiated from physical tiredness, low grade depression, or lethargy and malaise. A complaint of excessive somnolence should be taken seriously. Persons in this group fear ridicule and rarely complain of somnolence until it is truly serious, often only after some near accidents or other unpleasant occurrences.

The Multiple Sleep Latency Test (MSLT) is currently used to objectively verify excessive daytime somnolence (Richardson, Carskadon, Flagg, Van den Hoed, Dement, & Mitler, 1978). It consists of requiring patients to lay down at two hour intervals throughout the day in order to measure how long it takes them to fall asleep each time. Excessive somnolence is defined as falling asleep, on the average, in less than five minutes whenever one lays down even after adequate bedrest the previous night.

Once help is sought for DOES, misdiagnosis is common. The differential diagnosis of DOES begins with the exclusion of primary organic pathology, such as brain tumors, kidney failure, liver failure, anemia, or endocrine disease (Zarcone, 1977). Following this, the clinician should inquire about attacks of muscular weakness which may be related to cataplexy or narcolepsy, symptoms of sleep apnea, and medications which may be related to DOES. Again, it should be emphasized that diagnosis of DOES requires competent medical attention (Guilleminault & Dement, 1977).

Narcolepsy. Narcolepsy is defined as a syndrome of excessive daytime sleepiness combined with manifestations of abnormal REM sleep. About 200,000 Americans suffer from this disorder, which seems to have a genetic component. The first sign of narcolepsy is often excessive daytime sleepiness in the second or third decade of life. The sufferer begins to experience a sudden and unavoidable need to sleep. These sleep attacks tend to last about five minutes. Full blown narcoleptics tend to feel sleepy throughout the day. In addition to irresistible sleep attacks, narcoleptics usually experience cataplexy (i.e., muscle paralysis without losing consciousness), which is often triggered by strong emotions such as laughing or anger. Sleep paralysis, (i.e., an inability to move when falling asleep or waking up), and hypnagogic hallucinations, (i.e., vivid dreams that occur while the person is still conscious but close to sleep), are also often associated with narcolepsy.

Narcolepsy is most frequently conceptualized as a disorder of the sleep-wake-REM systems. REM phenomena intrude into wakefulness either as a full blown REM period (sleep attack), as the muscle paralysis of REM sleep (cataplexy, sleep paralysis), or as the hallucination of a dream while awake (hypnagogic hallucination). Nocturnal sleep tends to be poor in narcoleptics. In the lab, the appearance of REM sleep within 10 minutes of sleep onset is considered diagnostic of narcolepsy, provided that the patient also complains of excessive daytime sleepiness and there is no other reason for the rapid onset of REM such as drug use or drug withdrawal. Narcolepsy does not appear to be a psychogenic disturbance, although strict control over one's emotions can often diminish the number of narcoleptic attacks.

The excessive daytime sleepiness and inappropriate need to nap in narcolepsy are usually treated with stimulants, mainly methylphenidate, amphetamines, (Zarcone, 1973), and pemoline (Schmidt, Clark, & Hyman, 1977). Dosages are kept as low as possible because the chronic use of stimulants sometimes aggravates the condition. "Drug-holidays" of a few weeks are prescribed when the patient becomes habituated to the stimulants. Cataplexy, on the other hand, is usually treated with imipraminic drugs (Shapiro, 1975) or by protriptyline (Schmidt et al., 1977).

DOES Associated with Sleep-Induced Respiratory Impairment. Sleep apnea refers to difficulty in breathing while asleep and is a potentially lethal condition. An apneic episode is usually defined as a cessation of air flow lasting 10 seconds or longer. Episodes of apnea during sleep are often terminated by brief arousals, but without the patient reaching full consciousness. Apneic sleep episodes may last from a few minutes to an entire night. Hundreds of apneic episodes can be observed during one night in severe cases. While a tentative diagnosis of sleep apnea syndrome can often be made by observation of the sleeper, by interviewing the bed partner, or by listening to a recording of the patient's snoring, assessing the severity of the problem requires the evaluation of blood gases during sleep. Therefore, sleep apnea is one of the few disorders that requires evaluation at a Sleep Disorders Center.

Obviously, respiratory depressants, such as sleeping pills, should be avoided in treating this patient. Death has resulted from the prescription of barbiturates to some patients with sleep apneas. Sleep apnea is a medical problem and requires a team of many different specialists. The severity of the daytime somnolence or nocturnal insomnia, the extent of the oxygen deprivation at night, and the status of the associated medical complications, such as cardiac problems, hypertension, and headaches, all need to be evaluated.

Guilleminault and Dement (1978) describe three types of sleep apnea:

1. The most common type, **Obstructive or Upper Airway Apnea**, is characterized by an absence of air flow despite persistent respiratory efforts and is caused by an obstruction in the airway which develops during sleep. A snoring pattern is usually associated with this syndrome. Inspiratory snores gradually increase as the patient falls asleep and an airway obstruction develops. Eventually, there is silence, followed, 10 to 60 seconds later, by a loud, choking, inspiratory gasp as the patient partially arouses and overcomes the occlusion. Violent body movements often accompany this type of apnea.

2. **Central Apnea** is a neurological condition characterized by the cessation of air flow as a result of a lack of respiratory drive. In many central apnea cases, however, breathing does not completely stop, but becomes excessively shallow, especially during REM sleep. Respiratory stimulants, mechanical breathing, or phrenic pacemakers have been successful in some cases of central apnea.

3. **Mixed Apnea** is marked by an initial central component (i.e., cessation of respiratory effort) followed by an obstructive component (i.e., no air flow despite respiratory effort).

There is considerable variation in the intensity of daytime somnolence associated with sleep apnea. Daytime sleep attacks lasting up to an hour or more affect many patients. Severe cases may also report disorientation, blackouts, and periods of automatic behavior associated with amnesia. In children, the most prominent presenting symptom is typically a reappearance of enuresis after successful toilet training. Learning difficulties and decreases in school performance are also often observed. Respiratory functioning during wakefulness is usually normal.

The etiology of the sleep apnea DOES is not clear in a majority of cases. They occur at all ages, but tend to appear with increasing frequency as age increases beyond 40. Actual anatomic abnormalities of the upper airway exist in a small proportion of sleep apnea patients. Hypertrophied tonsils and adenoids are often the source of the apnea in children. Medical complications of the sleep apnea syndrome include cardiac arrhythmias and hypertension. This condition carries an increased risk of sudden death during sleep and has been associated with the sudden infant death syndrome. For obstructive apneas, men outnumber women by a ratio of 30 to 1.

DISORDERS OF THE SLEEP-WAKE SCHEDULE

This classification includes disorders in which an individual's actual sleeping and waking behavior does not coincide with the time when sleeping and waking "should" occur. Such patients cannot sleep when they want or need to sleep, but sleep well during other times. Once this disorder is diagnosed, it is important to consider psychological causes for the disorder. For example, a patient may remain awake at night in order to avoid other people. There are, however, individuals who have a purely biological basis for their sleep-wake cycle abnormalities.

Some persons suffer from the **Non-24-Hour Sleep-Wake Syndrome** which is caused by a biological inability to squeeze circadian rhythms into a 24 hour day. As a result, they experience an incremental pattern of delays in sleep onset and wake-up time, typically 1 to 2 hours later each night. Most persons with this problem make intermittent attempts to conform to the 24 hour rhythm by getting up at conventional morning hours. However, episodic sleep deprivation results because they fall asleep later and later, but still force themselves to wake up at the same time. It is necessary to have the patient keep a sleep log of at least 2 weeks duration in order to diagnose the non-24 hour syndrome. Patients are rarely aware of this problem, but will typically complain of periodic difficulties in getting to sleep along with extreme arousal problems.

Another problem of the sleep-wake schedule is caused by **Irregular Sleep-Wake Patterns** which often occurs in individuals who are indifferent as to whether it is day or night. In the insomniac whose work or life style is not tied to a regular time clock, the need to oversleep after a series of poor nights often becomes overwhelming. In order to catch up on sleep, many of these persons take numerous daytime naps. As a result of this self-imposed, irregular sleep-wake pattern, sleep and waking frequently become evenly spread over the 24 hour day. The patient often becomes chronically weak and groggy, and is almost always sleepy. The major feature of this disorder is the loss of a clear sleep-wake rhythm.

The irregular sleep-wake pattern results in a desynchronization of circadian rhythms. Treatment of the irregular sleep-wake pattern consists of gradually imposing a regular day-night cycle. Many of these patients are weakened from chronic bedrest. Therefore, wake-up times during daytime hours should be gradually lengthened, naps gradually abolished, and bedtime gradually limited to the usual sleeping hours. Daily exercise is also recommended to help strengthen the circadian cycle. Measures such as body temperature can be graphed daily in order to provide the patient with feedback on changes in circadian rhythms. It should be noted, however, that it is rarely possible for individuals to regularize a seriously disturbed sleep-wake pattern on their own. Either an outside "enforcer" such as a spouse is required, or admission to an inpatient program which requires normal sleep-wake patterns and fills the waking hours with activity, is necessary in order to regularize the patient.

DYSFUNCTIONS ASSOCIATED WITH SLEEP, SLEEP STAGES, OR PARTIAL AROUSALS (PARASOMNIAS)

Parasomnias are problems that either occur exclusively during sleep or are exacerbated by sleep. Although there are many parasomnias, the most common parasomnias are sleepwalking (somnambulism), sleep terror (pavor nocturnus, incubus), and bed wetting (enuresis). It should be noted that parasomnias are occasionally a symptom of a nocturnal seizure disorder even though the daytime EEG is normal. Only sleep walking and sleep terror will be discussed here (enuresis is considered in some detail in another part of this volume). All three common parasomnias typically begin in delta sleep, usually about an hour after sleep onset. It has been suggested that the parasomnias are actually problems of incomplete arousal (Broughton, 1968). Rather than awakening fully when disturbed in delta sleep, such people seem to enter a confusional state in which sleep and waking brain waves are present. It is during this confusional state that sleepwalking, night terrors, and enuresis occur.

Sleepwalking (Somnambulism). Higher cortical functions are inefficient during sleepwalking episodes and coordination is typically poor. Senses also operate at a low level during sleepwalking and, although sleepwalkers are often able to avoid objects in their path, they are much clumsier when sleepwalking than during wakefulness. There is a danger of stumbling, losing balance, and falling down steps or out of windows. While somnambulism in adults is often associated with significant psychological problems, sleepwalking in children does not, in itself, indicate significant psychopathology (Kales, Soldatos, Caldwell, Kales, Humphrey, Charney, & Schweitzer, 1980). Indeed, occasional episodes of sleepwalking in children are normal, although stress and emotional tension seem to increase the frequency of sleepwalking. Sleepwalking needs to be differentiated from complex partial seizures which occur during sleep and from waking fugue states which are of longer duration and contain more purposeful behavior.

Initial concern in the treatment of somnambulism should be directed at helping the patient avoid injury. Adults who sleepwalk may benefit from psychotherapy, whereas sleepwalking in children usually can be handled by reassurance to the child and parents. Sleep habits are also important. The more sleep is deepened, such as by sleep deprivation, sedatives, or alcohol, the more likely are episodes of somnambulism. No universally helpful drug has been found, but some patients respond to imipramine, while others respond to stimulants.

Sleep Terrors (Pavor Nocturnus, Incubus). Sleep terrors almost always begin with a terrifying scream and are usually accompanied by signs of intense panic, including a frightened expression, profuse perspiring, and a quick pulse. It is difficult to awaken a person during a sleep terrors episode and full consciousness is usually not achieved for several minutes, even with severe shaking. If aroused, the patient may report a sense of terror, dread, or helplessness, or a feeling of paralysis, but detailed dream content is rarely remembered (Fisher, Byrne, Edwards, & Kahn, 1970).

Sleep terrors need to be differentiated from dream anxiety attacks (Kramer, 1979). In children, sleep terrors are typically a biological phenomenon and do not require psychotherapy, whereas dream anxiety attacks have a psychological basis and patients exhibiting such attacks frequently need psychotherapy or situational change in order to relieve stress. Diagnostically, sleep terrors usually occur early at night and show intense physiological agitation, but little dream content, while dream anxiety attacks usually occur later at night, show little physiological agitation, but are fairly vivid and detailed in dream content. The patient is usually easy to arouse and is quickly oriented to the environment during dream anxiety attacks. Sleep terrors should also not be confused with terrifying hypnagogic hallucinations which may occur in the twilight state between waking and sleeping in depressed patients, posttraumatic stress disorders, narcoleptics, and schizophrenics.

Sleep terrors in children usually disappear in adolescence. Like somnambulism, sleep terrors may be more frequent in times of stress, but are not associated with increased psychopathology, at least not in children. Benzodiazepines are often effective in decreasing sleep terror and dream anxiety attacks.

CONCLUSION

In this primer we have attempted to introduce information about the basic characteristics of sleep as well as present the more common sleep disorders. Various sleep disorders are frequently encountered in the patients of mental health clinicians, and it is essential for them to be able to make basic distinctions among these disorders. While certain forms of insomnia may be readily treated with psychotherapy, behavior therapy, and relaxation techniques, other sleep disorders, such as sleep apnea, represent serious problems which require prompt medical evaluation. Our goal here is to make some of the basic distinctions for clinicians who do not routinely evaluate sleep disorders. Readers who wish more detailed information and case examples are referred to Hauri (1982).

Peter J. Hauri, Ph.D., is currently Director of the Dartmouth-Hitchcock Sleep Disorders Center in Hanover, New Hampshire, Professor of Psychiatry, Dartmouth Medical School, and Adjunct Professor of Psychology, Dartmouth College. He has been involved in sleep and dream research since the early 1960's. He has published numerous articles on sleep pathology, particularly insomnia. Dr. Hauri may be contacted at the Sleep Disorders Center, Dartmouth Medical School, 703 Remsen Building, Hanover, NH 03756.

Terry S. Proeger, Ph.D., is presently in private practice in Sarasota, Florida. Prior to entering private practice, he was Chief Psychologist at the Sarasota Guidance Clinic. He received his Ph.D. from the University of Florida in June, 1969 and was a Fellow of The Center for Neurobiological Sciences while at the University of Florida. Dr. Proeger may be contacted at 635 S. Orange Avenue, Suite 4, Sarasota, FL 33577.

RESOURCES

Allison, T. & Van Twyver, H. The evolution of sleep. NATURAL HISTORY, 1970, **79**, 56-65.

Association of Sleep Disorders Centers. DIAGNOSTIC CLASSIFICATION OF SLEEP AND AROUSAL DISORDERS, First Edition, prepared by the Sleep Disorders Classification Committee, H. P. Roffwarg, Chairman, SLEEP, 1979, **2**, 1-137. Address correspondence to: Assoc. of Sleep Disorders Centers, P.O. Box YY, East Setauket, NY, 11733.

Baekeland, F. & Lasky, R. Exercise and sleep patterns in college athletes. PERCEPTUAL AND MOTOR SKILLS, 1966, **23**, 1203-1207.

Bixler, E. O., Kales, A., Vela-Bueno, A., Jacoby, J. A., Scarone, S., & Soldatos, C. R. Nocturnal myoclonus and nocturnal myoclonic activity in a normal population. RES. COMMUN. CHEM. PATHOL. PHARMACOL., 1982, **36**(1), 129-140.

Bonnet, M. H., Johnson, L. C., & Webb, W. W. The reliability of arousal threshold during sleep. PSYCHOPHYSIOLOGY, 1978, **33**, 412-416.

Bootzin, R. STIMULUS CONTROL OF INSOMNIA. Paper presented at the Symposium on the Treatment of Sleep Disorders, American Psychological Association Convention, Montreal, Canada, July 1973.

Bootzin, R. R. & Nicassio, P. N. Behavioral treatments for insomnia. In M. Hersen, R. Eisler, & P. Miller (Eds.), PROGRESS IN BEHAVIOR MODIFICATION. New York: Academic Press, 1978.

Borkovec, T. D. Pseudo (experiential)-insomnia and idopathic (objective) insomnia: Theoretical and therapeutic issues. ADVANCED BEHAVIORAL RESEARCH AND THERAPY, 1979, **2**, 27-55.

Borkovec, T. D. & Weerts, T. D. Effects of progressive relaxation on sleep disturbance: An electroencephalographic evaluation. PSYCHOSOMATIC MEDICINE, 1976, **38**, 173-180.

Brezinova, V. & Oswald, I. Sleep after a bedtime beverage. BRITISH MEDICAL JOURNAL, 1972, **2**, 431-433.

Broughton, R. J. Sleep disorders - disorders of arousal. SCIENCE, 1968, **159**, 1070-1078.

Church, M. W. & Johnson, L. C. Mood and performance of poor sleepers during repeated use of flurazepam. PSYCHOPHARMACOLOGY, 1979, **61**, 309-316.

Claparede, E. Esquisse d'une theorie biologique du Sommeil. ARCHIVES OF PSYCHOLOGY, 1905, **4**, 245-349.

Clift, A. D. (Ed.). SLEEP DISTURBANCE AND HYPNOTIC DRUG DEPENDENCE. Amsterdam: Excerpta Medica, 1975.

Coleman, R. M., Pollak, C. O., Kokkoris, C. P., McGregor, P. A., & Weitzman, E. D. Periodic nocturnal myoclonus in patients with sleep-wake disorders: A case series analysis. In M. H. Chase, M. Mitler, & P. L. Walter (Eds.), SLEEP RESEARCH, 1979, **8**, Brain Information Service/Brain Research Institute, UCLA, Los Angeles, 175.

Elson, R. B., Hauri, P., & Cunis, D. Physiological changes in yoga meditation. PSYCHOPHYSIOLOGY, 1977, **14**, 52-57.

Evans, F. J., Cook, M. R., Cohen, H. D., Orne, E. C., & Orne, M. T. Appetitive and replacement naps: EEG and behavior. SCIENCE, 1977, **197**, 687-689.

Fisher, C., Byrne, J., Edwards, A., & Kahn, D. A psychophysiological study of nightmares. JOURNAL OF THE AMERICAN PSYCHOANALYTIC ASSOCIATION, 1970, **18**, 747-782.

Foulkes, W. D. Dream reports from different stages of sleep. JOURNAL OF ABNORMAL PSYCHOLOGY, 1962, **62**, 14-25.

Foulkes, D. & Vogel, G. Mental activity at sleep onset. JOURNAL ABNORMAL PSYCHOLOGY, 1965, **70**, 231-243.

Frankel, B. L., Patten, B. M., & Gillin, J. C. Restless legs syndrome. Sleep-electroencephalographic and neurologic findings. JOURNAL OF THE AMERICAN MEDICAL ASSOCIATION, 1974, **230**, 1302-1303.

Globus, G., Friedmann, J., Cohen, H., Pearsons, K. S., & Fidell, S. The effects of aircraft noise on sleep electrophysiology as recorded in the home. In W. D. Ward (Ed.). PROCEEDINGS OF THE INTERNATIONAL CONGRESS ON NOISE AS A PUBLIC HEALTH PROBLEM. Washington, DC: U. S. Environmental Protection Agency, 1973.

Guilleminault, C. & Dement, W. C. 235 cases of excessive daytime sleepiness. Diagnosis and tentative classification. JOURNAL OF THE NEUROLOGICAL SCIENCES, 1977, **31**, 13-27.

Guilleminault, C. & Dement, W. (Eds.). SLEEP APNEA SYNDROMES. New York: Alan R. Liss, 1978.

Hartmann, E. L. THE FUNCTIONS OF SLEEP. New Haven and London: Yale University Press, 1973.

Hauri, P. Behavioral treatment of insomnia. MEDICAL TIMES, 1979, **107**, 36-47. (a)

Hauri, P. CURRENT CONCEPTS. The Upjohn Company, Scope Publication, 1977.

Hauri, P. A sleep disorders primer. In R. J. Gatchel, A. Baum, & J. E. Singer (Eds.), HANDBOOK OF PSYCHOLOGY AND HEALTH (Vol. 1). Hillsdale, NJ: Lawrence Erlbaum Assoc., 1982.

Hauri, P. Treating psychophysiologic insomnia with biofeedback. ARCHIVES OF GENERAL PSYCHIATRY, 1981, **38**, 752-758.

Hauri, P. What can insomniacs teach us about the functions of sleep? In Drucker-Colin (Ed.), THE FUNCTIONS OF SLEEP. New York: Academic Press, 1979. (b)

Hauri, P. & Hawkins, D. R. Individual differences in the sleep of depression. In Jovanovic, U. J. (Ed.). THE NATURE OF SLEEP. Stuttgart: Fisher, 1973. (a)

Hauri, P. & Hawkins, D. R. Alpha-delta sleep. ELECTROENCEPHALOGRAPHY AND CLINICAL NEUROPHYSIOLOGY, 1973, **34**, 233-237. (b)

Hauri, P. & Olmstead, E. Childhood-onset insomnia. SLEEP, 1980, **3**, 59-65.

Hauri, P., Percy, L., Hartmann, E., & Russ, D. Treating psychophysiological insomnia with biofeedback, a replication. SLEEP RESEARCH, in press, 1981. (Abstract)

Hawkins, D. R., Taub, J. M., Van de Castle, R. L., Teja, J. S., Greyson, B., Garland, F., & Talley, J. E. Sleep stage patterns associated with depression in young adult patients. In W. P. Koella & P. Levin (Eds.), SLEEP. Basel: Karger, 1977.

Institute of Medicine. SLEEPING PILLS, INSOMNIA, AND MEDICAL PRACTICE. Washington, DC: National Academy of Sciences, 1979.

Jacobs, B. I. & McGinty, D. J. Effects of food deprivation on sleep and wakefulness in the rat. EXPERIMENTAL NEUROLOGY, 1971, **30**, 212-222.

Johnson, L. C., Burdick, J. A., & Smith, J. Sleep during alcohol intake and withdrawal in the chronic alcoholic. ARCHIVES OF GENERAL PSYCHIATRY, 1970, **22**, 406-418.

Jones, H. S. & Oswald, I. Two cases of healthy insomnia. ELECTROENCEPHALOGRAPHY AND CLINICAL NEUROPHYSIOLOGY, 1968, **24**, 378-380.

Kales, A., Kales, J. D., Bixler, E. O., & Martin, E. Common shortcomings in the evaluation and treatment of insomnia. In F. Kagan, T. Harwood, K. Rickels, A. Rudzik, & H. Sorer (Eds.), HYPNOTICS: METHODS OF DEVELOPMENT & EVALUATION. New York: Spectrum Publications, Inc., 1975.

Kales, A., Scharf, M. B., & Kales, J. D. Rebound insomnia: A new clinical syndrome. SCIENCE, 1978, **201**, 1039-1041.

Kales, A., Soldatos, C. R., Caldwell, A. B., Kales, J. D., Humphrey, F. J., Charney, D. S., & Schweitzer, P. K. Somnambulism. ARCHIVES OF GENERAL PSYCHIATRY, 1980, **37**, 1406-1410.

Karacan, I., Blackburn, A. B., Thornby, J. I., Okawa, M., Salis, P. J., & Williams, R. L. The effect of doxepin HCl (sinequan) on sleep patterns and clinical symptomatology of neurotic depressed patients with sleep disturbance. SINEQUAN (DOXEPIN HCl): A MONOGRAPH OF RECENT CLINICAL STUDIES, 1975. Amsterdam: Excerpta-Medica, 1975.

Karacan, I., Thornby, J. I., Booth, G. H., Okawa, M., Salis, P. J., Anch, A. M., & Williams, R. L. Dose-response effects of coffee on objective (EEG) and subjective measures of sleep. In P. Levin & W. P. Koella (Eds.), SLEEP. Basel: Karger, 1975.

Karacan, O., Williams, R. L., Finley, W. W., & Hursch, C. J. The effects of naps on nocturnal sleep. Influence on the need for stage 1 REM and stage 4 sleep. BIOLOGICAL PSYCHIATRY, 1970, **2**, 391-399.

Kay, D. C., Blackburn, A. B., Buckingham, J. A., & Karacan, I. Human pharmacology of sleep. In R. L. Williams & I. Karacan (Eds.), PHARMACOLOGY OF SLEEP. New York: Wiley, 1976.

Kramer, M. Dream disturbances. PSYCHIATRIC ANNALS, 1979, **9**, 336-376.

Kupfer, D. J. & Foster, F. G. EEG sleep and depression. In R. L. Williams & I. Karacan (Eds.), SLEEP DISORDERS. New York: Wiley, 1978.

McGinty, D. J. Encephalization and the neural control of behavior. In M. B. Sterman, D. J. McGinty, & A. M. Adinolfi (Eds.), BRAIN DEVELOPMENT AND BEHAVIOR. New York: Academic Press, 1971.

Moldofsky, H., Scarisbrick, P., England, R., & Smythe, H. Musculoskeletal symptoms and non-REM sleep disturbance in patients with "fibrositis syndrome" and healthy subjects. PSYCHOSOMATIC MEDICINE, 1975, **37**, 341-351.

Myrsten, A. L., Elgerot, A., & Edgren, B. Effects of abstinence from tobacco smoking on physiological and psychological arousal levels in habitual smokers. PSYCHOSOMATIC MEDICINE, 1977, **39**, 25-38.

Nicholson, A. N. Hypnotics: Rebound insomnia and residual sequelae. BRITISH JOURNAL OF CLINICAL PHARMACOLOGY, 1980, **9**, 223-225.

Oswald, I. SLEEP. Harmondsworth, Middlesex: Penguin Books, 1974.

Otto, E. Physiological analysis of human sleep disturbances induced by noise and increased room temperature. In W. P. Koella & P. Levin (Eds.), SLEEP. Basel: Karger, 1973.

Rechtschaffen, A., Hauri, P., & Zeitlin, M. Auditory awakening thresholds in REM and NREM sleep stages. PERCEPTUAL AND MOTOR SKILLS, 1966, **22**, 927-942.

Rechtschaffen, A. & Kales, A. (Eds.). A MANUAL OF STANDARIZED TERMINOLOGY, TECHNIQUES AND SCORING SYSTEM FOR SLEEP STAGES OF HUMAN SUBJECTS. Los Angeles: Brain Information Service/Brain Research Institute, UCLA, 1968.

Richardson, G. S., Carskadon, M. A., Flagg, W., Van den Hoed, J., Dement, W. C., & Mitler, M. M. Excessive daytime sleepiness in man: Multiple sleep latency measurement in narcoleptic and control subjects. ELECTROENCEPHALOGRAPHY AND CLINICAL NEUROPHYSIOLOGY, 1978, 45, 621-627.

Roth, T., Kramer, M., & Lutz, T. The effects of hypnotics on sleep, performance, and subjective state. DRUGS AND EXPERIMENTAL CLINICAL RESEARCH, 1977, 1, 279-286.

Schmidt, H. S., Clark, R. W., & Hyman, P. R. Protriptyline: An effective agent in the treatment of the narcolepsy-cataplexy syndrome and hypersomnia. AMERICAN JOURNAL OF PSYCHIATRY, 1977, 134, 183-185.

Schmidt-Kessen, W. & Kendel, K. Einfluss der Raumtemperatur auf den Nachtschlaf. RES. EXP. MED. (BERLIN), 1973, 160, 220-233.

Shapiro, W. R. Treatment of cataplexy with clormipramine. ARCHIVES OF NEUROLOGY, 1975, 32, 653-656.

Stuss, D. & Broughton, R. Extreme short sleep: personality profiles and a case study of sleep requirement. WAKING AND SLEEPING, 1978, 2, 101-105.

Vogel, G. W. A review of REM sleep deprivation. ARCHIVES OF GENERAL PSYCHIATRY, 1975, 32, 749-761.

Ware, J. C. The symptom of insomnia: causes and cures. PSYCHIATRIC ANNALS, 1979, 9, 353-366.

Webb, W. B. Sleep as an adaptive response. PERCEPTUAL AND MOTOR SKILLS, 1974, 38, 1023-1027.

Webb, W. B. Theories of sleep functions and some clinical implications. In R. Drucker-Colin, M. Shkurovich, & M. B. Sterman (Eds.), THE FUNCTIONS OF SLEEP. New York: Academic Press, 1979.

Wever, von R. (Problems of circadian periodicity and its disorders). Probleme der zirkadianen Periodik und ihrer Stoerungen. DRUG RESEARCH, 1976, 26, 2-6.

Zarcone, V. Narcolepsy. NEW ENGLAND JOURNAL OF MEDICINE, 1973, 288, 1156-1166.

Zarcone, V. P. Diagnosis and treatment of excessive daytime sleepiness. In H. L. Klawans (Ed.), CLINICAL NEUROPHARMACOLOGY. New York: Raven Press, 1977.

Zorick, F., Roth, T., Salis, P., Kramer, M., & Lutz, T. Insomnia and excessive daytime sleepiness as presenting symptoms in nocturnal myoclonus. In M. H. Chase, M. Mitler, & P. L. Walter (Eds.), SLEEP RESEARCH. Los Angeles: Brain Information Service/Brain Research Institute, UCLA, Vol. 7, 1978, p. 256 (abstract).

STRATEGIES FOR FACILITATING CLIENT'S PERSONAL PROBLEM SOLVING

P. Paul Heppner

A number of writers have conceptualized counseling as a problem solving process (e.g., Heppner, 1978; Krumboltz, 1965; Weitz, 1964), and books have appeared which discuss problem solving processes aimed at clients (Borck & Fawcett, 1982; Carkhuff, 1973). Yet, Horan (1979) observed that psychologists have not developed a technology for helping clients with regard to problem solving and decision making. A number of investigations have examined variables associated with training in problem solving skills (e.g., Dixon, Heppner, Petersen, & Ronning, 1979; D'Zurilla & Nezu, 1980; Nezu & D'Zurilla, 1979, 1981; Wagman, 1980; Wagman & Kerber, 1980). At this time, however, it remains unclear precisely what the essential problem solving skills are, how such skills can best be facilitated, and how individual skill differences affect the problem solving process.

The purpose of this contribution is to describe a number of methods that facilitate the problem solving process of clients. The methods will consist of strategies aimed at general problem solving skills previously identified in the professional literature (i.e., defining the problem, generating alternatives, decision making), as well as a number of techniques designed to affect one's general problem solving appraisal (e.g., confidence, approach-avoidance). The methods described in this article will be client-oriented, self-help techniques that could also be utilized as tools clinicians employ with clients in conjunction with typical counseling interventions.

PROBLEM DEFINITION

Although people can usually recognize when they have a problem, most do not fully understand their problem. Some evidence suggests that good problem solvers "understand" the essence of problems (Bloom & Broder, 1950). After reviewing the literature, this author (Heppner, 1978) concluded that successful problem solvers seem to gather information, operationalize vague elements, and identify relationships among environmental events that facilitate a more accurate understanding of the problem.

An individual may be unable to adequately define a problem because of a deficit in any of a number of requisite skills (e.g., unable to identify self-statements, feelings, obstacles, and beliefs, unable to gather relevant information, unable to identify relationships between problem elements). To adequately define a personal problem, the problem solver typically needs to examine at least three areas: (a) assessing oneself, one's behaviors, knowledge, emotions, and feelings relevant to the problematic situation, as well as the consequences of these events, (b) assessing one's environment relevant to the problematic situation, and (c) delineating the problematic situation, including goals, expectations, and conflicts (Heppner, 1978).

The Problem Analysis Grid (Figure 1, following page), presents a method to assist clients in defining elements of the problematic situation. The top section of the grid is designed to elicit information about the problem itself. How does the client view the problem, what goals does he or she have, and what are the areas of conflict, if any? The center section is designed to help the client gather essential information about internal contingencies and discriminative stimuli which surround the problem. Given the problem elements previously identified, what feelings, self-statements (positive or negative), and fears is the person aware of that relate to various aspects of the problem? And very importantly, what is the outcome (or consequence) of the feelings, self-statements, or fears? For example, does the person end up avoiding the problem (perhaps procrastinates) because of a fear of failure, or feelings of inferiority. Finally, the bottom of the grid is designed to cue the client to consider elements of the environment which may interact with the problem. What do other people expect him or her to do in this situation, especially significant others? Are there environmental demands or pay-offs (reinforcers) for acting one way or another? And again, what is the consequence on the problem solver of the environmental events. For example, do parental expectations (e.g., achievement) lead to avoidance of selecting a major, or ambivalent feelings about certain career paths?

The Problem Analysis Grid seems to be consistent with the Problem Definition and Formulation Training described by Nezu and D'Zurilla (1981). These authors found that specific training in problem definition activities enhanced the problem solving process, rather than provided global guidelines. Additional research is needed which examines the long term effects of such analyses or training, as well as differential treatment effects across individual differences of clients. Practitioners may also consider utilizing the Problem Analysis Grid in conjunction with other interventions used in the problem definition activities of counseling (cf. Heppner, 1978; Horan, 1979).

GENERATING ALTERNATIVES

After a problem solver has defined the problem, typically the person then contemplates what alternatives might solve the problem. While generating alternatives might seem like a simple task, any one of several events can provide cues which trigger incompatible or restrictive responses. In short, evidence seems to suggest that people may reduce the number of alternatives they consider due to negative transfer effects, emotional components, or a narrow perspective of the problem (Heppner, 1978). An important problem solving skill may be the ability to maximally benefit from one's past experiences and awareness to generate a wide range of feasible alternatives. How can this skill be developed or enhanced?

Perhaps the most widely discussed method of generating alternatives is Osborn's (1963) brainstorming technique. Evidence suggests that brainstorming

PROBLEM ANALYSIS GRID

ASSESSING THE PROBLEM:	
Problem	
Goals	
Conflicts	

ASSESSING ONESELF:	
Feelings	
Self-Statements	
Fears	
Consequences	

ASSESSING THE ENVIRONMENT:	
Others' Expectations	
Environmental Demands	
Consequences	

Figure 1.

is more likely to produce effective responses than attempting to generate only good alternatives (Brilhart & Jochem, 1964; Meadow & Parnes, 1959; Parnes & Meadow, 1959). Table 1 (Brainstorming Plus) presents a technique which combines Osborn's brainstorming with a series of questions designed to cue consideration of additional alternatives.

TABLE 1: BRAINSTORMING PLUS

I. Your first task is to brainstorm or generate as many solutions as possible. In brainstorming, keep the following four rules in mind:

   A. **Withhold judgment.** Criticism is ruled out. Evaluation and final judgment of the ideas produced during this phase is withheld until the "brainstorming" procedure is completed. The advantages arising from the application of this principle of deferred judgment maximize the release of creative potential and prevent the hampering effects of premature judgment. All judgment is suspended until the evaluation and decision making phase is begun. Allowing yourself to be critical at the same time you are being creative is like trying to get hot and cold water from the same faucet at the same time. The results are tepid!

   B. **Free-wheeling is welcomed.** The wilder the idea, the better; it is easier to tame down than to think up. Even offbeat, impractical suggestions may "trigger" in others practical suggestions which might not otherwise occur to them. The key is to think with the "brakes off."

   C. **Quantity is wanted.** The greater the number of ideas, the greater the likelihood of useful ideas. Quantity breeds quality.

   D. **Combination and improvement are sought.** The combining of two or more ideas into still another idea is indicated by this rule as well as the taking of others' ideas and suggesting how they could be improved.

Now brainstorm as many solutions to your particular problem as you can generate. Be creative.

Now use the following questions to help spark more ideas.

II. Some ways of increasing the number of alternative problem solving strategies is to look at the conditions or things which contribute to the problem. Many times, things that occur immediately **before, during,** or **after** the desired behavior are the things that we need to change in order to solve the problem. Therefore, you might want to ask yourself the following questions:

   A. Is there something occurring before the desired behavior that is influencing the behavior, such as the environment (e.g., the posters in my room distract me from studying; when I study in my dorm room, friends stop by and interrupt me)? In other words, is there something which triggers behaviors which are interfering or incompatible with your desired goal related behavior? This suggests that other possible alternatives are:

B. Is there something occurring during the desired behavior which is preventing you from achieving that behavioral goal, such as anxiety (e.g., I get so tense and nervous when talking to my supervisor that I don't understand her)? This suggests that other possible alternatives are:

C. What occurs or does not occur after the desired behavior? A behavior that gets reinforced with a reward tends to be strengthened, or will occur again. Therefore, is there an adequate reward. This suggests that other possible alternatives are:

III. To make the most of your past achievements as well as those by your friends, ask yourself the following questions:

A. How is this similar to previous situations? What worked in those situations? This suggests that other possible alternatives are:

B. How might a friend, who is a good problem solver, respond to this problem? Ask a friend how he or she might respond. This suggests that other possible alternatives are:

An earlier version of the Brainstorming Plus technique was developed as a written handout utilized in problem solving training by Dixon et al. (1979). Essentially, the client (in this case a student) is first instructed in the rules of brainstorming: (a) judgment is withheld while trying to generate alternatives, (b) free-wheeling is welcomed, (c) quantity is wanted, and (d) combinations and/or improvements of alternatives are encouraged. Subsequently, the client is asked to generate as many alternatives as possible or, in other words, to brainstorm. The client is then asked to contemplate two series of questions, which may also help generate other alternatives. The first set of questions inquires about the antecedent and consequential events which contribute to the problem; the second set attempts to alter the problem solver's perspective by comparing this problem to previous but similar problems, as well as to how a friend might solve the problem. The primary function of both sets of questions is to focus on or compare different elements of the problem which in turn may cue additional alternative solutions.

This technique has been useful in helping clients consider a broader range of alternatives. This seems important given that there is some speculation that unsuccessful problem solvers generate fewer alternatives (Heppner, 1978). Recent evidence also suggests that the quantity rule is a critical component of brainstorming which facilitates the generation of alternatives (D'Zurilla & Nezu, 1980). Brainstorming or Brainstorming Plus could also be used in conjunction with a variety of clinician responses and strategies which also serve to generate new alternatives to client problems (cf. Heppner, 1978; Horan, 1979).

DECISION MAKING

Decision making is the process of selecting one action from a number of alternative courses of action (Bross, 1953). The "goodness" of a decision has been defined in several ways (Dilley, 1967), such as if the decision maker (a) chooses the alternatives that have the expected outcomes with the highest probability coupled with the highest desirability (Dilley, 1965; Edwards, 1961), or (b) is internally consistent (Cronbach & Gleser, 1957), or (c) is willing to assume personal responsibility for the decision (Tyler, 1969), or (d) reaches a solution involving the maximum number of positive consequences and a minimum of negative ones (D'Zurilla & Goldfried, 1971). Research suggests, however, that individuals often are not able to identify the "best" alternative (e.g., Arnkoff & Stewart, 1975; Johnson, Parrott, & Stratton, 1968; Nezu & D'Zurilla, 1979).

Clients often enter counseling because they are troubled with a particular decision (e.g., to marry, to divorce, to have children, which academic major, which career, whether to have premarital sex). Difficulties in real life decision making often involve problems with accurately (a) assessing the probabilities of success for each alternative, (b) assessing utilities, preferences, or values related to each alternative, and (c) assessing consequences for each alternative. Whereas some evidence suggests that instruction in the specific decision making criteria (utility, probability, and consequences) facilitates effective decision making (Nezu & D'Zurilla, 1979), surprisingly little evidence exists to identify techniques which facilitate generalizable, real life decision making skills across time. Two models of decision making will be presented, either of which can be used for immediate client decisions as well as for a more generalizable, self-management tool for future client decisions.

The first model is that proposed by D'Zurilla and Goldfried (1971), and utilized in later investigations (e.g., Nezu & D'Zurilla, 1979). The Decision Making Grid is a form developed to facilitate the utilization of the D'Zurilla and Goldfried (1971) model, and is presented in Figure 2. Essentially, this

Alternatives	Short-Term Consequences		Long-Term Consequences		Personal Consequences		Social Consequences		Probability of Success
	+	−	+	−	+	−	+	−	
Alternative #1									
Alternative #2									
Alternative #3									

Figure 2. Decision Making Grid

Innovations In Clinical Practice: A Source Book

model involves four activities: (a) a rough screening of alternatives, (b) identification of consequences, (c) estimating probabilities of success, and (d) assessing preferences or values. The client is initially asked to screen the list of alternatives to eliminate the obviously inferior options, which consequently reduces the alternatives to a humanly manageable number. Second, the client is instructed to consider a range of consequences for each alternative: personal consequences (own feelings, needs, desires), social consequences (reactions of others), short-term consequences (immediate consequences in one's life), and long-term consequences (e.g., long range personal goals). The various consequences are briefly identified and listed as either positive or negative on the Decision Making Grid. After delineating consequences, the client is asked to examine the activities involved within each alternative, and determine the likelihood of success by considering three broad categories (highly likely, likely, and unlikely). The client is then asked to examine the consequences listed in the Grid, and circle the consequences which are most important with regard to his or her own values and preferences. The value clarification process is often highlighted if the client restricts himself or herself to circling only two or three consequences that are most important. Finally, the client is asked to make a decision by weighing the pros and cons of each alternative through examination of consequences, probabilities, and values. From my clinical experience, commonly reported client outcomes are an increased awareness of the various consequences, a thorough but succinct summary of the client's deliberations, values clarification, and reduction in anxiety about the decision making process.

The second model is that proposed by Janis and Mann (1977) and called the Balance Sheet (depicted in Figure 3, following page). The procedures involved with this model are to first specify at least three alternatives, then to identify the positive and negative consequences for each of the types of anticipation: gains or losses for self, gains or losses for others, self-approval or disapproval, and social approval or disapproval. For example, depending on the particular decision, gains or losses for oneself might include personal income, amount of vacation time, life style, and long-term relationships. Gains or losses for significant others might include social status, reducing racism, and ecological considerations. Self-approval or disapproval relates to a number of internal comparisons, such as moral considerations and events which contrast the real self to the ideal self; social approval or disapproval relates to judgments from external sources, such as spouse, family, friends, and employers. The primary purpose of this method is to examine the positive and negative consequences of alternatives along certain anticipation events and reduce the possibility of overlooking important information (Horan, 1979). Janis and Mann (1977) provide empirical evidence suggesting that subjects utilizing the balance sheet experience less postdecisional regret and have increased adherence to the decision (e.g., Hoyt & Janis, 1975).

In short, clients often experience difficulty making a variety of decisions. Both the D'Zurilla and Goldfried model and the Janis and Mann model present a grid to facilitate the decision making process by either depicting consequences, probabilities, and/or preferences or values. The overall goal of both of these models is to help clients make decisions based on more information. Whereas some empirical evidence exists to support the utility of both of these models for the more immediate decisions, it is still unclear what models, training experiences, and client individual differences will affect clients' real life, generalizable decision making skills.

TYPES OF ANTICIPATION	Alternative Courses of Action					
	Alternative 1 (e.g.,)		Alternative 2 (e.g.,)		Alternative 3 (e.g.,)	
	+	-	+	-	+	-
A. Utilitarian gain or losses for self. 1. 2. 3. 4. 5. 6. 7.						
B. Utilitarian gains or losses for significant others. 1. 2. 3. 4. 5. 6. 7.						
C. Self-approval or disapproval. 1. 2. 3. 4. 5. 6. 7.						
D. Social approval or disapproval. 1. 2. 3. 4. 5. 6. 7.						

Figure 3.   Balance Sheet

GENERAL PROBLEM SOLVING STYLE

In addition to specific problem solving activities (e.g., decision making), writers have noted that the general orientation or mental set of the problem solver affects the problem solving process (e.g., Bloom & Broder, 1950; D'Zurilla & Goldfried, 1971). A set is an inferred predisposition that influences a client to behave in a certain manner, which can be either facilitative or disruptive, depending on whether it moves the client toward or away from an effective procedure or solution. Evidence suggests that there are some important differences within the problem solving process, such as confidence in a person's problem solving, accepting problems as a normal part of life, approaching versus avoiding problems, and personal control (D'Zurilla & Goldfried, 1971; Heppner, Hibel, Neal, Weinstein, & Rabinowitz, 1982).

The question is what interventions can be utilized to enhance or facilitate the development of a functional problem solving set or process. I will describe two techniques that my graduate students and I have developed to increase clients' awareness of their problem solving processes.* These techniques were developed and utilized in an eight week Applied Problem Solving class. Whereas we used the two techniques successively, the techniques could also be utilized separately or in conjunction with other intervention strategies.

The first technique was designed to aid students in beginning to examine the activities in which they engaged and obstacles they encountered while attempting to solve a particular personal problem. The major activity was the Problem Solving Worksheet, which is presented in Figure 4. Students were told

Stages	Activities	Obstacles
Defining the Problem		
Coming up with Alternatives		
Choosing one Alternative		
Acting on that Alternative		
Evaluating		

Figure 4. Problem Solving Worksheet

to select a recent personal problem, and record the activities and obstacles that occurred in the various stages. For example, a typical analysis might involve the student identifying a number of activities that were used to define the problem: being aware of feeling hurt and depressed, talking to a friend who confirmed that the student's roommate has seemed angry lately and is acting passive-aggressively toward others. Obstacles that were encountered during the problem definition stage included: feeling afraid of being

---

*I would here like to acknowledge the insightful contributions of Ann Baumgardner and Lisa Larson in developing some of these techniques.

rejected by the roommate, negative self-statements about one's own interpersonal skills. In addition, we planned classroom activities which involved students discussing and re-examining their analyses with one other student. A counselor could also serve as the discussant and person who probed, identified, and suggested other activities and obstacles. The outcome of utilizing the Problem Solving Worksheet seemed to be enhanced awareness of the problem solving process and identification of obstacles or self-defeating patterns.

The second technique was designed to aid students' examination in greater detail of the specific obstacles that they tend to encounter while solving personal problems. The stimulus to accomplish this goal was the Obstacle Analysis Worksheet (Figure 5). Definitions and examples of various obstacles were initially given, such as specific self-statements (e.g., I am a klutz), fears (e.g., I am afraid nobody likes me), beliefs (e.g., I must be liked by everyone on my residence hall floor), and feelings (e.g., feeling uncomfortable, embarrassed, depressed). In addition, examples were given of how people respond to various obstacles, particularly the negative consequences (e.g., avoiding the problem, blaming the cause of the problem on someone else). Students then selected a problem and analyzed various events that occurred in the problem solving process by recording specific obstacles and the subsequent outcomes. We also found peer dyads useful for discussing and re-examining the students' initial analyses; again a clinician could be well suited to fulfill this role.

Various Parts of the Situation	Self-Statements	Fears?	Beliefs?	Feelings?	Outcomes or Consequences

Figure 5. Obstacles Analysis Worksheet

We found that these and similar techniques were effective in increasing students' awareness of their problem solving set and subsequently enhancing a more functional problem solving set. It seemed that by reflecting on their problem solving processes, students became more cognizant of the interrelationship of problem solving activities, and would succumb to fewer self-defeating patterns. Given that a person's problem solving style tends to be well engrained, repeated awareness enhancing trials seem warranted. The previously mentioned techniques or similar activities could be well suited for clients' homework assignments in which a shaping process would occur over eight to ten counseling sessions. Since research is needed to examine the utility and comparative effectiveness of various techniques for affecting people's general problem solving processes, practitioners who systematically collect process and outcome data from clients regarding problem solving activities could make significant contributions to the applied problem solving area.

DISCUSSION AND SUMMARY

This contribution has described a number of client oriented, self-help techniques that facilitate the problem solving process. The methods can be utilized as self-help techniques or tools that counselors employ with clients in conjunction with typical counseling interventions. Since psychologists have not developed a technology for helping clients with regard to problem solving and decision making (Horan, 1979), research is needed to examine the comparative effectiveness of various problem solving techniques.

Practitioners who attend to clients' problem solving processes are in a unique position to examine how clients proceed in coping with personal problems, and particularly what effect various intervention strategies have on those problem solving processes across different clients. For example, recent research suggests that clients' self-appraisal of their problem solving skills subsequently affect a range of cognitive, affective, and behavioral problem solving activities (Heppner et al., 1982). Would intervention strategies directly aimed at the more general self-appraisal variables (e.g., problem solving confidence) have more therapeutic impact than strategies focused on specific problem solving skills (e.g., generating alternatives)? Practitioners who collect data regarding clients' problem solving processes either on a case study or group study basis have the potential of providing very important insights into applied problem solving. In addition, few methods or techniques have been published that are designed to facilitate client's personal problem solving. Creativity is needed in developing a broader range of methods, tools, and training programs that facilitate problem solving. Finally, the effect of important individual differences (e.g., self-appraisal variables, specific problem solving skills) on various intervention strategies have not been examined. Again practitioners could make significant contributions in the applied problem solving area by collecting data (perhaps most easily through intensive, single case studies) on how various intervention strategies differentially interact with client attributes.

P. Paul Heppner, Ph.D., is currently an Assistant Professor in the Department of Psychology and a senior staff psychologist in Counseling Services at the University of Missouri, Columbia. With a background in counseling psychology, he has published several articles on the applied problem solving process and the interpersonal influence process in counseling. Dr. Heppner may be contacted at the Department of Psychology, 210 McAlester Hall, University of Missouri-Columbia, Columbia, MO 65211.

RESOURCES

Arnkoff, D. B. & Stewart, J. The effectiveness of modeling and videotape feedback on personal problem solving. BEHAVIOR RESEARCH AND THERAPY, 1975, **13**, 127-133.

Bloom, B. S. & Broder, L. J. PROBLEM SOLVING PROCESSES OF COLLEGE STUDENTS. Chicago: University of Chicago Press, 1950.

Borck, L. E. & Fawcett, S. B. LEARNING COUNSELING AND PROBLEM SOLVING SKILLS. New York: Haworth Press, 1982.

Brilhart, J. K. & Jochem, L. M. Effects of different patterns on outcomes of problem-solving discussion. JOURNAL OF APPLIED PSYCHOLOGY, 1964, **48**, 175-179.

Bross, I. D. DESIGN FOR DECISIONS. New York: Macmillan, 1953.

Carkhuff, R. R. THE ART OF PROBLEM SOLVING. Amherst, MA: Human Resource Development Press, 1973.

Cronbach, L. J. & Gleser, G. C. PSYCHOLOGICAL TESTS AND PERSONAL DECISIONS. Urbana: University of Illinois Press, 1957.

Dilley, J. S. Decision-making ability and vocational maturity. PERSONNEL AND GUIDANCE JOURNAL, 1965, **44**, 423-527.

Dilley, J. S. Decision-making: A dilemma and a purpose for counseling. PERSONNEL AND GUIDANCE JOURNAL, 1967, **45**, 547-551.

Dixon, D. N., Heppner, P. P., Petersen, C. H., & Ronning, R. R. Problem solving workshop training. JOURNAL OF COUNSELING PSYCHOLOGY, 1979, **26**, 133-139.

D'Zurilla, T. J. & Goldfried, M. R. Problem solving and behavior modification. JOURNAL OF ABNORMAL PSYCHOLOGY, 1971, **78**, 107-126.

D'Zurilla, T. J. & Nezu, A. A study of the generation of alternatives process in social problem solving. COGNITIVE THERAPY AND RESEARCH, 1980, **4**, 67-72.

Edwards, W. Behavioral decision theory. ANNUAL REVIEW OF PSYCHOLOGY, 1961, **12**, 473-499.

Heppner, P. P. A review of the problem-solving literature and its relationship to the counseling process. JOURNAL OF COUNSELING PSYCHOLOGY, 1978, **25**, 366-375.

Heppner, P. P., Hibel, J. H., Neal, G. W., Weinstein, C. L., & Rabinowitz, F. E. Personal problem solving: A descriptive study of individual differences. JOURNAL OF COUNSELING PSYCHOLOGY, 1982, **29**, 580-590.

Horan, J. J. COUNSELING FOR EFFECTIVE DECISION MAKING: A COGNITIE-BEHAVIORAL PERSPECTIVE. North Scituate, MA: Duxbury Press, 1979.

Hoyt, M. F. & Janis, I. L. Increasing adherence to a stressful decision via a motivational balance-sheet procedure: A field experiment. JOURNAL OF PERSONALITY AND SOCIAL PSYCHOLOGY, 1975, **31**, 833-839.

Janis, I. L. & Mann, L. DECISION MAKING: A PSYCHOLOGICAL ANALYSIS OF CONFLICT, CHOICE, AND COMMITMENT. New York: The Free Press, 1977.

Johnson, D. M., Parrott, G. R., & Stratton, R. P. Production and judgment of solutions to five problems. JOURNAL OF EDUCATIONAL PSYCHOLOGY MONOGRAPH, 1968, **59**(6, Pt. 2).

Krumboltz, J. D. Behavioral counseling, rationale and research. PERSONNEL AND GUIDANCE JOURNAL, 1965, **44**, 383-387.

Meadow, A. & Parnes, S. J. Evaluation of training in creative problem solving. JOURNAL OF APPLIED PSYCHOLOGY, 1959, **43**, 189-194.

Nezu, A. & D'Zurilla, T. J. An experimental evaluation of the decision-making process in social problem solving. COGNITIVE THERAPY AND RESEARCH, 1979, **3**, 269-277.

Nezu, A. & D'Zurilla, T. J. Effects of problem definition and formulation on decision making in the social problem-solving process. BEHAVIOR THERAPY, 1981, **12**, 100-106.

Osborn, A. F. APPLIED IMAGINATION: PRINCIPLES AND PROCEDURES OF CREATIVE PROBLEM-SOLVING (3rd ed.). New York: Scribner's, 1963.

Parnes, S. J. & Meadow, A. Effects of "brainstorming" instructions on creative problem solving by trained and untrained subjects. JOURNAL OF EDUCATIONAL PSYCHOLOGY, 1959, **50**, 171-176.

Tyler, L. THE WORK OF THE COUNSELOR (3rd ed.). Englewood Cliffs, NJ: Prentice-Hall, 1969.

Wagman, M. Plato DCS: An interactive computer system for personal counseling. JOURNAL OF COUNSELING PSYCHOLOGY, 1980, **27**, 16-30.

Wagman, M. & Kerber, K. W. Plato DCS, an interactive computer system for personal counseling: Further development and evaluation. JOURNAL OF COUNSELING PSYCHOLOGY, 1980, **27**, 31-39.

Weitz, H. BEHAVIOR CHANGE THROUGH GUIDANCE. New York: Wiley, 1964.

THE TREATMENT OF ENURESIS

Suzanne Bennett Johnson

Most children are reliably continent during the day by 2 years of age and are dry at night by 3 years. If a youngster who is 4 years or older continues to wet and there is no organic pathology to account for the wetting, he or she is described as enuretic. Most of these children are bedwetters (nocturnal enuretics) although a few have day wetting problems as well (diurnal enuretics). The child's enuresis is termed primary if he or she has never had a prolonged period of dryness. Secondary enuresis refers to wetting that occurs after some substantial period of complete urinary continence. Secondary enuresis is sometimes associated with psychological trauma in the child or significant upheaval in the child's environment (e.g. birth of a new baby; separation from mother; hospitalization or serious injury to the child). It is generally less common than the primary form of the disorder.

Available prevalence estimates suggest that enuresis is a very common problem affecting 15-20% of 4 and 5 year olds, 5% of 10 year olds, and 1% of 15 year olds. It is significantly more common in boys than in girls. Given time, most enuretic children will ultimately become dry. However, in any given 1 year period, only 15% of all enuretic children attain complete daytime and nighttime control. Waiting for enuretic children to spontaneously become dry is one alternative to treatment. However, this approach may demand substantially longer than a 1 year waiting period (Johnson, 1980).

THEORETICAL FORMULATIONS

A variety of intrapsychic, behavioral, and biological explanations of enuresis have been proposed. These are outlined below.

PSYCHODYNAMIC OR INTRAPSYCHIC FORMULATIONS

From the intrapsychic or psychoanalytic point of view, enuresis is a symptom of an underlying emotional disorder. Repression is the defense mechanism typically involved although different theorists emphasize different feelings as the focus of the child's repression. For example, feelings of sexuality, fear or anxiety, hostility toward the parent, or desire to return to or maintain an infantile relationship with the mother, have all been proposed as underlying enuretic symptomatology (Johnson, 1980).

BEHAVIORAL OR LEARNING THEORY FORMULATIONS

From the behavioral or learning theory perspective, enuresis is the result of faulty learning. To be dry, a child must learn to discriminate a full bladder as the physiological cue that he needs to void. The youngster must also learn where micturition is appropriate (i.e., the toilet). Finally, the child must learn to postpone voiding until reaching the bathroom and appropriately preparing to urinate (e.g., removing underwear and sitting on the toilet). Since most enuretic children are dry during waking hours, the faulty learning is presumed to be in the area of discriminating full bladder cues when asleep as a signal that the child needs to void. While energetic youngsters are usually able to make this discrimination when awake, they have not yet learned to wake to such cues when asleep (Johnson, 1980).

BIOLOGICAL OR MEDICAL FORMULATIONS

Diurnal or nocturnal wetting can be caused by illness or organic pathology (e.g., uropathological obstruction or lesions, diabetes, spina bifida). Children with such disorders are not considered "true" enuretics and account for less than 5% of all youngsters presenting with wetting problems (Campbell, 1970). Some physicians believe that organic pathology is often overlooked in children with continued wetting problems; they claim that such pathology accounts for symptoms in over 95% of the cases (Arnold & Ginsburg, 1973; Mahoney, 1971). However, this is currently a minority view and has been criticized as leading to potentially dangerous urethral instrumentation and surgical intervention (Kendall & Karafin, 1973; Scott, 1973).

Assuming that most bedwetters have no organic pathology to account for their poor bladder control, several biological theories have been proposed to account for their nighttime wetting. These include profoundness of sleep or poor arousal mechanisms, small bladder capacity and/or bladder spasms, and maturational or developmental delay, suggesting some sort of neuropsychological immaturity (Barbour, Borland, Boyd, Miller, & Oppe, 1963; Gerrard & Zaleski, 1969).

ASSOCIATED CHARACTERISTICS

Enuretic children have been the subject of much empirical scrutiny. Their personalities, behavior, developmental level, toilet training histories, sleep patterns, bladder capacities, and families have all been the subject of numerous investigations. Highlights from this extensive literature will be summarized here.

PERSONALITY AND BEHAVIOR

Efforts to assess enuretic youngsters' personalities and behavior stem primarily from intrapsychic formulations that these children suffer from an underlying emotional disorder. Despite a large quantity of studies on this subject, it is difficult to draw firm conclusions due to numerous methodological flaws in the studies' design and execution. Data are frequently gathered from parents or by examiners aware of the child's enuresis, making the information obtained highly susceptible to bias. The enuretics studied often come from populations with a higher known incidence of deviance than the normal population (e.g., outpatient clinics, schools for delinquents). Measures selected are typically global in nature and consequently highly susceptible to bias, or are without evidence of reliability or validity. It is probably safe to conclude that there is no one personality or behavior problem that is characteristic of the enuretic child.

Most children with bedwetting problems do not present with clinically significant psychopathology. However, individual children may need assistance with problems other than bedwetting. When emotional or behavioral problems do exist in conjunction with the child's enuresis, no causal inferences can be drawn. Since the data are entirely correlational, existant problems may have been the result of the enuresis rather than its cause, or both the enuresis and the child's behavior problems may be the result of some third variable, such as family disorganization (Johnson, 1980).

DEVELOPMENTAL LEVEL

A number of studies have assessed intelligence, neuropsychological and other developmental characteristics of the enuretic child, primarily as an outgrowth of the biological theories suggesting that maturational and developmental delay plays a causal role in enuresis. Most investigators now agree that enuretic children are of normal intelligence and evidence little in the way of developmental delay. If maturational differences do exist, they do not seem to be readily apparent from currently available behavioral tests of intelligence or development (Johnson, 1980).

TOILET TRAINING HISTORY

An interest in the toilet training histories of enuretic children stems from both the intrapsychic and behavioral formulations of this disorder. Psychodynamic theorists postulated that very early or punitive toilet training practices may have led to the underlying emotional disturbance presumed to be at the root of the child's enuretic behavior. Learning theorists were more interested in the length of time it took to train the child, how completely the child was trained, and any associated problems that occurred when the child was taught this new behavior. Unfortunately, all available data on the subject are entirely retrospective. Most investigators report no differences between enuretics and nonenuretic controls as to what age toilet training was initiated or the general procedures used (Couchells, Johnson, Carter, & Walker, 1981; Johnson, 1980). However, some studies suggest that enuretic children were more uncooperative during training (Cust, 1952; Dimson, 1959) and that mothers experienced more frustration and anger during training (Murphy, Nickols, & Hammer, 1970). Given the retrospective nature of this data, it is difficult to assess its validity. It is possible that some children are difficult to train, leading to frustration and impatience in their mothers with ultimate incomplete learning by the child. Initial impatience of the mother in handling the child may lead to uncooperative behavior on the child's part and, again, incomplete learning. Still another possibility is that the parent will remember interactions with her child during toilet training as particularly difficult solely because of the negative halo effect the child's current enuresis may create. Until better prospective data is collected on this issue, the role of toilet training practices in enuresis will remain unclear.

SLEEP AND AROUSAL PATTERNS

Parents often report that their enuretic child is unusually difficult to arouse. However, controlled studies suggest that enuretic children are no more difficult to wake than their nonenuretic counterparts. Studies using EEG sleep recordings also suggest that there are no consistent differences between enuretics and controls. One of the few replicated findings in this literature is the absence of wetting episodes during dreaming or REM sleep. In fact, children's wetting episodes seem to occur in every sleep stage except REM sleep. These data seem to counter some psychoanalytic interpretations which postulate that wetting occurs during the child's dream-work (Johnson, 1980).

BLADDER CAPACITY

In 1950, Hallman reported that enuretics had smaller functional bladder capacities than normals. Since that time, a number of investigators have replicated this finding and discussed what causal role bladder capacity may play in enuresis.

Maximum functional bladder capacity (MBC) is usually measured by one of two methods. The child may be given an oral waterload of 30 ml/kg body weight (maximum volume of 500 ml) and told to refrain from voiding until he or she feels discomfort. When the child voids, the urine output is measured. Usually the larger of two voided specimens is taken as the MBC. The second method is to have the child's parents measure and record every time the child micturates at home for up to 1 week. The largest volume of urine passed at any one time is taken as the MBC (Zaleski, Gerrard, & Schokier, 1973).

Carefully controlled studies by Starfield (1967) and Starfield and Mellits (1968) demonstrated quite conclusively that enuretics do have smaller bladder capacities than nonenuretics. This leads to more frequent micturation even during their waking hours. Troup and Hodgson (1971) measured enuretics' urine volumes when they wet at night. They found day and nighttime volumes to be equivalent, and both were less than nonenuretic controls. They also report that the child's "true" bladder capacity, measured under mild anesthesia, was not different between the groups. A recent study by Zaleski et al. (1973) replicated Starfield's findings, but also noted that enuretics with daytime urgency or wetting have even smaller MBC's than enuretics with nighttime symptoms only. There is some evidence that primary enuretics have smaller MBC's than secondary enuretics (Starfield, 1967). Also of interest is the increase in MBC that has been found with treatment cures (Esperanca & Gerrard, 1969; Starfield & Mellits, 1968; Zaleski et al., 1973).

While the data on MBC is compelling, we do not yet know the exact role small MBC plays in enuresis. On the average, enuretics have smaller MBC than nonenuretics but there is overlap between groups (i.e., not all enuretics have small MBC and some nonenuretics do). Further, even if enuretic children must urinate more often, why do they not awake in response to their more frequent urgency? Although a larger MBC may help a child sleep through the night without ever needing to use the toilet, normal children and adults are able to awake and go to the bathroom if need be. Finally, it is worth noting that small MBC could very well be the result rather than the cause of enuresis.

FAMILY CHARACTERISTICS

Enuresis seems to be a familial disorder. Enuretic children are more likely to have siblings, parents, or other relatives who are or have been enuretic as well. Parents who were enuretic often have children with bedwetting problems and if **both** parents were enuretic during childhood, 77% of their offspring will suffer the same symptomatology (Bakwin, 1973). Although these data are often viewed as supportive of a biological basis for the disorder, an environmental explanation cannot be ruled out (e.g., parents who were enuretic may be more accepting of enuresis in a child).

Enuresis is also more prevalent in lower socioeconomic populations. The meaning of this association is not entirely clear. Some authors have suggested that family deviance, particularly mother-child separation, may be causally linked to continued bedwetting in the child (Cust, 1952; Douglas, 1973; Umphress, Murphy, Nickols, & Hammar, 1970). Both of these factors may be more common in lower socioeconomic classes.

Few studies have attempted to assess parent-child interactions in enuretic and nonenuretic comparison groups. A number of investigators have reported that mothers of enuretic children seem to view these children more negatively than mothers of nonenuretic youngsters (Couchells et al., 1981; Nilsson, Almgren, Kohler, & Kohler, 1973; Oppel, Harper, & Rider, 1968). It is difficult to know whether these mothers' perceptions are colored by the children's enuresis or whether the children are, in fact, difficult children who exhibit bedwetting in addition to a number of other problems. In the study by Couchells et al. (1981), child-rearing practices were examined. Mothers of enuretic youngsters reported using more rule-oriented, controlling practices than mothers of nonenuretic controls. In this correlational study, it is impossible to separate the effects of the mother's behavior on the child's enuresis from the effect of the child's bedwetting on the mother's selection of child-rearing practices. Although some interesting hypotheses may be delineated, the relationship between specific parent-child behaviors and enuresis remains unknown.

TREATMENT

Treatment for enuresis is usually not initiated until the child is 5 years of age or older. There is some evidence that enuretic children for whom treatment is requested differ from enuretic youngsters whose parents do not seek such treatment. Parents who request treatment for bedwetting seem to have children who are older and who wet the bed more frequently. Treatment-seekers are also parents who report less tolerance of the child's wetting. In other words, mothers with children who have wet the bed frequently, for long periods of time, and who feel frustrated or irritated with the child's continued wetting are more likely to seek treatment (Couchells, et al., 1981).

A number of intervention approaches are available. Some are more effective than others. Probably the most common-sense approach is to wake the child during the night in order to urinate in the toilet. However, such a procedure has been used in four controlled studies with only minimal success (Johnson, 1980). Another tact is to have the child self-record wet and dry nights, praising dry nights and ignoring wetting incidents. Dische (1971) and White (1968) have reported good success with this approach in about a third of the cases. We recommend that all children keep a calendar of wet and dry nights for 1 to 2 weeks before treatment is initiated. If a child becomes dry during this baseline recording period, no treatment is necessary other than following the child while strongly encouraging him or her to do the record-keeping. If the child does not become dry or is unable to maintain nighttime continence, treatment can begin. The baseline data already collected will be most helpful in evaluating any treatment program selected.

The two primary methods of treating enuresis are medication and the use of a conditioning alarm device. Insight-oriented psychotherapy or play therapy has not proved to be particularly successful in the few controlled studies that have assessed this approach (Johnson, 1980). Consequently, it will not be reviewed here. Two additional approaches, Retention Control Training and Dry Bed Training, will also be discussed, since they may be of some assistance to the interested therapist.

MEDICATION

Tofranil or imipramine has been used extensively with enuretics. In fact, it remains the most common treatment for this disorder today. Its popularity is probably the result of several factors. It is a medical treatment and consequently is likely to be the treatment of choice for physicians who are medically trained and who may not be familiar with other nonmedical approaches to bedwetting behavior. Physicians, of course, see the vast majority of enuretic youngsters, and medication offers a relatively simple treatment for this sometimes annoying but hardly life-threatening disorder.

Imipramine is a tricyclic antidepressant medication. Its use with bedwetters was first suggested by a psychologist, Hugh Esson, who noted difficulty in urination by many depressed patients treated with imipramine (MacLean, 1960). A variety of other types of drugs have been tried, but only the tricyclics have shown any consistent effectiveness (Blackwell & Currah, 1973).

There are numerous published, well-controlled studies comparing one of the tricyclics to a placebo. The drug appears to be most effective with childhood outpatient populations, less effective with institutionalized children, and of questionable utility with adult enuretics. Although medication seems to help many nocturnal enuretic children, this treatment approach is not without problems. First, although many youngsters' bedwetting improves (i.e., they have fewer wet nights), very few youngsters are actually cured (i.e., become completely dry for a prolonged period). Relapse remains a significant problem. Most children who show improvement while taking the drug return to high rates of wetting once medication is withdrawn (Johnson, 1980). Side effects of imipramine ingestion include dryness of mouth, dizziness, drowsiness, irritability, difficulty concentrating, and appetite and sleep disturbances. The general consensus seems to be that imipramine is safe if it is given under proper supervision and is not taken for prolonged periods of time (Blackwell & Currah, 1973).

The mechanism by which imipramine affects enuresis is not completely understood. Some studies suggest that its anticholinergic properties increase bladder capacity and thereby reduce the number of nighttime wetting episodes. Although this is the most compelling of the available explanations, it is not considered entirely satisfactory. The use of other anticholinergic medications has not proved to be as effective as imipramine for the treatment of enuresis (Blackwell & Currah, 1973).

In summary, tofranil may offer some relief to bedwetters seen on an outpatient basis. However, cure rates are low and most children return to pre-medication frequencies of wetting once the drug is terminated. Consequently, long-term use of this medication is not recommended.

In 1938, Mowrer and Mowrer introduced a device which they believed would enhance a child's learning of nocturnal urinary control. In their view, enuretics suffered from faulty learning and could be cured by presenting the discriminative cues and contingencies necessary for learning in a more precise and consistent manner. To this end, they developed a device which has been popularly referred to as the "bell and pad," the "urine alarm," or the "bed-buzzer." Although a number of modifications have been made since its original development and several different devices are now currently available (Dische, 1973), the basic mechanism has remained the same. The child sleeps on a pad or pads which are connected to a buzzer. When the child wets, the urine completes an electrical circuit and the alarm sounds. The most common type of detector consists of two wire mesh or aluminum foil pads kept separate by a layer of cloth. Each pad remains connected to the alarm, but the circuit is only completed if the child urinates, wetting the separation cloth and thereby "connecting" the two pads (see Figure 1).

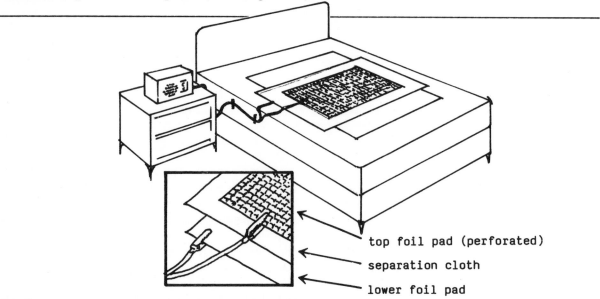

top foil pad (perforated)

separation cloth

lower foil pad

Figure 1. Urine alarm properly positioned on a bed (adapted from instructions for use of the "Wee Alert" distributed by Sears, Roebuck & Company).

A very similar device was developed as early as 1904 by a German pediatrician, Pfaundler. His purpose was to alert the nursing staff caring for a hospitalized child when that child had wet the bed and needed changing. He was somewhat surprised to note that the device, which was designed for convenience, seemed to have some therapeutic effect as well (Mowrer & Mowrer, 1938).

Mowrer and Mowrer explained the learning mechanism by which Pfaundler's device and their own urine alarm "cured" enuresis as classical conditioning. The bell and pad's alarm served as an unconditioned stimulus (US) producing waking, the unconditional response (UR). Through repeated trials, feelings of bladder distention which occurred prior to the alarm, became a conditioned stimulus (CS) leading to arousal. When learning was complete, bladder distention (CS) would lead to waking prior to urination and the subsequent onset of the alarm. The child would then use the toilet instead of wetting the bed.

This formulation, however, is not entirely adequate. Responses to conditioned stimuli, for example, rapidly drop out if the CS is not repeatedly paired with the US. In other words, once the child is waking to his or her own bladder cues (CS), the alarm (US) no longer sounds and the CS-US pairing is eliminated. This, in turn, should lead to extinction of the arousal response to the CS (bladder distention) and a return to wetting. Other theories involving instrumental learning (e.g., models of active or passive avoidance; models of social learning) have been proposed as more parsimonious explanations of mechanisms involved (Azrin, Sneed, & Foxx, 1974; Lovibond, 1964; Turner, Young, & Rachman, 1970).

Although the urine alarm was developed in the 1930's, it was not used extensively until the 1960's. Since it treated the child's "symptoms," it was not held in very high regard by those who had a more psychoanalytic view of the disorder (O'Leary & Wilson, 1975).

Since the 1960's, a large number of studies have assessed the effectiveness of this device. There is overwhelming evidence that this method is effective in reducing or eliminating bedwetting in most children. In fact, many controlled studies report cure rates (i.e., complete elimination of bedwetting) of 75% or higher in outpatient childhood populations (Johnson, 1980). A recent study by Wagner, Johnson, Walker, and Carter (1982) compared medication treatment with tofranil to conditioning treatment with the urine alarm to a waiting-list control condition. The superior effectiveness of the conditioning treatment was clear with 83% of the youngsters cured compared to 33% in the medication group and 8% in the control condition. All of the medication treatment youngsters that were cured relapsed after the drug was withdrawn.

Despite the positive results using the conditioning device reported in this study and others, some problems remain. Considerable effort and patience is required to appropriately use the alarm. Treatment often takes up to 16 weeks to complete. Poor parental cooperation seems to be the most common reason for failure. Parents either quit using the device altogether or use it inconsistently.

The therapist must decide whether to simply suggest the parent buy the conditioning device and use it without further supervision or whether weekly contact with the child and parent is indicated. We find that compliance seems to be improved and treatment more successful if weekly contact with the therapist is maintained. This permits the therapist to be aware of and intervene quickly should problems arise. This approach can be made more cost effective by seeing patients in groups and by "renting" the alarms instead of asking each parent to buy one. In our Enuresis Clinic we "rent" the Sears Wee Alert. However, the latest Sears model of this device uses a delayed alarm. We have not found this to be as effective and recommend purchase of conditioning devices through Penney's or Montgomery Ward's. Other manufacturers offer similar instruments. It is wise to test these with a few patients before purchasing a large number of them to make sure they can withstand the physical abuse the treatment procedure requires.

Steps for carrying out the procedure are provided in Table 1, on the next page. We recommend that these steps be thoroughly discussed with the parent and child and a copy be sent home with the family. Helping the child set up the device on a "bed" in the therapist's office is often a good idea.

TABLE 1: INSTRUCTIONS FOR USING THE URINE ALARM

GENERAL INSTRUCTIONS

1. Your child's bed should be as firm as possible. This may require the use of a "bed board" beneath the mattress.

2. It is important that the perforated foil pad be placed on top with the solid pad and cloth layer underneath. Be certain that the cloth layer completely eliminates any direct contact between the foil pads.

3. Center the pads in the middle of the mattress in the area where your child is most likely to wet.

4. When the wire clips are attached to the foil pads, be sure the clips are placed at least 6 inches apart on the side of the pad adjacent to the bedside unit.

5. Cover the pads with a regular flat sheet. It will help to tuck the sheet tightly under the mattress in order to keep the foil pads in place. Do not have your child sleep directly on top of the foil pads.

6. It will help if your child sleeps without pajama bottoms and if he or she begins each evening by sleeping face down on the mattress.

7. On a weekly basis it will be necessary to test the strength of the battery in the bedside unit. Do this by turning the switch on the unit to "ON" and then touch the two wire clips together to get a sound.

8. Turn on a dim night light each evening in your child's bedroom.

BEFORE THE CHILD RETIRES:

9. Make certain that a change of dry sheets is available in the room.

10. Make certain that a paper shopping bag is available for the disposal of any wet sheets that might result during the night.

11. Check the foil pads to make certain that the pads are completely separated by the cloth layer. Make sure that the wire clips are attached to the pads and are at least 6 inches apart from each other.

12. Place the regular flat sheet on the mattress and tuck it under tightly.

13. Switch the buzzer unit to "ON."

14. Have the child go to bed by lying face down on the mattress.

WHEN THE CHILD WETS, HE OR SHE SHOULD:

15. Awaken, when the alarm sounds, STAND UP alongside the bed, and turn on a bedside lamp before turning the alarm switch to "OFF."

16. Go to the lavatory and splash water on his or her face to be sure of actually being awake.

17. Walk to the toilet and finish urinating.

18. Return to the bedroom, remove the wet sheet from the bed, and place the sheet in the paper bag located nearby.

19. Separate the foil pads, remove the wet cloth layer and put it in the paper bag.

20. Take a dry cloth and wipe any moisture from the foil pads.

21. Replace the bottom foil pad on the mattress, insert a new layer of dry cloth, placing the perforated foil pad on top. Be sure the foil pads are not touching.

22. Attach a wire clip to each pad. Be sure the clips are at least 6 inches apart.

23. Place a dry flat sheet over the foil pads and tightly tuck under the mattress.

24. Turn the alarm switch to "ON."

25. Return to bed and lie face-down on the mattress.

It is important to test the strength of the battery on a weekly basis (Step 7) so that the alarm is sure to go off when the child wets. "Buzzer ulcers," or small sores, may occur if the batteries become so weak that the alarm does not sound and the child continues to sleep while remaining in contact with a weak electrical current. Buzzer ulcers are very rare but can be eliminated altogether if the strength of the batteries is checked on a regular basis. We also recommend that the child sleep without underpants or pajama bottoms (Step 6). This will permit the alarm to sound as soon as the youngster begins to wet, enhancing the conditioning effect. It is important for the child to take as much responsibility as possible for the management of this program. His or her exact responsibilities should be age-appropriate. However, the child should be made to understand that the therapist and parent are there to assist in solving the problem. If the parent takes all the responsibility, it is the parent's behavior that is trained and not the child's. Most children participate willingly but some may need to be encouraged by giving them small rewards (e.g., stars or stickers) for following each step in the program. Sometimes the child is motivated but does not wake up to the alarm. Placing the alarm inside a tin can may increase the decibel level sufficiently to arouse the child. If this is not effective, the parent might apply a cold washcloth to the child's face, conditioning the sound of the alarm to a more aversive waking procedure and thereby teaching the youngster to respond to the alarm. It is important that the child learn to wake up to the alarm. If the parent rushes into the child's room, turns off the alarm, attempts to arouse the child and carry him or her to the bathroom, the youngster may never become sufficiently awake to learn anything.

It is often helpful to have the child keep a graph or chart of the number of wetting episodes per week. This is usually completed during the therapist's session by having the youngster bring a daily record of wet or dry nights for the preceding week. Number of wetting episodes is a good behavior to chart because many children wet the bed more than once a night. The high frequency of wetting on a nightly basis is usually not apparent until the child starts using the alarm. Often, the first sign of treatment success is a reduction in the number of nightly wetting episodes rather than a dry night. Charting the number of wetting episodes often permits the therapist to socially reward the youngster for improvement sooner than if dry nights were the only criteria for success.

Occasionally, a child will show good improvement using the alarm but does not become completely dry (e.g. continues to wet twice a week). Sometimes such children can be motivated to improve their performance by using a simple operant reinforcement program in addition to the alarm device. The best approach is to offer a reward for a specified number of consecutive dry nights. The criteria can be increased as the youngster demonstrates the ability to go for longer and longer periods without wetting the bed.

Relapse can be a problem, occurring in as many as 50% of children initially cured using the device. Usually, these youngsters are successfully treated by re-introducing the alarm. Relapse rates also can be reduced by introducing an overlearning procedure. Once the child reaches a cure criterion of 14 consecutive dry nights, he or she is asked to increase fluid intake an average of 1 to 1.5 pints each night before retiring to bed. This precipitates a relapse in many children although most are able to regain full bladder control despite the increased fluid intake. Approximately 9% of initially cured youngsters do very poorly on an overlearning protocol and the procedure should be discontinued if the child continues to wet without any improvement (Morgan, 1978).

Combining medication with conditioning seems to be contraindicated. Although youngsters may be cured more quickly, they frequently relapse when this combined treatment is withdrawn (Johnson, 1980).

Almost all studies addressing the treatment of enuresis have focused on nighttime wetters. Consequently, the cure rates and relapse rates presented here are relevant for this population only. There is some evidence that youngsters who wet both during the day and at night are more difficult to treat. Their cure rates seem to be lower and they relapse more quickly following treatment (Fielding, 1980).

RETENTION CONTROL TRAINING

In Retention Control Training (RCT), the child is rewarded for holding urine for longer and longer periods of time. The desired behavior is the expansion of bladder capacity so that the child may sleep through the night without needing to urinate. The training procedure is carried out during the day by having the child inform the parent or trainer when he or she has to micturate. Initially the youngster is asked to hold his or her urine for 5 additional minutes. A reward is given for this and then permission is given to use the toilet. Gradually the holding time is increased up to 45 minutes after the child feels a need to void. As bladder capacity increases, the enuresis should be eliminated. Although this procedure is attributed to Kimmel and Kimmel (1970), it was suggested earlier by Muellner (1960) and Starfield and Mellits (1968). These latter researchers reported 19% of their children were cured and 66% improved. They also reported that increases in bladder capacity were associated with improvement, although this was not true for every child. In Kimmel and Kimmel's (1970) initial report, three children were all cured using RCT and no relapses occurred within 12 months. In a subsequent larger study (Paschalis, Kimmel, & Kimmel, 1972), 48% of the children were cured although one child required added involvement by the therapist. None relapsed within a 3 month follow-up. Good success has been reported in several individual cases, but controlled studies have not found RCT to be particularly effective (Fielding, 1980; Johnson, 1980). Although children often increase their bladder capacity with RCT, a subsequent improvement in enuresis does not always or even typically occur.

DRY BED TRAINING

Dry Bed Training (DBT) is a fairly complicated procedure initially developed and used with institutionalized retarded adults (Azrin, Sneed, & Foxx, 1973). Later, it was modified slightly and applied to normal children. It involves one night of intensive training in which the child is encouraged to drink large amounts of fluid before retiring. The youngster is then given "Positive Practice" in which he or she lies in bed with the light off for about 1 minute, gets up and goes to the bathroom and tries to urinate. After 20 practice trials of this kind, the youngster is permitted to go to bed but has to sleep on a urine alarm. That evening, the child is aroused every hour by the trainer and sent to the bathroom. At the bathroom door, the trainer asks the child if he or she can hold the urine for another hour. If the child says yes, the youngster is returned to bed. If the answer is no, the child is asked to inhibit urination for a few minutes and then is permitted to micturate. Praise is given for holding the urine and having a dry bed. Should the child accidentally wet, the alarm sounds and the child is sent to the bathroom to finish urinating. He or she is given "Cleanliness Training" which involves changing the wet sheets and pajamas, wiping off the mattress and disposing of the wet sheets in the appropriate place. Another 20 trials of Positive Practice are given before the child is allowed to go back to sleep. On the evening following an accident, the child must perform another 20 Positive Practice trials before going to bed. After this initial intensive training, the child continues to sleep on the urine alarm but is not repeatedly aroused except when the parents go to bed. However, should an accident occur, the youngster must carry out Cleanliness Training and Positive Practice. All dry nights are socially reinforced. After a number of consecutive dry nights, the urine alarm is removed. In the initial study (Azrin et al., 1973), all 12 of the retarded subjects reached criterion of 7 consecutive dry nights. One resident relapsed within 3 months. With normals, Azrin, Sneed, and Fox (1974) also report 100% initial cures, although 29% had to be re-treated. Similar data have been reported by Bollard and Woodroffe (1977). However, results of a study published by Doleys, Ciminero, Tollison, and colleagues (1977) are not as favorable. Only 38% of their subjects became dry within 6 weeks of treatment and one-third of these children relapsed.

A great deal is involved in DBT including punishment through Positive Practice and Cleanliness Training, social reinforcement for a dry bed, training in inhibiting urination, the use of the urine alarm, and intensive initial involvement with an outside "trainer." It is not yet clear which variables are crucial to treatment success. Bollard and Woodroffe (1977) and Bollard, Nettelbeck, and Roxbee (1982) reported that parents could be successfully trained to carry out the entire procedure, thereby eliminating the necessity of an outside trainer entering the home for the child's initial intensive training session. They also report, however, that using the procedure without the urine alarm reduced its effectiveness considerably. In contrast, recent studies by Azrin and his colleagues (Azrin, Hontos, & Besalel-Azrin, 1979; Azrin & Thienes, 1978) described excellent success with DBT procedures even when the urine alarm component was eliminated.

SUMMARY

Enuresis is defined as continued wetting after the age of three when there is no organic pathology to account for the disorder. It is a common problem affecting 15-20% of 4 and 5 year olds, 5% of 10 year olds, and 1% of 15 year olds. Over time, most enuretic children will ultimately become dry. However, in any given one year period only 15% of all enuretic children attain complete day and nighttime control.

A variety of intrapsychic, behavioral and biological explanations for enuresis have been proposed. These theories have resulted in a wealth of descriptive studies assessing the personalities, behavior, developmental level, toilet training histories, sleep patterns, bladder capacities, and families of enuretic youngsters. Although some children who are bedwetters also have behavioral or emotional problems, most do not exhibit any clinically significant difficulties of this sort. There is little evidence to date that enuretic children differ from their nonenuretic counterparts in developmental level, toilet training history, or sleep and arousal patterns. As a group, enuretic children do have smaller bladder capacities although this characteristic could be a consequence as well as a cause of enuresis. Enuresis seems to be a familial disorder. However, the genetic and environmental components of this relationship are not well understood.

The two primary methods of treating enuresis are medication with imipramine (tofranil) and the use of a conditioning alarm. Controlled studies suggest that conditioning results in higher cure rates and lower relapse rates than medication. Most studies report cure rates (i.e. complete elimination of bedwetting) of 75% or higher in outpatient childhood populations who exhibit nighttime wetting only. However, this treatment approach is not without problems. It often requires up to 16 weeks for treatment to be completed and continued parental cooperation may be difficult to obtain in all cases. Relapse may occur in up to 50% of initially cured children. Re-treatment with the alarm or the use of an overlearning procedure is usually successful.

Other behavioral methods available to the interested therapist include Retention-Control Training (RCT) and Dry-Bed Training (DBT). Neither approach has been studied as extensively as treatment with medication or the urine alarm. RCT holds little promise as a primary treatment for enuresis but may prove to be helpful as an adjunctive procedure when combined with conditioning for certain populations (e.g., enuretics with small bladder capacities). DBT appears to offer better results than RCT but is a very complicated procedure that may be difficult for some parents to follow. Its effectiveness over and above the use of the urine alarm alone remains to be seen.

Suzanne Bennett Johnson, Ph.D., is currently a clinical psychologist and Associate Professor in the Departments of Psychiatry, Pediatrics, and Clinical Psychology at the University of Florida's Medical Center. She is also Director of the Diabetes Project Unit, and conducts research in the area of behavioral pediatrics. She has published numerous articles on enuresis, psychological aspects of juvenile diabetes, and the assessment and treatment of children's fears. Dr. Johnson may be contacted at the Division of Child and Adolescent Psychiatry, Box J-234, J. Hillis Miller Health Center, Gainesville, FL 32610.

RESOURCES

Arnold, S. & Ginsburg, A. Enuresis: Incidence and pertinence of genitourinary disease in healthy enuretic children. UROLOGY, 1973, 2, 437.

Azrin, N., Hontos, P., & Besalel-Azrin, V. Elimination of enuresis without a conditioning apparatus: An extension by office instruction of the child and parents. BEHAVIOR THERAPY, 1979, 10, 14-19.

Azrin, N., Sneed, T., & Foxx, R. Dry bed training: A rapid method of eliminating bedwetting (enuresis) of the retarded. BEHAVIORAL RESEARCH AND THERAPY, 1973, 11(4), 427-434.

Azrin, N., Sneed, T., & Foxx, R. Dry-bed training: Rapid elimination of childhood enuresis. BEHAVIORAL RESEARCH AND THERAPY, 1974, 12(3), 147-156.

Azrin, N. & Thienes, P. Rapid elimination of enuresis by intensive learning without a conditioning apparatus. BEHAVIOR THERAPY, 1978, 9, 342-354.

Bakwin, H. The genetics of enuresis. In I. Kolvin, R. MacKeith, & S. Meadow (Eds.), BLADDER CONTROL AND ENURESIS, CLINICS IN DEVELOPMENTAL MEDICINE, 1973, 48-49.

Barbour, R., Borland, E., Boyd, M., Miller, A., & Oppe, T. Enuresis as a disorder of development. BRITISH MEDICAL JOURNAL, 1963, 2, 787-790.

Blackwell, B. & Currah, J. The psychopharmacology of nocturnal enuresis. In I. Kolvin, R. MacKeith, & S. Meadow (Eds.), BLADDER CONTROL AND ENURESIS, CLINICS IN DEVELOPMENTAL MEDICINE, 1973, 48–49.

Bollard, J., Nettelbeck, T., & Roxbee, L. Dry-bed training for childhood bedwetting: A comparison of group with individually administered parent instruction. BEHAVIOR RESEARCH AND THERAPY, 1982, **20**, 209–217.

Bollard, R. & Woodroffe, P. The effect of parent-administered dry-bed training on nocturnal enuresis in children. BEHAVIOR RESEARCH AND THERAPY, 1977, **15**(2), 159–165.

Campbell, M. Neuromuscular uropathy. In M. Campbell & H. Harrison (Eds.), UROLOGY. Philadelphia: Saunders, 1970.

Couchells, S., Johnson, S. B., Carter, R., & Walker, D. Behavioral and environmental characteristics of treated and untreated enuretics and matched non-enuretic controls. JOURNAL OF PEDIATRICS, 1981, **99**(5), 812–816.

Cust, G. The epidemiology of nocturnal enuresis. LANCET, 1952, **2**, 1167–1170.

Dimson, S. Toilet training and enuresis. BRITISH MEDICAL JOURNAL, 1959, **2**, 666–670.

Dische, S. Management of enuresis. BRITISH MEDICAL JOURNAL, 1971, 2(752), 33–36.

Dische, S. Treatment of enuresis with an enuresis alarm. In I. Koern, R. MacKeith, & S. Meadow (Eds.), BLADDER CONTROL AND ENURESIS, CLINICS IN DEVELOPMENTAL MEDICINE, 1973, 48–49.

Doleys, D., Ciminero, A., Tollison, J., Williams, C., & Wells, K. Dry-bed training and retention control training: A comparison. BEHAVIOR THERAPY, 1977, **8**(4), 541–548.

Douglas, J. Early disturbing events and later enuresis. In I. Kolvin, R. MacKeith, & S. Meadow (Eds.), BLADDER CONTROL AND ENURESIS, CLINICS IN DEVELOPMENTAL MEDICINE, 1973, 48–49.

Esperanca, M. & Gerrard, J. Nocturnal enuresis: Comparison of the effect of imipramine and dietary restriction on bladder capacity. CANADIAN MEDICAL ASSOCIATION JOURNAL, 1969, **101**(12), 65–68.

Fielding, D. The response of day and night wetting children and children who wet only at night to retention control training and the enuresis alarm. BEHAVIOR RESEARCH AND THERAPY, 1980, **18**, 305–317.

Gerrard, J. & Zaleski, A. Nocturnal enuresis. PAKISTAN MEDICAL REVIEW, 1969, **4**, 77.

Hallman, N. On the ability of enuretic children to hold urine. ACTA PAEDIATRICA, 1950, **39**, 87–93.

Johnson, S. B. Enuresis. In R. Daitzman (Ed.), CLINICAL BEHAVIOR THERAPY AND BEHAVIOR MODIFICATION (Vol. I). New York: Garland Press, 1980.

Kendall, A. & Karafin, L. Editorial: Enuresis. JOURNAL OF UROLOGY, 1973, **109**(137).

Kimmel, H. & Kimmel, E. An instrumental conditioning method for the treatment of enuresis. JOURNAL OF BEHAVIOR THERAPY AND EXPERIMENTAL PSYCHIATRY, 1970, 1, 121–123.

Lovibond, S. CONDITIONING AND ENURESIS. New York: Macmillan, 1964.

MacLean, R. Imipramine hydrochloride (tofranil[R]) and enuresis. AMERICAN JOURNAL OF PSYCHIATRY, 1960, **117**, 551.

Mahoney, D. Studies of enuresis: I. Incidence of obstructive lesions and pathophysiology of enuresis. JOURNAL OF UROLOGY, 1971, **106**(6), 951–958.

Morgan, R. T. Relapse and therapeutic response in the conditioning, treatment of enuresis: A review of recent findings on intermittent reinforcement overlearning and stimulus intensity. BEHAVIOR RESEARCH AND THERAPY, 1978, **16**, 273–279.

Mower, O. & Mower, W. Enuresis: A method for its study and treatment. AMERICAN JOURNAL OF ORTHOPSYCHIATRY, 1938, 8, 436-459.

Muellner, S. Development of urinary control in children. JOURNAL OF THE AMERICAN MEDICAL ASSOCIATION, 1960, 172, 1256-1261.

Murphy, S., Nickols, J., & Hammer, S. Neurological evaluation of adolescent enuretics. PEDIATRICS, 1970, 45(2), 269-273.

Nilsson, A., Almgren, P. Kohler, E., & Kohler, L. Enuresis: The importance of maternal attitudes and personality. A prospective study of pregnant women and a follow-up of their children. ACTA PSYCHIATRICA SCANDINAVIA, 1973, 49(2), 114-130.

O'Leary, K. & Wilson, G. BEHAVIOR THERAPY: APPLICATION AND OUTCOME. Englewood Cliffs, NJ: Prentice-Hall, 1975.

Oppel, W., Harper, P., & Rider, R. Social, psychological, and neurological factors associated with nocturnal enuresis. PEDIATRICS, 1968, 42(4), 627-641.

Paschalis, A., Kimmel, H., & Kimmel, E. Further study of diurnal instrumental conditioning in the treatment of enuresis nocturna. JOURNAL OF BEHAVIOR THERAPY AND EXPERIMENTAL PSYCHIATRY, 1972, 3, 253-256.

Scott, J. A surgeon's view of enuresis. In I. Kolvin, R. MacKeith, & S. Meadow (Eds.), BEHAVIORAL CONTROL AND ENURESIS, CLINICS IN DEVELOPMENTAL MEDICINE, 1973, 48-49.

Starfield, B. Functional bladder capacity in enuretic and non-enuretic children. JOURNAL OF PEDIATRICS, 1967, 70(5), 777-781.

Starfield, B. & Mellits, E. Increase in functional bladder capacity and improvements in enuresis. JOURNAL OF PEDIATRICS, 1968, 72, 483-487.

Troup, C. & Hodgson, N. Nocturnal functional bladder capacity in enuretic children. WISCONSIN MEDICAL JOURNAL, 1971, 70(7), 171-173.

Turner, R., Young, G., & Rachman, S. Treatment of nocturnal enuresis by conditioning techniques. BEHAVIOR RESEARCH AND THERAPY, 1970, 8, 367-381.

Umphress, A., Murphy, S., Nickols, J., & Hammar, S. Adolescent enuresis. ARCHIVES OF GENERAL PSYCHIATRY, 1970, 22, 237-244.

Wagner, W., Johnson, S. B., Walker, D., & Carter, R. A controlled comparison of two treatments for nocturnal enuresis. JOURNAL OF PEDIATRICS, 1982, 101(2), 302-307.

White, M. A thousand consecutive cases of enuresis: Results of treatment. MEDICAL OFFICER, 1968, 120, 151-155.

Zaleski, A., Gerrard, J., & Schokier, M. Nocturnal enuresis: The importance of a small bladder capacity. In I. Kolvin, R. MacKeith, & S. Meadow (Eds.), BLADDER CONTROL AND ENURESIS, CLINICS IN DEVELOPMENTAL MEDICINE, 1973, 48-49.

F

AMILY THERAPY

a model of therapy developed at the Philadelphia
der the leadership of Salvador Minuchin, M.D.,
pproach to the problems of individuals in their
based on the assumption that the emotional and
behavioral p   lividuals are maintained by patterns of thinking and
behaving in their context, and that the amelioration of those problems is
through a change in the patterns. Prior to the application of a systemic
approach, the major paradigm for the treatment of psychological problems was
an intrapsychic approach. Therapy based on an intrapsychic model entails a
process by which the individual evaluates his or her way of thinking, based on
early learnings, with the anticipation that insight will lead to new ways of
responding. From a general systems perspective, a focus on the individual
psyche is a limited one which excludes the influence of the individual's
current context in maintaining a particular view of the world. A systems
approach defines the individual as part of a dynamic interactive process, and
not as an isolated unit. Individuals are reliant on their context, constantly
in communication with other individuals, with their boundaries being
"permeable" or receptive to input by others. It is through a process of
feedback (the interchange of information, nurturance, and so on) that
individuals "grow." Growth is interpreted as the individual's ability to
respond with increased complexity to the challenges of living. The greater
the alternatives that individuals and groups have in responding to challenging
events, the greater their flexibility, and hence their power. In contrast,
rigid systems and rigid individuals have a limited repertoire of alternative
responses to new situations. They become "stuck" in the increasingly complex
demands of living, repeating a limited repertoire of responses to new
situations.

Systems tend to be conservative and maintain familiar ways of functioning
(homeostasis). Changes resulting from internal biological adjustments (e.g.,
during adolescence) or through external social pressures (e.g., changes of job
or moves) challenge a family's homeostasis. These changes are experienced as
stressful since it requires new and different responses to replace the more
familiar ones. The responses of family members to given situations serve as
the "rules" by which the family members operate. These rules may be explicit
(e.g., a child's bedtime); however, for the most part, family rules emerge as
the myriad unspoken patterns which form the rituals of everyday life. The
family is deemed functional to the degree that their rules of interaction can
change to allow members to meet the normal challenges of child and adult
development.

The dysfunctional family resists change in its patterns, adhering to a limited repertoire of emotions, behaviors, and ways of perceiving the world. The lack of responsiveness of the dysfunctional family to changing situations comes to the attention of the helping professional in the form of a "problem" or symptomatic person. An individually oriented approach to treatment would begin with the identified patient as its frame of reference, while a family-oriented approach would evaluate how all of the members of a family are contributing to maintain patterns of behavior which support the presenting problem.

FAMILY TRANSITIONS

The application of systemic thinking to the individual's psychological development assumes that families go through developmental stages, and that functional interactional patterns for each stage are different. Hence, the childless couple has typically different tasks and different ways of responding (rules) than families of young children. Similarly, families of adolescents must reorganize their rules of interaction to allow for growth on the part of each of its members.

The concept of family transitions is more than an elaboration of traditional concepts of individual development. It recognizes the normal developmental stages that children, as well as adults, typically go through during their lives. Also, it assumes that the ability to respond to those tasks is a function not only of the individual's resources, but the ability of those most involved with him or her to adjust in supporting change. The unit of intervention then becomes the individual-in-context.

The concept of "structure" is inherent in the concept of developmental transitional patterns. Since behaviors are considered patterned and not random, the rules of a family's behaviors are a manifestation of its structure. For example, in a patriarchal family where the father is the executor in dealing with the outside world, but mother functions as the nurturer and manager of the home, there may be a family "rule" that children share their daily needs and thoughts with mother while financial matters are father's domain. The structure of this family may reveal more intense proximity between mother and children, while, in areas of executive decision making, father serves as ultimate authority. For purposes of simplification, structural family therapists present the structural "map" of the family based on two parameters: (a) proximity and distance (how close and how distant family members are from one another); and (b) hierarchy (the power relationship between those members). In the preceding example, the map of the family would indicate a close relationship between mother and children, with the father less close, but higher in the hierarchical structure of the family (Figure 1).

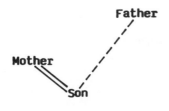

Figure 1.

A family's structure changes according to its developmental stage. These changes vary in degree; some are incremental, evolving gradually over time, while other changes are abrupt, requiring major revisions of usual family relationships.

The abrupt shifts require major adjustment of roles among family members whereby the child, through increased competence, gains stature in the family decision-making process, and develops greater equality with parents. Major (second order) changes shift the relationships of parent to child and parents to each other and reorganize the rules regulating the proximity and hierarchy of family interactions. It is the response to the inevitable stresses of those changes that distinguish flexible and adaptive family patterns from rigid, dysfunctional ones. A family's difficulties in effecting the normal transitional changes may become manifested by symptomatic behavior in one of its members. The goals of change become the reorganization of the family system in a way that will allow alternate responses (growth) in each of its members.

STRUCTURAL FAMILY THERAPY

The structural family therapist approaches the goal of changing dysfunctional patterns of interaction through changing the family's structure. While one member of a family or one individual comes, or is brought, to a psychiatric clinic as the symptomatic person, or identified patient, the therapist assumes that all members closely involved with this person are necessary for the remediation of the problem. The structural family therapist will attempt to assess the patient's role in the family context through interviewing the family, noting patient and family interaction patterns that maintain the presenting problem. The structural diagnosis, or family map, becomes a precondition for developing a treatment plan for changing the structure.

The skills required of the structural family therapist in diagnosing and intervening in families are conceptual as well as interpersonal. The ability to think systemically entails an orientation to conceptualizing behavior as part of a sequence of behaviors. For example, focus on a child described as "uncontrollable" will yield an orientation which punctuates the observers' frame of reference with the behavior of the child. Broadening that frame of reference to include, for example, the pleading responses of the child's mother in response to the child's aggressiveness, shifts the focus of the problem from the child to the "dance" between mother and child. If we further expand our frame of reference to include the father's punitive response to the child, we may find that what starts as ineffectiveness on the mother's part may be her attempt to balance out father's harshness by being reasonable. Hence, our system includes the sequence of interactions among mother, father, and child to maintain an "out-of-control" child. The ability to think in terms of sequences of behaviors, and observe behaviors as complementary to one another is a critical part of systems thinking.

TECHNIQUES OF STRUCTURAL FAMILY THERAPY

For the clinician, theory finds its application to practice in the techniques of psychotherapy. In structural family therapy, techniques can be classified into two categories: those that maintain family members' sense of themselves and the way they operate, and those that challenge them.

Joining, an essential part of any psychotherapy, is a process by which a therapist, who is foreign to the family system, becomes more acceptable and more familiar to the family. Joining techniques include those responses that confirm and support family members' sense of themselves. Minuchin refers to three sets of operations which characterize joining behaviors of the therapist: maintenance, tracking, and mimesis.

Through **maintenance operations** the therapist highlights the positive connotations of family members' behaviors, reinforcing certain ideas, behaviors, and emotions, as well as highlighting the person's strengths. For example, the intensely involved mother referred to above may be described as extremely patient and responsive to the needs of her child. Similarly, the therapist may defer to the father as the head of the family, maintaining the family's traditional hierarchy, rather than challenging it through the use of a privileged position. Joining occurs at all levels of communication, through words, feelings, as well as behaviors, and is experienced by the family as the empathic responses of the therapist.

Tracking is the process by which a therapist follows both content and process of family members' contributions in the session. By following the train of thought or content of the family members, utilizing their metaphors, eliciting expansion on some of their ideas, and reinforcing others, the therapist not only becomes less threatening and more familiar to the family, but they become more familiar to the therapist. A form of natural "induction" becomes part of the joining process, by which the therapist and family, beginning as separate entities, become more responsive to each other, more like each other.

Mimesis is the nonverbal component of the process of joining. It is the means by which the therapist is captured and responds to the affect, pace, mood, and posture of the family. This becomes manifest in the way the therapist communicates, rather than the content of that communication. A therapist engaged with a family that has a staccato pace, active and emotionally intense, would be experienced as somewhat foreign and unfamiliar if he or she maintained a detached and intellectualized response. Mimetic operations are often unconscious, a facet of the therapist's responsiveness to the context. However, mimetic operations can be utilized skillfully, as when, for example, a therapist chooses to join the pace of the identified "hyperactive" child, challenging the more depressed mood of the rest of the family, or when the therapist goes into a session in shirt sleeves as a way of maintaining a more casual and relaxed atmosphere. It is the public representation of ourselves that constitutes one of the most powerful forms of communication with others.

Separating joining operations from the techniques that challenge the family structure is an arbitrary task, useful only for purposes of highlighting the craft of the family therapist. In practice, the therapist cannot challenge or be critical of family members without having recognized and communicated understanding and respect for those members. Conversely, empathy and compassion are essentials to the understanding and treatment of emotional problems, but in themselves do not produce change.

Techniques of challenging the family's way of dealing with problems are all predicated on the notion of complementarity of interaction. The punctuation of a sequence of events into units, labeled cause and effect, is part of our Western scientific tradition. A family is a group, well rehearsed in the intricacies of its interactive network, each member stimulating reciprocal responses from the other. This family dance can be seen in its totality, or may be broken down to the various solo performances. The problem of approaching a therapeutic situation with too narrow a focus is that, in neglecting the gestalt, the therapist may give undue importance to the role and ability of any one person or event in effecting change. This limits the therapist's alternatives in initiating change.

For example, in an interview with a young single parent who had difficulty managing her 4 year old daughter, an emphasis which focuses on the daughter as the unit of change, negates the fact that the girl is responding to the mother's ambivalent directives. Similarly, a focus on the complementarity of the mother-daughter dyad, in which mother's ambivalence evokes daughter's challenge which escalates mother's ambivalence, may itself prove to be too narrow a focus. We may find the maternal grandmother, with whom mother and daughter live, typically steps in to "settle" escalating conflicts between the two, and in that way keeps both mother and daughter on the level of peers, and maintains grandmother as the sole authority.

The therapist's ability to see behavior in terms of sequences (Haley, 1976) allows him or her to choose the optimal point of reference for challenging the way the family members respond to their situation. The **reframing** of the patient's sense of reality is a basic therapeutic intervention of all therapists. The patient's limited conceptualization of a situation, usually contributes to the problem. A limited perspective allows fewer possible responses to any given situation. For example, if the concern of the single parent, cited above, was limited to her child's responses, the only alternative for change would be in altering her child's way of behaving, or changing the girl's attitude. Expanding the problem to the mother-daughter interaction allows the potential for change to include a more firm and assertive stance on the part of the mother.

The therapist typically challenges the way the patient is viewing situations, providing alternative ways of considering it. The technical aspects of the intervention are based on the assumption that most people, in their growing experiences, categorize certain sensory information in a way that makes daily living predictable. However, when these categories become too limited or too rigid, the range of responses also become limited. Reframing interventions then challenge the patient's (and family's) typical ways of categorizing an experience or event, offering an alternative way of thinking about it, which yields alternative responses.

In the struggle between mother and child cited earlier, the mother might "frame" the daughter's behavior as belligerent, thinking she gets perverse satisfaction in upsetting her mother. This leads the angry mother into an escalating symmetrical struggle with her child. The therapist may offer an alternative perspective in suggesting the daughter's behavior as signaling her need for mother to emerge as confident, particularly in relation to maternal grandmother. This reframe salvages the daughter's behavior as potentially productive and challenges mother to expand her view of the problem, as well as move out of a position of dependency and helplessness. While reframing challenges the family's cognitive frame of reference, techniques of **enactment** provide the behavioral counterpart of this reframing. Put differently, where reframing corrects the patient's thinking, enactment directs an appropriate response.

Individuals within the family develop their way of seeing themselves in relationship to each other and the world around them through years of accumulated interpersonal experiences. For example, a two-parent family with two adolescent children, Alan, age 14, and Gayle, age 13, came for help because of Alan's withdrawn behavior at school and with peers, and his general shyness. Gayle, on the other hand, had the reputation of being outgoing and social. In the therapy session, Gayle maintained centrality through her talkativeness which, because of its liveliness, was eagerly responded to by the parents. However, to the degree Gayle was talkative, Alan remained silent. The therapist's consistent efforts at attending to Alan, and being inattentive to Gayle, yielded a different experience for the family. Alan became a source of interest. His style, though slower, was reframed as being pensive and profound. This reframing allowed Alan, in the course of treatment, to become more outgoing and personable. Alan's shifting position in the family created a challenge to Gayle's position. The "reality" of Alan being somewhat withdrawn and slow was supported by the complementary patterns of family members in relation to Alan. The family's intent was, of course, to help Alan who was having trouble socially and academically; but their ways of responding to him served to maintain the problem that they had hoped to solve.

Through the actualization of the family transactional patterns within the session, the therapist develops the diagnostic information which helps place the problem within its context. This knowledge is then utilized to expand the family's awareness of not just the presenting symptoms, but the problem as it involves all of them. The family is challenged to change their patterns within the session, allowing alternative, more adaptive, ways of relating to emerge. The therapist moved from defining an entity (withdrawn, slow Alan) to a process (withdrawing response to talkativeness, or slow response to being pushed). This transformation of entity into process (noun to verb) is enhanced by the technique of **enactment**, which typically appears spontaneously within the session, or may be induced by simply directing any two or more family members to interact with each other. The goals of the enactment are diagnostic as well as therapeutic. It elicits relevant data on the way the family functions; data of which the family is usually unaware. This data is then used to both challenge their view of the problem and test the family's ability to expand their repertoire of responses, allowing greater interpersonal flexibility.

The concept of **boundaries** in families is at once theoretical and concrete, one reflecting the other. As family members negotiate positions with one another over time, they negotiate rules delineating who is close to whom, who maintains distance from whom, who has greater privileges in given areas, and who makes given decisions. This process is evolutionary, changing over time in an ordered way. At times, families become stuck in their process of negotiating appropriate boundaries. In the preceding family, Gayle maintained a rather overinvolved position with her parents, while Alan was in a more disengaged one. This pattern was problematic because it did not allow alternatives for any of the family members, though Alan's behaviors were the ones that most drew the parents' negative attention, bringing the family to treatment. By the therapist protecting Alan's space and encouraging his participation in the family process, Gayle was challenged to learn to listen as part of her repertoire of skills. Marking boundaries, which is done by setting simple rules of interaction (e.g., persons talking for themselves, or family members talking to each other rather than about each other) makes a profound statement to the individuals in the session. Through it, the therapist communicates to the family its need to realign their priorities in terms of the changing needs of each of its members. The consistent redefining of boundaries of individual family members, and between subsystems within the family provides an orderly process of growth and development, and a context for "individuation."

Though each of the techniques of challenging a family's reality is described in terms of their idiosyncratic nuances, they are, of course, interdependent. Just as the technique of **unbalancing** refers to a certain set of concepts and applied skills aimed at disequilibriating family patterns, all restructuring techniques serve that end. As I noted in the preceding family, although the parents were genuinely interested in Alan's becoming more assertive and productive, their preferential styles of interaction maintained his passivity and peripherality. The intervention described as marking boundaries (i.e., protecting Alan's right to talk for himself) could have been intensified in degree to create a major shift in the family's organization if the therapist consistently aligned with Alan, no matter what his position, while ignoring Gayle's or the parent's attempt to return to their usual ways. Unbalancing the system seeks to change the hierarchal order of relationships through the creation of a crisis within the system. Given that families maintain order through their customary feedback process, a therapeutic intervention that successfully blocks the feedback process, not allowing the usual responses to occur, puts the system into crisis and forces new potentially productive processes to emerge.

A dramatic example of unbalancing occurred in a session with a 14 year old boy, Glen, who had experienced a phobia about going to school for over a year. At a critical juncture in therapy, approximately 6 weeks into treatment, the therapist successfully framed the boy's behavior as manipulating mother and taking advantage of her kindness to him, thus temporarily affiliating with the mother in a coalition against the identified patient. The coalition was maintained and intensified in the session, allowing mother to move from a position of failure and hopelessness to a firm conviction that she would not be victimized by her son. The unbalancing of the system, though highly stressful, eventuated in the boy's return to school the next day (A PROCESS OF CHANGE, videotape by W. Silver, therapist). Unbalancing techniques require an intense personal involvement by the therapist, utilizing the privileged position as therapist in maintaining a coalition with family members which, at a linear level (the level of content), seems unfair. That Glen manipulated his mother was only partially true. Also true was the fact that mother was manipulating Glen by maintaining his presence in the home in order to fulfill her own needs for caring. However, in emphasizing only one aspect of the complementarity, the therapist can create enough stress to counteract the family's extreme and chronic resistance to change. What is experienced as unfair at a linear level, may be valid at a systemic one.

The use of interpersonal **intensity**, though not a specific set of techniques in and of itself, is an important facet of a therapist's use of self and will ultimately determine the effectiveness of any of the therapist's technical interventions. Intensity emerges from the therapist's ability to arrest the attention of his or her patients. Each therapist maintains a particular style of engendering intensity. Some do it through projecting themselves as bright or insightful, while others use their ability to be emphathetic, warm, and nurturing. Others may use their authority in a convincing way.

Critical for therapists is the ability to expand their repertoire of interpersonal skills to effectively overcome the family's ability to filter out or reject what it chooses to ignore. People attend to what is novel in their context. Change in movement, voice tone, posture, or kinesthetic environment may all serve to reinforce a message. Effective communicators can call on a range of interpersonal responses that will enhance their therapeutic effectiveness. The constant repetition of a certain message is often used to bring a message into the family's awareness. For example, in one 3 hour session a therapist worked at establishing intensity around a husband's responsibility for not initiating a move into his new home with his wife by repeating multiple variations of the same question, "Why didn't you move?" (MAD COUPLE, videotape by, C. Fishman, therapist).

Similarly, manipulations of time in which family transactions occur achieve an intensity within the session. For example, in one two-parent family in which most of the nurturant interactions with the children involved the mother, the therapist maintained a task for father and son to engage in a playful interaction, without mother's assistance. The intensity of the intervention was maintained through extending the amount of time the members were engaged in this new pattern.

The integration of techniques within the personal style of the therapist is the essence of effective psychotherapy. Defining the various steps of treatment provides the basic notes of the composition. However, the artistry of the performance comes from the uniqueness of the therapist's individual interpretation of those notes.

THE INITIAL SESSION

The intricate interplay of theory, practice, and personal use of self is best illustrated in the model for a first family session originally developed by Jay Haley and the staff of the Philadelphia Child Guidance Clinic. The intent of the model is to provide a simple and clear outline for the therapist applying the concepts of systems thinking to the therapy situation. Beginning with the definition of each members' view of the presenting concern, the process of the interview is organized to move from a linear perspective to an interactional one. This allows for the reinterpretation of the problem and the solution as one involving the participation of the entire family.

The session is divided into five stages: the social stage, defining the problem, enacting the problem, mapping the structure, and restructuring interventions. The session begins with a social stage which enhances the joining process, followed by the therapist eliciting each members' view of the problem as he or she sees it, or a sense of what each would like changed within the family. The social and problem stages are often combined in the therapist's attempts to join with the immediate concerns of the family. The information elicited from each member's description of the family's current situation needs to be enhanced by a view of the problem involving the entire family, a broader view than the diverse individual perspectives available to the family. The problem of being a family member who is emotionally involved in the process makes objectivity difficult. It is difficult, if not impossible, to be a participant in a process while at the same time being an observer to that process. At times it seems as if family therapists must tackle the impossible: They must spontaneously engage with the family, allowing themselves to experience what it feels like to be a part of the family, while at the same time assessing and evaluating their responses to the family, and process that data as part of their diagnosis. Therapists accomplish this task by alternately being proximal to the family's emotional field and distancing, giving a more cognitive perspective.

Distancing may be enhanced by having the therapist function as observer to the family through initiating an enactment of family interaction around the presenting problem. This involves supporting an interaction between key members of the family to allow the family to "dance its dance" rather than talk about it. The enactment can be initiated simply by asking the principals involved in a relevant issue to discuss their views with one another rather than with the therapist. This allows the therapist the freedom to be observer rather than participate in the family's process. Enactments may evolve spontaneously through the normal interchange among family members or may be initiated by the therapist. In either case, observing and assessing the family's interactional patterns provides the therapist with enough emotional distance to make some assessment of the rules as they pertain to the presenting concern.

The assessment of these rules provides the therapist with some hypothetical assumptions regarding the family structure. For example, in a two-parent family with a 7 year old son who presented a range of somatic complaints without any organic cause, the therapist asked the boy to discuss his concerns with his mother. Being outside of the interaction, the therapist was able to observe the way the boy would offer his list of physical complaints to his mother, which elicited a rapid succession of remedies from her. This process involved both mother and son in an escalating cycle which was only interrupted by the father's frustrated and ineffective attempts to get the boy to attend to mother. The conflict between father and son was followed by an attempt on mother's part to rescue her son from father's intervention which then initiated conflict between father and mother. Father's response to his wife's attack was to withdraw, leaving mother feeling isolated and frustrated, and allowing the boy to again engage her in his endless list of somatic complaints (A CASE OF NERVES, videotape by W. Silver, therapist).

Observation of the family's process from a decentralized position allows the family to transact in their typical fashion and permits the therapist to develop a hypothetical map of the family's structure. This map serves as a temporary blueprint by which the therapist plans interventions. In the example cited previously, the therapist's map suggested an intense overinvolvement between mother and son (Figure 2), and a conflictual involvement between father and son (Figure 3).

Figure 2.   Figure 3.

This pattern of shifting coalitions repeats itself throughout the initial part of a session, preventing resolution of conflict between any two members. The pattern captures the attention of the therapist. The therapist's restructuring interventions include blocking the mother's intrusion into the interchange between father and son, protecting the boundary of the subsystem, and supporting the resolution of their conflict. The therapist then reframes father's involvement as his attempt to teach his growing son independence, while congratulating mother for her patience in allowing the two men in her life to work things out between them. In this way the therapist supports a more active position by the father and engages the mother in a way that will support that process.

In following a map, the therapist utilizes a series of structural interventions (joining, enactment, boundary making, and reframing), to challenge the family's repetitive patterns. The interplay of content and process finds its most effective expression in the dance that includes the family and the therapist, which constitutes the therapeutic system.

Resistance to a therapist's probes and challenges are not only expected, but are considered healthy responses from people confronted with change. The artistry of therapy is the ability to work with these resistances to effect the goals of treatment. In the last example, the therapist, in the interest of initiating a positive interchange between father and son, suggests that the father teach his son how to effectively arm wrestle, while again encouraging mother to relax and observe her husband's teaching technique with their son. Though the parents accommodated the therapist's request, the son became helpless with his father, again drawing in his mother to coach him.

Despite the family's intention to change, resistance to change is the family system's attempt to maintain their more familiar ways. This is the family's way of letting the therapist know its concern about entering into new and unknown ways of operating. The therapist acknowledges the concern around change. In this case, mother was asked if she felt the boy was ready to learn to be more autonomous. The therapist then asked father to be the boy's coach, answering any of his questions related to the task. With the guidance of the therapist, the family was able to successfully effect the task within the session. Both father and son enjoyed the boy's more assertive and playful side, while mother, though anxious, allowed her son the autonomy she knew he needed.

The structural map of the family now shows a closer, more productive involvement of father and son, and a more appropriate distance between mother and son.

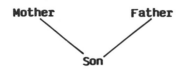

Figure 4.

However, the resolution of the parental differences is essential for the task to generalize itself to the family's interactions outside the session. The task is a symbolic representation of the family's problem of an overburdened, overfunctioning mother and a peripheral father maintaining a pattern of dependence and helplessness on the part of the son. In order for change to be maintained, each parent must feel supported by the other in their common goal. To this end, the therapist attends to the mother's sense of isolation and loneliness, a precondition of her overinvestment with her son. The therapist asked the husband, who he had supported throughout the session, to attend to his wife's need, reframing her challenges of him and her nagging as her clumsy way of flirting with him.

At first glance, this unbalancing maneuver appears to be unfair. It seemed the wife's nagging was justified on the basis of her husband's chronic inaccessability to her and to their two children. The goal of therapy, however, is change; what seems unfair at the level of content ultimately becomes fair at the overarching systems level. The practice of disequilibriating an enmeshed system stresses each of the members, not just the one made most vulnerable. The temporary alliance with the father will also serve the more long range needs of the mother in having her husband more accessible to her and more dependable. Hence, the map of a family pattern shifts to more involvement between father and son, and greater proximity between husband and wife.

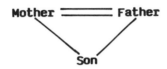

Figure 5.

The evolution of the session begins with a focus on a fearful dependent boy but becomes refocused as the transitional process which involves the boy's need for his father's involvement and mother's need for emotional support from her husband. The focus also includes father's need to be reinvolved in the everyday management of the family's affairs. The reframing of the problem is complete and is made concrete enough that each member has clarity on what he or she needs to do in order to help resolve the problem. It is also made personal and intense enough to involve and motivate each of the members to change. The process of the interview translates the family's overfocused (linear) concern about the character of one of its members to a dynamic process involving all of them. Reframing the problem as a process implies that its solution involves the participation of all the family members. The reframing of the problem becomes a metaphor for the complex interplay of individual traits that characterize the family, concretely defining those traits in a way that promotes change and growth. Structural Family Therapy becomes a useful shorthand for the intricate operations of therapist and family engaged in a process of change.

William Silver, D.S.W., is currently a senior faculty member of the Training Center, and Director of Social Work Training at the Philadelphia Child Guidance Clinic. He is also a Clinical Associate in Psychiatry at the University of Pennsylvania School of Medicine and a faculty member of the Rutgers University School of Social Work, and maintains a private clinical practice in Philadelphia. Dr. Silver may be contacted c/o Philadelphia Child Guidance Clinic, 34th & Civic Center Blvd., Philadelphia, PA 19104.

RESOURCES

Haley, J. PROBLEM SOLVING THERAPY. San Francisco: Jossey Bass, 1976.

Minuchin, S. FAMILIES AND FAMILY THERAPY. Cambridge, MA: Harvard University Press, 1974.

Minuchin, S. & Fishman, H. C. FAMILY THERAPY TECHNIQUES. Cambridge, MA: Harvard University Press, 1981.

Videotapes rented through the Philadelphia Child Guidance Clinic, 34 Civic Center Boulevard, Philadelphia, PA 19104:

Fishman, C., therapist, THE MAD COUPLE.

Silver, W., therapist, A CASE OF NERVES.

Silver, W., therapist, A PROCESS OF CHANGE.

PRACTICAL ISSUES AND APPLICATIONS IN FAMILY THERAPY

Terry M. Levy

It is virtually impossible to understand behaviors apart from the context in which they occur. This is the basic notion of family therapy. It is an attempt to redefine the focus of therapy from the individual to the family system. In doing so, family therapy becomes more than just another therapeutic technique, for it is based on new ideas of behavior and interpersonal transactions.

There are many models of family therapy which vary greatly in their definition of dysfunction and methods of treatment. Regardless of how one conceptualizes the family system, though, it undeniably plays a primary role in psychosocial development. In almost all societies, the family serves several cardinal functions for spouses, children, and the society itself. First, through marital bonds, the family completes and stabilizes the lives of adults. Second, it provides a context for physical and emotional nurturance of children and for their personality development. Third, it satisfies a crucial societal need by maintaining and transmitting the culture (Lidz, 1963, 1967). In order to fulfill these functions, the family must operate with rules, structure, and a viable method of leadership. One task of the family therapist is to assess and understand how the family operates, dynamically and structurally, in order to determine what patterns of behaving and relating need to be changed for the benefit of all family members. Another task is to understand how individuals in the system influence and are influenced by that system.

It is often said that family therapy is a tedious and perplexing task, especially for the less experienced practitioner. Numerous questions arise: Who should be included in the session? How do you maintain order? What is the "real" problem when everyone has a different opinion? How do you get all family members to participate? These and other questions bring about confusion when the practitioner lacks a solid foundation of theory and method. Although one unified theory of family functioning and treatment does not exist, there is a growing body of relevant ideas and effective techniques available. In this contribution, I will endeavor to provide practical guidelines for approaching generic issues in working with families, and present an eclectic and holistic framework as the foundation of clinical work.

THE HOLISTIC APPROACH

The major clinical models of family therapy are: (a) structural (Aponte & Van Deusen, 1981; Minuchin, 1974); (b) psychodynamic/multigenerational (Ackerman,

1958; Bowen, 1978; Framo, 1976; Paul & Paul, 1975); (c) experiential (Satir, 1967, 1972; Whitaker & Keith, 1981); (d) strategic (Haley, 1976; Madanes, 1981; Watzlawick, 1974); and (e) behavioral/social exchange (Liberman, 1970; Patterson, 1975; Weiss, 1979). In my work with families, I have found it most advantageous, in terms of both diagnosis and treatment, to integrate major contributions within these models into a blended or eclectic approach. I have included the additional element of an increased emphasis on the historical emotional development and current condition of the individual (i.e., "intrapsychic"). This holistic approach focuses on both systems and individual variables.

It is my belief that even when working clinically with one person, family therapy is still being done. This is because any intervention into the emotional, cognitive, or behavioral aspects of one's life must take into consideration the current and historical family influences. The clinician must always be ready to approach the problem from a variety of levels, based upon treatment goals and patient(s) needs. Individual and systems factors will receive different emphasis at varying points in treatment, but they both must be considered.

SYSTEMS/INTERPERSONAL FOCUS

Systems theory is the study of the relationship of interactional parts in context (Von Bertalanffy, 1969). It forms the basis for much of family therapy in that it emphasizes the ways in which interacting parts (i.e., family members) affect one another. The major dimensions of systems theory are circular causality, family structure, communication processes, and developmental adaptation.

CIRCULAR CAUSALITY

Rather than viewing behavior in a linear or cause and effect manner ("billiard ball" model), it is viewed as circular. Family members each provoke, maintain, and reinforce one another's behaviors. Bateson, Jackson, Haley, and Weakland (1956) coined the term schismogenesis to describe this aspect of human relationships. It is also referred to clinically as vicious circles, negative feedback loops, mutual reaction processes, or interpersonal games. For example, a daughter who feels unloved and insecure may act out by being defiant and hostile. The mother responds with hostile criticism and rejection, increasing the child's feeling of insecurity, and provoking a continuation or increase in the symptomatic acting out. They keep each other going in a repetitive, circular, never-ending pattern. The child in this example is called the "identified patient" by a family therapist, because working with her alone would ignore the interpersonal context and processes which must be addressed for positive change to occur. The "patient," then, becomes the mother-child dyad or the whole family unit. There is a force in the family system, called homeostasis, to maintain the status quo. Therapists must be cautious as they move into the system to encourage new patterns, or they may provoke excessive resistance.

STRUCTURE

Family structure is defined as "the invisible set of functional demands that organizes the ways in which family members interact" (Minuchin, 1974, p. 51).

Patterns of relating repeated many times become "rules" and define how family members will relate in the future. In the previous example, the child defied her mother who responded in a childish and ineffectual way. A transactional pattern or rule was established in which the mother lacked effective parental control and the child lacked respect for the mother's parental position. Let us add father, who is more lenient and understanding of the daughter, to this case example. Now a larger, triangular process emerges. When daughter and mother are doing their mutually hostile dance, father steps in and tells his wife not to be so hard on the daughter. In structural terms, he forms a "coalition" with his daughter and invites a "breach of generational boundaries." That is, by siding with his daughter, he adds strength to her position and undermines both the mother's parental position and the sanctity of the parental team (i.e., "executive subsystem").

Understanding structural concepts is crucial when doing family therapy because it provides insight into how the system operates. The basic structural aspects to be understood are hierarchy of power and control, boundaries, coalitions, and subsystems.

In dysfunctional families, the power is typically in the wrong hands. In the previous example, the daughter had more clout than the mother because her father gave her power by affiliating and forming a parent-child coalition. The issue of power and control is very important. Healthy families share and negotiate for power, with an awareness that the parents are in charge. When it is clear that the parents are on top of the hierarchy of power (but not in an authoritarian or rigid way), the children feel more secure and learn, by modeling, to use power in appropriate ways.

There are three subsystems in a family, parental (executive), marital, and sibling, with each having a particular function. The role of the parental subsystem is to nurture and manage the young, the marital subsystem is to fulfill the needs of the spouses, and the sibling subsystem provides a context in which the young learn about peer relationships (e.g., communication, negotiation, sharing). Problems can occur within or between each of these subsystems.

Boundaries, the rules defining who participates and how, are of three types: diffuse, rigid, and clear. Each type of boundary has an interpersonal consequence regarding closeness. Diffuse boundaries are those that are too permeable and ill-defined, likened to a screen where water flows easily. The interpersonal consequence is overaffiliation, as with the father and daughter in our clinical example. Rigid boundaries are not permeable enough; they are too limiting, likened to a brick wall. Virtually no meaningful contact is possible (i.e., underaffiliation), as with the mother and daughter. Clear boundaries occur when there is a proper balance between closeness and limits. The parent who sets limits with a child and allows communication about those limits is creating a clear boundary. Well-functioning families achieve a balance between closeness and separateness, rules and openness, and structure and flexibility. Dysfunctional families do not achieve a balance; the scale tips either one way (too rigid) or the other (too unstructured).

COMMUNICATION

The means by which family members send and receive information, both verbally and nonverbally, is communication, which occurs on two levels (Satir, 1967).

The denotative level refers to the literal content (what is being said). The second level, metacommunication, is much more important to the family therapist because it gives clues as to the family dynamics and structure. Metacommunication is a "message about the message"; it is a comment on the literal content and on the nature of the relationship (how people relate, the process). For example, when the mother responds to her child in a hostile, vindictive manner, the metacommunication is: (a) I cannot express anger in an effective, adult way; (b) I am helpless in my efforts to manage your behavior; and (c) our relationship is one in which mutual hostility is the rule as we fight for power and control. These messages are communicated through the use of words, the tone and pace of voice, facial expressions, and body tonus and position.

Satir (1975) described five styles of communication often found in families: placating, blaming, super-reasonable, irrelevant, and congruent. Each style, except the last, is based on the inability of family members to share thoughts and feelings in a clear, direct, and authentic way. (See Satir, 1975, for a detailed description of these styles.) One of the most destructive communication methods is called the "double-bind," first discovered during a research project on schizophrenics and their families (Bateson, et al., 1956). A double-bind occurs when two distinct messages are given which both lead to trouble for the receiver. A good example is offered by humorist Dan Greenburg (1964): "Give your son two sports shirts as a present. The first time he wears one of them look at him sadly and say, 'The other one you didn't like?'" (p. 74). For the son no choice is possible. If he wears a shirt it is no good, and if he does not wear a shirt it is no good. Recipients of double-binds become frustrated and hopeless.

Family therapists must be able to assess, teach, and model communication. Assessment involves the ability to observe and understand the ways in which messages are conveyed. Teaching involves providing structured methods of improving how family members send and receive messages (see Tables 1 and 2 at the end of this chapter), and encouraging them to practice these skills both in the office and at home. Modeling involves the active and on-going demonstration of effective communication skills by therapists. This aspect must be emphasized, for it is the behavior of the therapists as they relate to family members that is perhaps the most powerful of all therapeutic tools to promote positive change.

DEVELOPMENTAL ADAPTATION

Family problems often emerge as a function of developmental or transitional changes. Individuals must learn to cope with life transitions (e.g., the shift into adolescence, adulthood, or marriage), and the family system must somehow adapt to these internal pressures. Haley (1973) describes five stages in the family life cycle and suggests that it is the interruption or dislocation of the natural unfolding of these cycles which cause family members to develop problems. Carter and McGoldrick (1980) offer an extensive description of the family life cycle stages and the process of change required at each step (see Table 3 at the end of this chapter).

All families must cope with developmental changes and the stresses they bring. Well-functioning families can respond with flexibility, a safe context to share feelings and thoughts, and mutual support. Families that are dynamically and structurally unsound, however, will not fare well at these times. As Minuchin (1974) suggests, "The strength of the system depends on its ability to mobilize alternative transactional patterns when internal or external conditions of the family demand its restructuring....If a family responds to stress with rigidity, dysfunctional family patterns occur" (p. 156).

INDIVIDUAL FOCUS

Systems theorists and practitioners often ignore individual intrapsychic and psychodynamic factors in favor of here-and-now relationship variables in their efforts to understand and treat family problems. Conversely, those who are individually oriented tend to ignore current interpersonal and systemic factors in favor of a historical and analytical emphasis. The holistic approach, as described in this chapter, focuses on both aspects.

The primary relationship is that of parent-child. It is in this context that the infant and young child forms his or her personality and social style. The individual personality dynamics of the parent(s), the structure of the family, and the psychosocial quality of family relationships all contribute to the formation of the developing child. Individual factors, having their roots at this early developmental time, are object-relations, differentiation, needs, introjection, unconscious material, repression, and transference. Individuals manifest themselves on three levels that must be addressed by the therapist: (a) cognitive (beliefs, perceptions, and "cognitive maps"), (b) affective (how emotions are experienced and expressed), and (c) behavioral (overt patterns of coping and responding).

The notion of object-relations, reduced to its basic premise, is that early parent-child transactions determine later adult relationships in regard to needs, expectations, and fears. In other words, we act, feel, and think toward significant others in adult life based on our "unfinished business" in early relationships. For example, a child with a passive, overprotective mother may develop the expectation that her needs and wishes will always be met by others. She becomes self-centered and demanding as an adult and searches for a partner who is passive and nonthreatening. She has internalized her mother-child relationship and developed a "map" or model that she now follows. Friedman (1980) writes, "As each person grows, he/she develops a model of the personally significant aspects of human experience, including representations of self and other people that becomes a map of inter- and intra-personal reality....I believe that mapping is primarily a non-dominant hemisphere function, later overlaid with verbal process, and suppressed to varying degrees" (p. 64).

The concept of introjection is important in understanding how early relationships are transferred to later family life. The child identifies with the parent and, in essence, "becomes" that parent. Thus, a boy who despises his hostile, critical father becomes similarly destructive with his own son. He is said to have a "critical father introject" operating at an unconscious and repressed level. Paul and Paul (1975) describe how unresolved issues in one generation inevitably distress subsequent generations. Framo (1965) describes similar forces in a family and recommends a combination of interpersonal and intrapsychic approaches to solving family problems.

The extent to which a child's primary needs (e.g., nurturance, safety, security, love) are met or unmet is a critical factor in understanding and treating an individual family member. Unmet needs produce emotional distress for the youngster and, consequently, for the family system, which lead to problematic and symptomatic behaviors. A thorough discussion of needs and psychopathology can be found in Horney (1950). Children are not able to develop an adequate self-identity when their basic needs are not met. They tend to act out aggressively or passively in a counterproductive effort to be cared for and loved. Bowen (1978), in his discussion of unfulfilled needs for validation, acceptance, and support, refers to the process of differentiation and individuation as crucial to healthy psychosocial development. He describes well-differentiated people as those able to assert their thoughts and feelings; they are autonomous but also able to be close and intimate. Less-differentiated individuals are emotionally needy and insecure, tend toward enmeshment and fusion (i.e., dependency) in their relationships, and fear being alone even though seeking relationships is anxiety-provoking. Situations in which parents discourage differentiation to an extreme can produce problems of psychotic proportions in the young adult.

THE "HEALTHY" FAMILY

Before discussing the practical aspects of family therapy, it is important to develop a model of family health. What is a healthy family? Can one isolate the qualities which contribute to effective family functioning?

Following a lengthy and detailed study of family life, Lewis, Beavers, Gossett, and Philips (1976) concluded, "We found no single quality that optimally functioning families demonstrated and that less fortunate families somehow missed" (p. 205). They did find, however, a number of factors that contribute to effective family functioning. Based on the work of these researchers, as well as others who work with families, it is possible to describe qualities which promote health. It is important for practitioners to keep these qualities in mind as goals toward which to work, in relation to realistic limits and circumstances with different family systems.

1. **Affiliative Attitude.** Family members demonstrate trust and openness in how they relate, rather than oppositional attitudes and guarded, distant, hostile behaviors.

2. **Subjective Views Respected.** Family members show respect for their own and others' ideas and perceptions. There is empathy and, therefore, people can be open and honest. Authoritarian and domineering power plays are absent; power is shared and/or negotiated.

3. **Options Considered.** Rather than being rigidly fixed, family members can explore alternatives in approaching problems. They are flexible and adaptive.

4. **Strong Initiative.** Constructive reaching out is demonstrated, rather than a passive, controlled, or contained style. Thus, family members are likely to be involved in the community and in one another. They are not isolated, but receive a variety of stimuli.

5. **Family Structure.** There is a balance between clear, firm rules and flexibility when needed. The parents are definitely in charge, but

do not utilize their power in an overly authoritarian manner. Leadership and power are shared by the marital partners, which provides the children with a model for healthy relationships. Children's opinions are considered and negotiation is allowable, within the framework of clear generational boundaries. Children cannot manipulate parents.

6. **Closeness and Autonomy.** Both closeness and separateness are encouraged. Family members have a high degree of personal autonomy and clear ego boundaries ("differentiation"). Communication is clear, with each person able to share his or her own thoughts and feelings. Self-responsibility is encouraged. Without the damaging effects of enmeshment and dependency, family members can be emotionally close, intimate, and meet one another's needs.

7. **Reality-based View.** The family perceives itself in a way that is congruent with how others see them. There is little need to deny painful realities (e.g., family conflicts) as in less healthy families.

8. **Feelings.** There is an atmosphere of warmth, affection, and caring. Family members are encouraged to express their feelings openly. Empathy is a well-developed skill. Due to this open and caring atmosphere, the quantity and severity of conflicts are minimized. Problems are handled as they come up, and there is no need for chronic, destructive resentments and conflicts.

9. **Additional Factors.** A high degree of spontaneity is found, with humor both acceptable and apparent. There is a belief that basic needs and drives are normal. Sexuality is dealt with openly. The passage of time is not denied; change is a part of life. Thus, issues of aging and death are approached in a realistic way.

PRACTICAL CONSIDERATIONS

WHEN IS FAMILY THERAPY INDICATED AND CONTRAINDICATED?

Family therapy is not a panacea but it is an appropriate mode of treatment for a multitude of situations. It is almost always indicated when the identified patient is a child or adolescent. It is necessary to have the family present in order to diagnose and modify the interpersonal influences which provoke and reinforce the symptomatic behaviors. It is often possible to reduce childrens' symptoms by only addressing the parents' child-management techniques. Family therapy is indicated for intergenerational conflicts (e.g., parent-adolescent conflict), marital disharmony (including separation, divorce, and remarriage), and situational crises (e.g., death of a family member). It is typically the primary approach to emotional problems of the poor and disadvantaged. It satisfies their need for immediate support and concrete, practical interventions, especially when utilizing the "eco-structural" approach (Aponte, 1981; Auerswald, 1968; Minuchin, Montalvo, Guerney, Rosman, & Shumer, 1967), which focuses on the use of tasks and basic structural modifications of the family system. Family therapy is also well suited for the management of severe psychosocial disorders, such as schizophrenia. As a part of a comprehensive treatment plan, which may include medication and individual intervention, the family approach focuses on the symbiotic relationship which prevents the patient from differentiating. Family sessions are conducted in the hospital and as outpatient follow-up. Other conditions such as alcoholism, where the individual's symptom is intertwined with marital and family dynamics, are amenable to family therapy (Albon, 1976; Berenson, 1976; Dulfano, 1978; Wegscheider, 1981).

Family therapy is contraindicated in situations where working with a person individually provides a valuable message about needed separation from parent(s). With some young adults who suffer from extreme dependency, it is counterproductive to involve the parents on a regular basis. Parental intervention is sometimes necessary, however, to reduce their attempts to sabotage the growth and independence of the young adult. For example, with a 27 year old drug abuser, it was necessary to meet several times with the father, sister, and brother-in-law to help them stop rescuing and protecting the patient. When they stopped, he finally admitted himself to a hospital for detoxification, and later received follow-up therapy on his own.

WHO SHOULD BE INCLUDED IN THE SESSIONS?

Twenty years ago, when family therapy was still in its infancy, many practitioners believed that all family members must attend all sessions. This is no longer so. Successful family therapy involves creative and flexible participation as orchestrated by the therapist. The entire family unit should be present during the initial part of treatment so that a systems diagnosis can be made. After that, parts of the system (dyads, triads, individuals) are seen intermittently with the whole family. For example, the marital dyad may be seen one time, a parent-child dyad the next, and the siblings the following time. The choice of who comes in should be determined on the basis of clinical goals. For example, if the goal is to unhook a child from the detouring of tension in the marital dyad, the therapist may ask the husband and wife to come in without the child. If the goal is to provide support to an overwhelmed single parent, the therapist may work with just the parent one time and the siblings the next. If the goal is to reduce enmeshment between a mother and son, the therapist may request that the father and son come in without the mother. If the goal is to provide extra help to one child who feels inadequate and peripheral (usually the identified patient), the therapist may see this child individually. Some practitioners believe that meeting alone with the identified patient only serves to reinforce his or her position as family scapegoat. It is my experience, however, that this practice, when done properly at the right time, facilitates both individual and family change and is not counterproductive.

Anyone who is influential in the life of the family can be made a part of the therapeutic process. The grandparent who may or may not live in the home but plays a role in the family, the school counselor who has developed a rapport with a child, or the probation officer who is resented by an acting-out teenager are good examples. These people may play a part in perpetuating the symptoms of a family member, in maintaining a dysfunctional family pattern, or in helping to solve a family problem.

WHAT IS THE ROLE OF THE FAMILY THERAPIST?

Family therapists have the reputation of being very active and direct, often utilizing strategic and manipulative methods. This is so in some situations, either due to the type of therapy practiced (e.g., Haley's strategic approach) or the specific clinical goal, regardless of one's basic model. The holistic model, described here, is both flexible and adaptive. Thus, at one point in time, it may be appropriate to modify structural elements of the family system through a strategic task (e.g., changing seating arrangements), and, at another time, an individually oriented, insight-type approach might be used. There is not one role. The practitioner must be firm yet flexible, in control yet responsive, objective yet involved, organized yet spontaneous. Minuchin (1981) writes, "The therapist is in the same boat as the family, but he must be the helmsman....Like every leader, he will have to accommodate, seduce, submit, support, directly suggest and follow in order to lead" (p. 11).

The most powerful therapeutic tool is the use of self. The therapist is powerful as a psychosocial influence, and must know how to handle and utilize this power. Therapists must guard against imposing their own cultural standards and value systems on families. Clinical goals must be generated by the family members based on their own needs and cultural context.

WHEN DO YOU EXCLUDE THE CHILDREN FROM SESSIONS?

It is sometimes appropriate to excuse younger family members (children and adolescents) during a session or, more effectively, plan meetings with only the adult(s) present. Specific areas of concern to the adult(s), such as sexual, financial, and family management issues, should not include the younger members, unless for a specific purpose. Often the message given is more important than the content area under discussion. That is, by working exclusively with the parents, a powerful statement is made: "Mom and Dad have a boundary around their marital relationship and are unified as an executive team to manage the children." It is especially important to provide this message when working with parents who exhibit ineffectual or insufficient limit-setting with their young. It is also necessary at times to exclude the children in order to facilitate family-of-origin work with one or both parents. For example, a father who is chronically distant and peripheral with his wife and children may need to explore the unresolved pain from his own childhood before becoming more emotionally available. It is typically most facilitative to work with the father individually for several sessions before involving other family members. This enables rapport to develop and issues to surface in a less threatening context.

HOW DO YOU HANDLE RESISTANCE?

When working with families it is common to confront resistance in one or more family members. Often the identified patient is reluctant or absolutely refuses treatment. The therapist can advise the parent(s) or spouse about how to respond to the resistance over the phone or in an initial session. Advising them to be firm but understanding, rather than either hostile or passive, is often effective. It is also often effective for the therapist to speak to the resistant family member on the phone. A warm, caring, and accepting attitude often goes a long way towards "taking the wind out of the sails" in a resistant person.

Often the parent(s) will not want to get involved directly but is desirous of having the therapist "fix the child." It is not productive to challenge the parent(s) with threat ("Don't you care about your child?"), guilt ("Your child will not make it without you."), or intellectual analysis ("Don't you know that you are a part of the problem?"). Rather, the therapist must "join" the resistance, accept it as real, and allow it to be. I believe that "what one resists, persists," and if you fight against the resistance it will grow. It is often effective to tell the parent(s) that you will make every effort to help their child, and would they be willing to help toward that goal? Telling a parent, "I need your help in my effort to help your son," is often less threatening and more effective than saying, "You are a part of the problem so you must come to the session." The therapist can meet with the child alone several times while consulting with the parent(s) on the phone. Once a positive and nonthreatening relationship is established between the therapist and parent(s), they are likely to accept more direct participation.

HOW DO YOU CREATE ORDER IN THE MIDST OF CHAOS AND CONFUSION?

Family sessions can become chaotic and nonproductive if not managed properly. It is crucial for the therapist to provide a firm, clear, and realistic framework (e.g., rules and limits). This structure is necessary for several reasons. It is important for family members to develop respect for the therapist, which is impossible if he or she can be manipulated. Second, family members often feel hopeless and lose motivation if they do not experience the therapeutic context as a place where change can occur. An unstructured atmosphere encourages repetition of dysfunctional patterns, thereby reducing expectation of success and discouraging positive change. Third, the therapist who manages the session properly provides a valuable model for the parent(s) who typically are deficient in this area. Rules should be made explicit (one person speaks at a time while others try to listen and understand; each one takes responsibility for his or her own thoughts, feelings, and actions - no blaming; everyone's viewpoint is valid and needs to be heard; all feelings are acceptable, but cannot be acted out in destructive ways in the session; sessions have a starting and ending time; if you are late that is not the therapist's responsibility). Rules are enforced consistently, not for the purpose of rigidity, but to teach limit setting, consequences, responsibility, and accountability.

One or more family members may challenge the therapist's leadership position by being directly defiant or passive-aggressive (e.g., argumentative). This is to be expected, because the process of change always involves resistance and fear. The therapist should not get "sucked into the system" by particpating in a struggle for power and control. This would prove counterproductive because the therapist would then be responding in the same ineffectual way as other family members. Rather, it should be handled therapeutically and, as in the previous discussion of resistance, the therapist can (a) allow and accept the show of force ("You are certainly entitled to your feelings."), (b) comment on the behavior in process terms ("It seems you become angry when things don't go your way."), and (c) turn the focus back to the family ("What do others feel about this?"). The therapist's leadership position cannot be taken away, only given up. The practitioner who is not comfortable handling the family therapy context will fight for power and inevitably lose.

WHAT ARE THE GOALS AND PROCEDURES FOR CONDUCTING A FAMILY INTERVIEW?

The effective family practitioner is like a well-trained athlete; he or she has trained so long and hard that the basic skills have become second nature.

Thus, the practitioner is able to respond spontaneously while keeping goals and therapeutic skills in mind. It is necessary to move into the family system with specific individual and systemic clinical goals, but also allow for spontaneity. The following outline can serve as a guide for conducting initial (as well as subsequent) family sessions, but it must be approached with flexibility.

Define the Problem. The task of the therapist is to sort out the issues and determine on what problem areas to focus. There must be some specific direction to follow. For example, in the family with a learning disabled youngster, it was determined that the problem was the parents' overprotectiveness rather than the youngster's symptomatic behaviors.

Collect Data. The therapist draws together data relevant to the problem defined. Data is collected from (a) family members' verbal reports of prior and current situations, (b) reports of others involved (e.g., a school counselor), and (c) observation by the therapist of current transactions in the session. The latter type of data is most useful in determining interventions.

Generate Hypothesis. It is now necessary to develop a specific idea (hypothesis) regarding the nature of the family conflict. Again, in the family with a learning disabled youngster, the hypothesis may be that mother overprotects son as a compensation for an unfulfilling marriage. She forms a coalition with son and the husband/father is emotionally peripheral to both mother and son. The hypothesis provides a specific framework for the therapist. It provides direction and leads directly to the development of clinical goals.

Goals. Short-term and long-term goals must be determined, based on the hypothesis. Short-term goals define the clinical methods used. Long-term goals define the desired outcomes toward which to work. In the latter case example, the goals may be to (a) create communication between husband and wife to reduce the mother-son coalition and to create a more effective management team, (b) help mother accept the reality of her child's impairment and "let go" of her symbiotic attachment, (c) help father to become a more active part of the family, and (d) help the child individuate by developing support systems and resources outside the home.

Intervention. The therapist moves into the system in light of all the above. He or she uses an array of therapeutic techniques in order to (a) facilitate an awareness of or change in some individual or transactional condition, (b) test the system and individual family members regarding their readiness and ability to change, and (c) increase both leadership credibility and positive rapport by managing the situation effectively.

Feedback. The therapist observes the family members' reactions to the intervention in order to validate, modify, or reject the initial hypothesis. Then the cycle starts again from the second step. Thus, working on the assumption that an overattachment between mother and son prevents the youngster from growing, the therapist would observe what happens after that coalition is reduced. If son does not improve, a new hypothesis must be formulated.

WHAT ARE THE SPECIAL CONSIDERATIONS OF FAMILIES WITH TRANSITIONAL-TYPE PROBLEMS (DIVORCE, SINGLE-PARENT, AND STEPFAMILIES)?

Less than 10% of families in the United States currently fall into the category of the traditional nuclear family (working husband, housekeeping wife, two children). One in seven children are raised in a single-parent home (one in four in urban areas). Of all children in the United States, 25% are living with "blended" (remarried) families. The number of unmarried couples living together has doubled in the past ten years (Toffler, 1980). These statistics reflect a trend toward alternative family forms. The family practitioner must be equipped to handle these common and often difficult situations.

Divorce. Divorce is now a socially acceptable solution but it provides immense disorganization in the family system and for individual family members. Family therapy is most effective if initiated as soon as possible (e.g., during the time of separation prior to the divorce) because this is when the system is most fluid or open to change. The therapist must approach the divorce situation as a family crisis, which means that a concrete, here-and-now, task oriented, approach to assessment and intervention is appropriate. The following areas are focused on:

> **Child-centered.** The primary emotional issue is that of loss; the loss of a parent, an intact family unit, and a hope for need fulfillment. Children need explanations to reduce confusion and guilt, immense emotional support, help in dealing with difficult feelings like anger and hurt, and a stable environment to continue functioning.

> **Relationship-centered.** It is necessary to focus on the significant relationships, including the custodial parent-child, the noncustodial parent-child, the ex-spouses, and extended kin. Issues of communication and negotiation must be addressed. Children must be extricated from the burdened position of "conduit" (message carrier) between parents.

> **Adult-centered.** The focus on individual adults can occur both in the context of family sessions and separately with one-to-one sessions. The custodial parent must be helped through the transition to single-parent status. The noncustodial parent (if available and willing to participate) needs help in finding ways to maintain both a positive relationship with the child(ren) and communication with the ex-spouse regarding that child.

Additional resources in the area of divorce and family therapy are Gardner (1976), Haynes (1981), Kaslow (1981, 1983), and Kessler (1975).

Single-Parent Families. The single-parent family is a common family form seeking help in both private and community based mental health settings. As with the divorce situation, the clinical focus is on the individuals, the relationships, and the community support systems. Children typically develop symptoms and act out due to the emotional strain (e.g., coping with loss, experiencing unexpressed rage) and the lack of effective family management. The single parent suffers from "executive burden" and the inability to handle overwhelming management tasks alone. The children are either overparented or underparented. This parent needs guidance in proper child management skills and support for his or her own need fulfillment as an adult. Often there is a surrogate parent, such as a grandparent or boyfriend, who takes on a management role with the children. This can provoke boundary and loyalty conflicts and undermine the parent's primary position. Enmeshed relationships between single parents and children are common, as they become overinvolved with their children to meet their own needs. One child, usually the oldest, might assume the role of "parental child," thereby sharing the family management role with parent. This can cause an array of problems. The parental child does not experience and express age-appropriate needs due to his or her adult-like role. There is too little contact between parent and other children because the parental child becomes a buffer or intermediary. An additional problem of the single-parent family involves the lack of a role model for the children. A boy in a family with an absent (noncustodial) father, for example, may act out his unmet needs for a father through hostile behaviors toward mother or siblings.

The primary clinical goals in working with the single-parent family are to (a) provide support to the overburdened parent (including emotional support and concrete help through community based resources), (b) facilitate clear and healthy boundaries between parent and children so that parental power is effective and the children can experience the sense of emotional stability which results, (c) address the emotional pain and needs of the children regarding loss, lack of a role model, confusion regarding their family situation, and other difficult feelings, and (d) encourage the parent to find ways to achieve need fulfillment outside of the family. This includes the emotional needs of companionship and peer contact as well as creating a positive future through career building and the development of competency skills.

Additional resources in working with the single-parent family include Gardner (1978), Stuart and Abt (1981), and Weiss (1979).

Stepfamilies. One out of every seven children is a stepchild and over twenty-five million adults must face the difficult and confusing task of stepparenthood every day (Visher & Visher, 1979). The role of stepparent is perplexing to most adults, just as that of stepchild causes conflict and confusion. The "blended" family, also referred to as the remarried (REM) or reconstituted (REC) family, is especially conflicted in that there is a coming together of two different systems without a necessary developmental unfolding. Stepfamilies have specific dynamic and structural problems. Loyalty conflicts occur where the children feel torn between their biological parent and stepparent. Parents often expect and demand "instant intimacy" without allowing for wounds to heal and trust to gradually develop. Children still mourning for their lost parent are expected to love the new parent figure. Marital pressures are enormous because the spouses often fear the possibility of another "failure," thereby placing too much pressure on themselves and one another, sometimes excluding the children in the process. For blended families there are often boundary problems. For example, battles between stepsiblings may be unknowingly encouraged by coalitions ("mother and her child against father and his child"). Children become fearful of any positive attachment to the new parent, often act out hostility towards this stepparent, and may develop an array of psychosocial symptoms. This becomes more damaging when children are asked to carry messages back and forth between households. Further, a remarriage may take place at a time in the life cycle of a spouse when family tasks are incompatible with his or her life cycle position. For example, a forty year old divorced woman with two children, ages seventeen and nineteen, married a man who had custody of the five year old daughter. This woman was not emotionally prepared to provide the necessary nurturance to the child. Severe resentments developed in the marriage and between the daughter and stepmother.

In working with stepfamilies, the following goals are important:

1. Evaluate the two systems that are now joined, regarding similarities and differences in their structure, needs, and expectations.

2. Help clarify roles. Each family member needs to understand his or her own and others' new roles. What is involved in changing from a mother to a stepmother, from a single man to an instant father, or from an only child to one of several siblings?

3. Boundaries must be clarified and modified. Coalitions which exist due to old loyalties need to change and firm lines of parental authority must be encouraged.

4. Each family member must face his or her own emotional conflicts and pain. A child may have unresolved resentment towards the custodial parent for "ruining" the original family, which is acted out towards the stepparent in the form of distance and rejection. A stepparent may feel guilt about not being with his or her biological child and, thereby, withhold love and caring for the stepchild.

5. The reality of stepfamily life must be considered. It takes time to develop family bonds, trust, and caring. All family members, especially the parents, must be aware of the complexities of the task and the emotional aspects of letting go of the old and allowing the new. With patience and fortitude, a viable and need-fulfilling family system can emerge.

Visher and Visher (1979) provide a comprehensive discussion of stepfamily issues and theirs is a worthwhile resource for practitioners to have.

HOW DO YOU RESPOND TO A FAMILY IN CRISIS (E.G., CHILD ABUSE)?

A crisis is a hazardous event, coming from inside or outside the family, which creates a state of disequilibrium, disorganization, and stress. This includes situations like death of a significant other, physical or sexual abuse of a child or spouse, or a youngster running away from home. During a crisis there are a number of predictable reactions. There is no structure for conflict and communication so family members are often isolated, alienated, and fearful because they lack the ability to respond effectively. Destructive patterns of relating increase. Family members rely on destructive and pathological modes of coping, such as scapegoating (blaming), side-taking, and denial, which only serve to exacerbate stress and turmoil. Disorganization occurs, lines of authority become unclear, power struggles occur, and family roles, rules, and problem-solving methods are ineffectual.

The therapist must respond to a family crisis with two central ideas in mind. First, the crisis should be dealt with immediately, using a concrete, reality oriented approach. People are most open to change during a crisis. Second, the crisis should be relabeled from an individual to a family problem. This promotes the possibility of interpersonal and systemic change.

The following specific clinical goals are recommended:

1. Clarify the situation and develop priorities and frameworks for coping. Help all family members to understand what they are dealing with to decrease confusion and helplessness.

2. Encourage the expression of emotion. Help family members express their feelings to reduce acting out and further turmoil.

3. Instill expectation of a positive solution. While being realistic and authentic, it is helpful to give family members something in which to believe.

4. Develop a plan of action. Providing structure helps to clarify the situation and the solutions.

5. Coordinate and utilize community resources. Help family members make contact with agencies or individuals who may provide further aid and support.

6. Suggest specific tasks and teach specific skills. Help family members respond to the crisis with new personal and interpersonal skills which may also be useful at a later time (prevention).

7. Modify the leadership position over time. Initially, the therapist must assume primary responsibility and a strong leadership role. Later, as the family develops its own effective coping abilities, the control and responsibility can be shifted.

A family crisis situation that is more common than many people think is that of child abuse. It was estimated in the year 1965 that approximately 5,000 cases per 100,000 children would occur. An estimate of 1.5 million cases of child abuse was given for the year 1973 (Justice & Justice, 1976). Three factors are important. First is the parent's personality dynamics and mode of interaction with the abused child. Abusing parents tend to lack impulse control, have a strong need for nurturing, show hostile and aggressive behaviors, have an underdeveloped ego structure (poor self image), and a confusion of the parenting role. They tend to "parentify" the child (i.e., they see the child as their own parent; demanding, having insatiable needs, and rejecting) and act out their hostility through physical or sexual abuse. They seek fulfillment of needs for comfort and nurturance through the child. They feel rejected and angry when the child does not deliver. The second factor involves the characteristics of the child. The child's behavior (e.g., aggressive, needy, attention getting) often provokes the parent. The children typically remain loyal to the abusing parent due to their fear of retaliation and loss of love, which serves to reinforce the abusive behavior. Third, the factor of stress is significant. External and internal stress, such as that from the burdens of raising a child as a single parent, tend to increase the likelihood of abuse.

Working with the abusive family is basically a long-term project. The parents need intensive help to work through their severe family-of-origin problems.

Limits must be set and maintained regarding the control of impulses, child management, and consistent therapy participation. Community resources are tapped, providing support and education to the parents. The courts and juvenile authorities may be called on for further structure and intervention. Many practitioners are not capable (practically and emotionally) of handling these situations, and referral to special agencies is often appropriate. Further information is found in the book, THE ABUSING FAMILY (Justice & Justice, 1976).

WHAT ROLE DOES THE FAMILY PLAY IN SUBSTANCE ABUSE?

During the early 1970's, when substance abuse became a national concern, the federal government began providing grants to study and clinically respond to the relationship between the family and drug abuse. Family therapy became an important part of a total treatment program, especially for adolescent substance abusers. The drug abuse symptom was found to serve a function within the family context: "They (the adolescent) are literally hanging around, mouths open, waiting to be fed. If they are not fed by human means within the context of a family setting, they will frequently resort to the use of chemicals to give them the illusion that their needs are being met pharmacologically" (Kaufmann, 1979, p. 71).

There are common dynamic and structural features in families where substance abuse occurs. There typically is a dependent, enmeshed relationship between the substance abuser and the parent(s), usually the mother. This is often paired with a distant, hostile relationship with the other parent, usually the father. The parents of young substance abusers often have drug or alcohol problems. The substance abuser becomes the family scapegoat, helping to prevent a focus on other severe problems in the family, such as marital conflicts. There are inadequate parenting skills and severe boundary problems between generations (e.g., cross-generational alliances which split the parental unit). Family members typically feel helpless and powerless, blame outside forces for the problem, and there is a lack of constructive pressure to change.

Similar features exist in families where alcoholism is the symptom. Based on extensive clinical experience, Ewing and Fox (1968) conclude that, "Alcoholism can no longer be seen purely in terms of intrapsychic dynamics....It is the family homeostatis which seems to perpetuate the drinking and it is this behavior which must be changed if the drinking is to be controlled" (p. 42). Steinglass and his colleagues (1977) have developed an "alcohol maintenance model" which suggests that the drinking behavior is deeply linked to family behavior and actually helps to stabilize the family system through repetitive patterns of relating.

In my work with alcohol and drug abusers utilizing the holistic treatment model, I have found that a combination of family therapy and individual intervention (e.g., out-patient psychotherapy, in-patient setting, AA groups) works best. The interested reader is referred to Kaufmann and Kaufmann (1979) for further information regarding substance abuse and the family.

WHAT TYPE OF SUPERVISION IS RECOMMENDED?

Since family therapy involves a switch in thinking from a linear to a circular systems model, it is necessary to have specific supervision even if the therapist has extensive experience in other therapeutic modalities. Valid supervision involves a combination of didactic and experiential learning formats. The most powerful learning tool is "live supervision," where the trainee is directly observed doing family therapy by a supervisor. The supervisor, observing from behind a two-way mirror, gives immediate feedback and suggestions to the trainee by phone. Videotaping the session is most useful. It allows the trainee(s) and supervisor to analyze and discuss the session in detail at a later time. Learning to observe, diagnose, and intervene on systems and process levels is like learning a new language; the longer one is immersed in it the more comfortable it becomes. It is realistic to allow a minimum of several years of supervision and experience before feeling confident as a family therapist.

TABLE 1: COMMUNICATION GUIDELINES

Family members are taught the specific skills of effective listening and sharing. They are encouraged to use these skills while discussing topics in the session and at home. Each family member is given his or her own guideline form to keep.

LISTENING SKILLS:

- Relax, absorb; do not censor or rehearse.
- Take a nonjudgmental attitude.
- Be empathic: place yourself in another's position.
- Send accepting, understanding, supportive messages.
- Be aware of yourself: nonverbal behavior such as posture, gaze, spacial alignment; thoughts, feelings, actions.
- Levels of listening:
  Top level: words, ideas, social games.
  Below level: needs, feelings, process.
  (Listening to the Below level gives information about individual needs and relationship rules.)

SHARING (including "feedback") SKILLS:

- Make statements rather than ask questions.
- Take responsibility for your own perceptions by saying "I," not "you," or "it."
- Be specific, clear, direct, brief.
- Share thoughts and feelings; they are separate.
- Be aware of yourself: What meta-messages do you send?
- Be nonjudgmental: Give feedback about behaviors observed rather than about intentions assumed.

TABLE 2: COMMUNICATION METHOD

Effective communication is the basis of nourishing, fulfilling relationships. It promotes acceptance, support, and understanding. The method outlined here can be used to foster effective, positive communication in dyads for any topic, issue, or content areas under consideration.

METHOD: (share/listen/restate/feedback/process)

1. SHARE (2 to 5 minutes)
   One person speaks while the other listens. The sharer is taught to:
   - Make "I" statements, instead of using "it" or "you".
   - Share statements not questions; this encourages the sharer to express himself or herself rather than placing responsibility on another.

- Be specific, direct, clear, and brief; generalities and lengthy speeches foster distance and are annoying.
- Be aware of yourself; eye contact, posture, voice, messages.
- Share thoughts and feelings.

2. LISTEN
While the sharer is expressing himself or herself, the other person's task is to listen by being:
- Empathic; put yourself in other's place in order to hear thoughts and feelings.
- Nonjudgmental; refrain from evaluating the other's comments to determine if they are right or wrong, but relax and absorb the other's comments. Keep from considering and rehearsing a response, but nondefensively accept the other's expression.
- Self-aware of nonverbal messages sent by posture, eye contact, and facial expression.

3. RESTATE (2 minutes)
After sharer is finished expressing himself or herself, the task of listener is to restate; to tell sharer what was heard. The sharer must now listen as the other person conveys "what I heard you say."

4. FEEDBACK (2 minutes)
After restating, the sharer gives the other person feedback as to the accuracy of his or her listening. If the listener restated accurately ("Yes, you really did hear me"), the sharer can reward by verbally or nonverbally showing appreciation. If the restating was inaccurate or partially accurate ("selective listening"), the sharer must clarify ("No, I didn't say what you heard, let me try again").

5. REVERSE ROLES
The sharer becomes the listener, and vice versa, so that both partners have a chance to express themselves.

6. PROCESS
After the above is completed, giving the partners a chance to take a good look at what they have just done with one another is usually very productive and positive. Suggesting to partners that they use the same method (share/listen/restate/feedback), have them consider such questions as:
- What was it like for you to communicate with one another in this way?
- How did you feel with your partner as "sharer" and as "listener"?
- In what ways will your relationship be enhanced by communicating in this way?
- What are some of the issues (relationship, parenting, and such) you would like to discuss at home using this way of communicating?

NOTE: Initially, using this method may seem artificial and tedious, but with practice it becomes natural, easy, and very rewarding. Emphasize that participants be brief and direct, and make sure they follow the method closely to insure success.

TABLE 3: THE STAGES OF THE FAMILY LIFE CYCLE*

Family life cycle stage	Emotional process of transition: Key principles	Second-order changes in family status required to proceed developmentally
1. Between families: unattached young adult	Accepting parent-offspring separation	a. Differentiation of self in relation to family of origin

Family life cycle stage	Emotional process of transition: Key principles	Second-order changes in family status required to proceed developmentally
		b. Development of intimate peer relationships c. Establishment of self in work
2. The joining of families through marriage: The newly married couple	Commitment to new system	a. Formation of marital system b. Realignment of relationships with extended families and friends to include spouse
3. The family with young children	Accepting new generation of members into the system	a. Adjusting marital system to make space for child(ren) b. Taking on parenting roles c. Realignment of relationships with extended family to include parenting and grandparenting roles
4. The family with adolescents	Increasing flexibility of family boundaries to include children's independence	a. Shifting of parent-child relationships to permit adolescents to move in and out of system b. Refocus on midlife marital and career issues c. Beginning shift toward concerns for older generation
5. Launching children and moving on	Accepting a multitude of exits from and entries into the family system	a. Renegotiation of marital system as a dyad b. Development of adult to adult relationships between grown children and their parents c. Realignment of relationships to include in-laws and grandchildren d. Dealing with disabilities and death of parents (grandparents)
6. The family in later life	Accepting the shifting of generational roles	a. Maintaining own and/or couple functioning and interests in face of physiological decline; exploration of new familial and social role options

Family life cycle stage	Emotional process of transition: Key principles	Second-order changes in family status required to proceed developmentally
		b. Support for a more central role for middle generation c. Making room in the system for the wisdom and experience of the elderly; supporting the older generation without overfunctioning for them d. Dealing with loss of spouse, siblings, and other peers, and preparation for own death. Life review and integration.

*By E. A. Carter & M. McGoldrick. Copyright 1980 by Gardner Press, Inc. Reprinted by permission.

Terry M. Levy, Ph.D., is currently in independent practice as a clinical psychologist and is Director of the Miami Psychotherapy Institute in Miami, Florida. He was formerly Clinical Director of the Family Life Center, a family systems oriented training and treatment program, and was associated with the Dade County Division of Human Resources. Dr. Levy can be contacted at the Miami Psychotherapy Institute, 7711 S.W. 62 Avenue, Miami FL 33143.

RESOURCES

Ackerman, N. W. THE PSYCHODYNAMICS OF FAMILY LIFE. New York: Basic Books, 1958.

Albon, J. Family structure and behavior in alcoholism. A review of the literature. In B. Kissin & H. Begleiter (Eds.), THE BIOLOGY OF ALCOHOLISM (Vol. 4). New York: Plenum, 1976.

Aponte, H. & Van Deusen, J. Structural family therapy. In A. Gurman & D. Kniskern (Eds.), HANDBOOK OF FAMILY THERAPY. New York: Brunner/Mazel, 1981.

Auerswald, E. H. Interdisciplinary vs. ecological approach. FAMILY PROCESS, 1968, 7, 202-215.

Bateson, G., Jackson, D. D., Haley, J., & Weakland, J. H. Toward a theory of schizophrenia. BEHAVIORAL SCIENCE, 1956, 1, 251-264.

Berenson, D. Alcohol and the family system. In P. J. Guerin, Jr. (Ed.), FAMILY THERAPY: THEORY AND PRACTICE. New York: Gardner Press, 1976.

Bowen, M. FAMILY THERAPY IN CLINICAL PRACTICE. New York: Jason Aronson, 1978.

Carter, E. A. & McGoldrick, M. (Eds.). THE FAMILY LIFE CYCLE: A FRAMEWORK FOR FAMILY THERAPY. New York: Gardner Press, 1980.

Dulfano, C. Family therapy of alcoholism. In S. Zimberg, J. Wallace, & S. Blume (Eds.), PRACTICAL APPROACHES TO ALCOHOLISM PSYCHOTHERAPY. New York: Plenum Press, 1978.

Ewing, J. A. & Fox, R. E. Family therapy of alcoholism. In J. H. Masserman (Eds.), CURRENT PSYCHIATRIC THERAPIES (Vol. 8). New York: Grune and Stratton, 1968.

Framo, J. Rationale and techniques of intensive family therapy. In I. Boszormenyi-Nagy & J. Framo (Eds.), INTENSIVE FAMILY THERAPY. New York: Harper and Row, 1965.

Framo, J. Family of origin as a therapeutic resource for adults in marital and family therapy: You can and should go home again. FAMILY PROCESS, 1976, **15**, 193-210.

Friedman, L. J. Integrating psychoanalytic object-relations understanding with family systems intervention. In J. Pearce & L. Friedman (Eds.), FAMILY THERAPY. New York: Grune and Stratton, 1980.

Gardner, R. THE BOYS AND GIRLS BOOK ABOUT ONE-PARENT FAMILIES. New York: G. P. Putnam, 1978.

Gardner, R. PSYCHOTHERAPY WITH CHILDREN OF DIVORCE. New York: Jason Aronson, 1976.

Greenburg, D. HOW TO BE A JEWISH MOTHER. Los Angeles: Price and Stern, 1964.

Haley, J. PROBLEM SOLVING THERAPY. San Francisco: Jossey-Bass, 1976.

Haley, J. UNCOMMON THERAPY. New York: W. W. Norton, 1973.

Haynes, J. M. DIVORCE MEDIATION. New York: Springer Publishing, 1981.

Horney, K. NEUROSIS AND HUMAN GROWTH. New York: W. W. Norton, 1950.

Justice, B. & Justice, R. THE ABUSING FAMILY. New York: Human Science Press, 1976.

Kaslow, F. W. Divorce and divorce therapy. In A. S. Gurman & D. P. Kniskern (Eds.), HANDBOOK OF FAMILY THERAPY. New York: Brunner/Mazel, 1981.

Kaslow, F. W. Stages and techniques of divorce therapy. In P. Keller & L. Ritt (Eds.), INNOVATIONS IN CLINICAL PRACTICE: A SOURCE BOOK (Vol. 2). Sarasota, FL: Professional Resource Exchange, Inc., 1983.

Kaufman, E. & Kaufmann, P. N. FAMILY THERAPY OF DRUG AND ALCOHOL ABUSE. New York: Gardner Press, 1979.

Kaufmann, P. N. Family therapy with adolescent substance abusers. In E. Kaufman & P. N. Kaufmann (Eds.), FAMILY THERAPY OF DRUG AND ALCOHOL ABUSE. New York: Gardner Press, 1979.

Kessler, S. THE AMERICAN WAY OF DIVORCE. Chicago: Nelson-Hall, 1975.

Lewis, J. M., Beavers, W. R., Gossett, J. T., & Philips, V. A. NO SINGLE THREAD. New York: Brunner/Mazel, 1976.

Liberman, R. P. Behavioral approaches to family and couple therapy. AMERICAN JOURNAL OF ORTHOPSYCHIATRY, 1970, **40**, 106-118.

Lidz, T. THE FAMILY AND HUMAN ADAPTATION. New York: International University Press, 1963.

Lidz, T. & Fleck, S. Some explored and partially explored sources of psychopathology. In G. Zuk & J. Boszormenyi-Nagy (Eds.), FAMILY THERAPY AND DISTURBED FAMILIES. Palo Alto: Science and Behavior Books, 1967.

Madanes, C. STRATEGIC FAMILY THERAPY. San Francisco: Jossey-Bass, 1981.

Minuchin, S. FAMILIES AND FAMILY THERAPY. Cambridge: Harvard University Press, 1974.

Minuchin, S. & Fishman, C. H. FAMILY THERAPY TECHNIQUES. Cambridge: Harvard University Press, 1981.

Minuchin, S., Montalvo, B., Guerney, B. G., Rosman, B. L., & Shumer, F. FAMILIES OF THE SLUMS. New York: Basic Books, 1967.

Patterson, G. FAMILIES: APPLICATIONS OF SOCIAL LEARNING TO FAMILY LIFE. Champaign: Research Press, 1975.

Paul, N. & Paul, B. A MARITAL PUZZLE. New York: W. W. Norton, 1975.

Satir, V. CONJOINT FAMILY THERAPY. Palo Alto: Science and Behavior Books, 1967.

Satir. V. PEOPLEMAKING. Palo Alto: Science and Behavior Books, 1972.

Satir, V., Stachowiak, J., & Taschman, H. A. HELPING FAMILIES TO CHANGE. New York: Jason Aronson, 1975.

Steinglass, P., Davis, D., & Berenson, D. Observations of conjointly hospitalized "alcoholic couples" during sobriety and intoxification. FAMILY PROCESS, 1977, **16**, 1.

Stuart, I. R. & Abt, L. E. CHILDREN OF SEPARATION AND DIVORCE. New York: Van Nostrand Reinhold, 1981.

Toffler, A. THE THIRD WAVE. New York: William Morrow, 1980.

Visher, E. B. & Visher, J. S. STEPFAMILIES. New York: Brunner/Mazel, 1979.

Von Bertalanffy, L. General systems theory - an overview. In W. Gray, F. Duhl, & N. Rizzo (Eds.), GENERAL SYSTEMS THEORY AND PSYCHIATRY. Boston: Little, Brown, 1969.

Watzlawick, P., Weakland, J. H., & Jackson, D. CHANGE: PRINCIPLES OF PROBLEM FORMATION AND PROBLEM RESOLUTION. New York: W. W. Norton, 1974.

Wegscheider, S. ANOTHER CHANCE: HOPE AND HEALTH FOR THE ALCOHOLIC FAMILY. Palo Alto: Science and Behavior Books, 1981.

Weiss, R. S. GOING IT ALONE. New York: Basic Books, 1979.

Whitaker, C. & Keith, D. V. Symbolic-experiential family therapy. In A. S. Gurman & D. P. Kniskern (Eds.), HANDBOOK OF FAMILY THERAPY. New York: Brunner/Mazel, 1981.

CREATIVE COMMUNICATION FOR CLINICIANS*

Charles M. Citrenbaum, William I. Cohen, and Mark E. King

During the average week, we teach at universities, work on books or journal articles, engage in the practice of medicine and psychotherapy, consult for a community agency of some kind or another, and often spend some time doing media work. We are able to integrate these diverse functions because we see ourselves as professional communicators. We also believe that most readers of this contribution are professional communicators in that, no matter what you do, your ability to do it effectively depends on your ability to communicate effectively. This does not mean that you do not need the requisite skill and knowledge in your field, but rather that, no matter how knowledgeable you are in professional areas, you will not be effective as a clinician unless you are also an effective communicator. In this brief chapter we will discuss some of the essential principles of effective communication. We will then try to demonstrate and discuss some unusual (and we believe creative) communication tools that you, as a clinician, might find useful. Examples from both psychotherapy and behavioral medicine will be included.

Let us start the discussion by briefly mentioning the concept of professional ethics relating to communication. We believe the job of a professional communicator is to change the attitudes or behaviors of the clients with whom they work. We have known many psychotherapists whose technique is to spend months having "authentic" dialogues with their clients about their "being-in-the-world." Unfortunately, although this may be the basis for a nice friendship, in many instances the client's status does not improve. We know other therapists who engage in behavior that might be called "inauthentic," in that they tell lies and use cool, almost disinterested behavior modification techniques, but often the result is effective treatment of the patient. There are also times when the exact opposite may be true, however, and each clinician needs to know which is the best treatment method for each particular client at any given time and which will produce the desired outcomes. We recognize that what we have said is clearly debatable and, even though it is beyond the scope of this particular presentation to discuss these issues in depth, we believe it is important that, at the very beginning, we present our personal viewpoint.

One of the major jobs of all clinicians is to change the reality strategy of their clients: to change the clients' views of themselves from sick to well, from being helpless victims to being active agents in their own recovery. Reality is not a truth outside of people but is that which is experienced by

---

*The content for this chapter was adapted from IRRESISTIBLE COMMUNICATION, by M. E. King, L. Novick, & C. M. Citrenbaum, published by Saunders, Inc., Philadelphia, 1983.

each person. The use of language in shaping our reality was understood quite profoundly by a major league umpire who, when confronted by a manager arguing over a call, said, "The pitch was neither a ball nor a strike. It was nothing but a small round ball flying through the air until I called it something, and then it was whatever I called it." That is the type of reality by which we all live, and it is also the type of reality that is easily modified by an effective communicator. In like manner, modifying reality is also the job of a teacher, and in that light right now we would like to modify your reality about the nature of communication by sharing with you a few basic and important principles of communication.

All clinicians should remember that, if they are effective communicators, their clients will believe whatever view of the world is presented to them. For example, it is difficult in a metaphysical sense to believe there is such a thing as an id, ego, or super ego, and yet for many psychoanalysts the existence of such is an existential reality that clearly gets passed on to their clients. People who have been psychoanalyzed talk as if they have an id, ego, super ego, Oedipal complex, transference, and so on. Thus, it is very important for clinicians to begin to examine their beliefs about the nature of therapeutic change. For example, one common belief we have is that change is often slow and almost always painful. Since we have this belief, we pass it on to our clients and then wonder why some of our clients are so hesitant to make changes. The idea that change is slow and painful is no more or less real than any other idea, but it is a dysfunctional idea in terms of encouraging change. Imagine what might happen if we began to believe and share with our clients the idea that all change was quick, easy, and for the most part enjoyable! It is necessary for you to examine all of your own attitudes about growth, change, therapy, and concepts not in terms of whether they are metaphysically correct (because no one will know), but in terms of how functional they are for you as a clinician and for your clients.

THE LAW OF REQUISITE VARIETY

There are two specific laws of communication which, if followed, will make any clinician an effective professional communicator. Essentially, these two principles are our "reality strategies" about communication. The first principle is called the "law of requisite variety." This is basically a principle of physics which states that in anything that operates systematically, the element in the system with the most variability will have the most control. A simpler way of saying this is that the more flexibility you have in your own approach to communication, the greater chance you will have of getting the outcomes you desire.

Most professional communicators learn one particular way to communicate. The problem is that when that one way does not work, they try the same approach again, longer and louder. If this still does not work then the communicators either call their clients names (the term "resistant" is one of the more common ones), or they call themselves names thinking of themselves as poor practitioners. The law of requisite variety presents the idea that you try an approach and then keep your sensory channels open to see if it is working. If it is, you continue in that way but, if it is not working, you try another approach. We believe that if you have flexibility, if you have enough requisite variety, then as a professional communicator you can get almost any outcome you wish from clients.

This concept allows us to consider the issue of patient compliance in a new way. We believe that it is up to the clinician to make sure that the messages are received and followed by the patient. For example, if a physician gives a particular prescription to a patient, or if a physical therapist gives a certain exercise routine to a client and the patient does not take the medicine or follow the exercise routine, we believe it is up to the clinician to change his or her approach in such a way as to assure patient compliance.

UTILIZATION OF BEHAVIOR

The second basic principle of communication was illustrated most clearly in the work of Dr. Milton Erickson, the father of clinical hypnosis and perhaps the most effective professional communicator who ever lived. This principle is called "utilization of behavior." Instead of viewing a client's symptoms as behaviors to discard or "resistance" as a negative trait in treatment, the principle of utilization suggests that these behaviors or traits be viewed as gifts to be used to reach therapeutic objectives.

Jay Haley points out in his book, UNCOMMON THERAPY (1973), that Erickson's metaphor for resistance was of a raging river with a great deal of energy. Engineers (professional treatment personnel) could attempt to construct a dam to impede the river, but the force of the river would most likely destroy such a dam. Instead, the engineers could channel the river to a place where its energy could be used constructively. Haley cites an elegant example of the principle of utilization when he tells how Erickson was assigned to work with a resistant paranoid schizophrenic patient who believed himself to be Jesus Christ. Erickson approached the patient and said, "I understand you have experience as a carpenter," and the patient responded affirmatively. Erickson continued, "And I heard that you liked to help people." Of course, the patient nodded affirmatively. Erickson then handed the man a hammer and said, "Good, we are having some construction done on the west wing and need help and would appreciate yours." Within two minutes this man was very involved in occupational therapy (something he had refused to do earlier) and, after several months of this "milieu" therapy with a group of hard hat construction workers (who did not care who he thought he was but only that he did his work), he was able to function more effectively and eventually was released from the hospital. (Haley, 1973, p. 28)

Another time, Erickson was consulted by a lonely and homely looking young woman who complained to him that she was ugly, especially because of a small gap between her front two teeth. The patient worked in an office, and, when Dr. Erickson asked her about men there, she said there was one fellow who was always at the water fountain but he certainly could not be interested in her since she was so ugly. The patient insisted she would kill herself in a few months unless her life changed significantly. Erickson did not argue with this patient or try to persuade her otherwise. Instead he told her that since she was going to kill herself anyway, she might as well spend some of the money for which she had worked so hard. He convinced her to buy some new clothes, and to change her hairstyle (perhaps he told her she might want to look nice for her funeral). Erickson also instructed the woman to go home and practice squirting water accurately through the gap in her front teeth. After his patient had followed these instructions, Erickson directed her to one day squirt water in the face of the young fellow who frequented the office water fountain. When she did so he squirted her back, they began a relationship, and were engaged. Of course, the woman withdrew her plans for suicide. While few of us can to be as elegant as Dr. Erickson, each of us would be considerably more effective as clinicians if we accept all the gifts a client gives us and utilize them in treatment.

An implication of the utilization principle is the concept that the client's symptoms are very helpful or beneficial to him or her in some way. "Reframing" one's view of symptoms as beneficial and purposeful will orient the clinician toward allying with the client, and it goes a long way toward defusing the "resistance" normally displayed. The next step would often be to help the client find other symptoms or patterns of behavior that are equally beneficial. For example, rebellious or delinquent youths could be sincerely congratulated on their independence and powerful stance and then helped to channel their power positively. One of the authors recently worked with an attractive but very overweight young married woman. This client refused to lose weight even though she had serious health complications. She finally was able to diet only when she became aware that her weight had been serving some very useful psychological functions related to sexuality and relationships, and then she learned alternative patterns of behavior to deal with those issues.

The principle of utilization refers to the use not only of the client's symptoms but also in treatment, to the use of the client's life and interests. For example, if you were working with a farmer in the hospital and he was discouraged by his slow progress, you could tell him stories about seeds and plants, noting the similarities between the patient's progress and the slow but steady growth of seedlings. One of the authors was recently asked to treat a middle aged man for alcoholism. This patient made several references to his prowess with "the ladies" and his softball skill, compared to the other men on his team. It was clear that it was very important that this patient prove his adequacy as a man. Keeping this in mind, the author talked about how difficult it was to stop drinking, that several patients had failed to do so recently, and that it took a "real man" to stop drinking and maintain sobriety. After this communication, the patient was eager to make a commitment toward sobriety, and his treatment had effectively begun.

A music teacher we knew was working with a 10 year old boy who was beginning to get bored with his lessons because of a growing interest in football. The music teacher decided to utilize her student's new interest and modified the music lessons in structure so that they resembled parts of a football game. Every time the student did well with a piece she raised her hand, blew a whistle, and put points on a scoreboard. Every time he made a mistake, she threw a flag down and marked off an imaginary penalty. She was able to utilize her student's interest in football to be a more effective music teacher. In like manner, you will be more successful as a clinician if you take the client's interests, beliefs, and even the so called symptoms and use them as part of the treatment.

PACING

An extension of the concept of utilization is a category of communication techniques called **pacing**. When a clinician paces a client, he or she meets that person at his or her view of the world before attempting to lead the client to a healthier experience. Pacing techniques can be verbal or nonverbal. Verbal pacing would use language that is understandable to the client. The clinician should pay particular attention to a client's use of symbols or metaphors ("My husband is such a headache to me," "I need to open up more doors for myself," "I feel like a volcano ready to explode") and use similar language in ongoing communication. Many clients will display a particular preference for visual, auditory, or kinesthetic predicates in their language indicating that they may experience the world primarily using that system. A psychotherapy client may come into your office and talk about how "dark" the world is and how he cannot "see" any solutions to his problems. It might be ineffective to ask this person how he "feels". Instead, an effective response would be to tell this client, who uses visual experience, that you are glad to see him and that you believe his world will be appearing brighter and clearer soon. An effective psychotherapeutic tool for this client would be guided fantasy since it utilizes visual experience. A more auditory client might state that she has talked to many clinicians, but no one has said anything that sounded right to her. An effective therapeutic response might be that you have a lot to say that will ring true for her. A kinesthetically oriented client would complain of how badly he feels, and the clinician can respond with a pat on the client's shoulder and an assurance that he can grasp the seriousness of the situation.

Nonverbal pacing involves mirroring various aspects of a client's body language, such as breathing rate, body posture, and hand and arm movements. Voice tone, tempo, and amplitude can also be mirrored. In using this approach, the communicator mimicks one or more of the client's nonverbal behaviors. At an unconscious level, the client has more of a sense that he or she is with a person who understands. Simply notice how two lovers or good friends mirror each other's bodily movements when they talk, and many aspects of nonverbal pacing will be illustrated.

INDIRECT COMMUNICATION TECHNIQUES

So far, we have discussed the two basic principles of good communication, the use of requisite variety and utilization of behavior. We now want to share with you some specific communication techniques for applying these principles. All of the techniques to be discussed are similar in that they are forms of **indirect communication**. That is, they bypass the conscious processes and the resistance which most clients bring into clinical situations. Another way to understand these techniques is to perceive them as directed toward the client's unconscious, right hemispheric brain processes as contrasted to the conscious left hemispheric brain processes. Most often, clients have already attempted to deal directly or consciously with their problems and this has failed. Clients have thought at length about problems or talked with friends, family, or other clinicians. The law of requisite variety dictates that the clinician not become another person to join in the fight with the client's consciousness, but instead use alternative approaches.

Since the indirect communication techniques to be discussed are all directed to the client's unconsciousness, we would like to clarify our view of what the concept of unconsciousness means. It is not the traditional Freudian model of the unconscious as the seat of forbidden impulses or hidden, unpleasant memories. We believe the unconscious to be a vast reservoir of resources, energy, and potential for problem resolution and it is the clinician's job to help the client tap into these resources. The use of indirect communication allows therapeutic suggestions to "sink into" the client's mind or to tap into unconscious resources and bypass defensiveness or resistance that would interfere with treatment or compliance.

One of our favorite indirect communication techniques is the use of the telephone. For example, one author was recently treating an 11 year old boy with hypnotherapy to help him overcome fears of being in the house alone. The secretary was requested to call 5 minutes after therapy had begun, and the author spoke over the phone as if she were another child who was calling to say he was going to return a magic rock that the author had lent to him. The author expressed delight at the quick and positive results and made arrangements to have the magic rock returned before the next therapy session with the youngster in his office. The author then told how he was given the magic rock by Indians and how it helped children to feel more safe and powerful. Of course, the phone call helped to establish the credibility of this situation. The following week, the client took the magic rock home and used it successfully to overcome his fears.

Another useful technique is to talk about other people or patients. Many physicians suspect that their patients may not be complying with the prescribed treatment regimen. Nevertheless, they may ask or interrogate the patient, perhaps only to throw up the evidence of noncompliance. One thinks of the diabetic patient who must juggle a complicated schedule of diet, medication, and self-assessment. A resourceful physician, aware that the patient being seen has not been faithful to the treatment plan might decide to avoid an open conflict and sadly comment on the last diabetic patient who was seen - a patient who was not compliant and for whom the physician had great concern over the consequences of noncompliance. He would then tell the patient how glad he was to be working with someone who had developed an understanding of the disease such that, in spite of the difficulty of the dietary restrictions and the need for urine testing, pills, or injections, was striving to optimize her health. In our experience, this almost casual remark would indeed serve as a vehicle to allow the patient to change her own behavior in the interval between that office visit and the next with the obvious advantage of not placing the patient in the position of being chastised.

Skillful parents know the effectiveness of the "illusion of choice" technique when they ask their son or daughter, "Shall I read you two stories or three before you go to bed tonight?" The child's attention is focused on the choice of "two or three stories" and, by making this choice, he or she accepts the premise that, after the stories (no matter how many), it will be time to go to bed. Likewise, the hospital-based pediatric nurse, in preparing an intravenous treatment for a child who needs cancer chemotherapy, will ask whether the youngster wants the intravenous started in the left arm or the right.

The use of "junko logic" is another appropriate tool for the clinician. "Junko logic" is putting two sentences together, the first of which is obviously true, while the second one is quite debatable but is really what you want to have happen. You make the second one true by hooking it up with the first sentence. For example: "Because you are highly trained and well motivated individuals, it will be easy for you to learn the important points of effective communication." The second half is what we want to have happen but we hook it into the first part of the sentence which is obviously true.

The clients (or readers) thus get into a set of agreeing and soon they will be agreeing to the second part of the statement also.

There are a group of patients who very strongly resist direct approaches to change behaviors, to the extent that they respond by doing the exact opposite of what they are asked or told to do (i.e., they give a polarity response). For these individuals, the use of paradoxical directives is particularly effective. A psychologist was working with a young woman with severe chronic pain and learned from her that one of the reasons she was experiencing so much pain was that she was attempting unsuccessfully to hold the pain inside; her family, which felt overwhelmed by her symptoms and unable to tolerate seeing her in agony, was urging her to resist the expression of the pain. Rather than using various relaxation or biofeedback training techniques to diminish the intensity of the perceived pain, the therapist gave her the prescription (homework assignment) to spend at least 1 hour every day, from 1:00 p.m. to 2:00 p.m., freely expressing her pain in any way which seemed appropriate to her (crying, yelling, drawing pictures, or whatever). The therapist quickly discerned the important pattern that this woman was showing: She was massively resentful of those people who were telling her not to express her pain. The therapist then encouraged her to do so more than she was already doing, expecting, correctly, that she would soon tire of expressing her pain and have difficulty doing what she was told to do, such that the focus of the interventions could move to her dysfunctional living situation.

One of the most elegant of the indirect techniques is the use of metaphors and stories in communicating ideas, outcomes, and the sense that the clinician has of his or her patient's resources. It will be apparent that this technique is similar to talking about another patient with a similar condition. These stories may be of two basic varieties: They may include the resolution to the problematic situation, or they may refer to a wise person or someone who has the resources or achieved the outcome, but the specifics of the outcome are not mentioned. In any event, it is important to create the story in such a fashion that it parallels the life situation of the individual.

A 12 year old boy was referred to one of us by his pediatrician because of cyclic vomiting, which began to increase in intensity to the point that he was evaluated in the hospital and given intravenous fluids. Evaluation of the family and the boy revealed a bright child who was the third of four boys. His older brothers excelled in aquatic athletics, and this boy was on a pre-Olympic training team. Although the parents did not pressure him to participate, he had already apparently internalized notions of successful performance as being of utmost importance. After several sessions, it was apparent that he was symptom-free when he did not engage in the sport. Consequently, he was given permission to attend a practice session, and the night after he was given permission to return to practice, he began to develop nausea, which was aborted when he was told that he should not go to practice. At the fourth session, he was told the following story about a family of musical individuals:

> The youngest of the four children was learning to play the violin, and the older family members (Katherine who played the cello, Vincent who played the viola, and Victor who played the violine) loved to play chamber music together, especially trios. However, they knew that the repertoire for string quartet was even more varied, and they looked forward eagerly to the time when their youngest brother would join them.

However, this boy developed a tingling, and then a soreness in his fingers, so that it became difficult to play. He was taken to various doctors who found that he seemed to react very strongly to the violin bows, and they wondered whether he was allergic to a chemical in the finish of the bow. In any event, the physicians were unable to find any treatment for the numbness and lack of strength, and they recommended that he abandon his plans to become a musical virtuoso. The interesting thing was that the boy found there were other activities that he could do which gave him a great sense of satisfaction; activities which he was unable to participate in because of all the time he had spent studying at the conservatory and practicing the violin. His parents were delighted at his personal growth in these new areas. After several years, he picked up the violin out of curiosity, and began to play very casually, just to see what it was like. To his surprise, he was able to make a very pleasing sound, and his fingers were able to find their way around the fingerboard nimbly. He started out playing for short periods of time, and realized how much enjoyment he received from these musical activities. He was able to enjoy it even more fully as time went by, for he found an opportunity to play the violin in various community musical organizations.

It is important to realize that the boy, to whom the story was told, understood this as an interesting story about a boy from a musical family. There was absolutely no effort to interpret this for him, inasmuch as that would interfere with the unconscious learning, which is the intent in using such indirect techniques.

If the exact nature of the solution was left to the individual's unconscious, the above story could be changed such that the protagonist would have a dream and, in the dream, meet a wise old man who would lean close to the boy and tell him a secret. Following the dream, the boy would find a satisfactory conclusion to the story, without the listener or the storyteller knowing what the solution is, but with the listener's own resources being called into play in order to find the most appropriate solution from his or her own experience.

In this type of treatment we normally do not end up finding out exactly, in terms of psychological processes, what the client does to cure himself or herself, nor does the client usually understand since the treatment is totally unconscious.

These communication techniques are best taught over a long period of time where they can be demonstrated and practiced. We hope that you can now begin to understand the principle that you as a clinician are also a professional communicator; that your ability to be successful with your client depends not only on your knowledge in your field, but also on your ability to communicate successfully; and that words can heal and the appropriate use of words can heal to a degree not previously thought possible.

Charles M. Citrenbaum, Ph.D., currently maintains a private practice, specializing in the use of hypnosis in brief and strategic psychotherapy. He is past president of the Baltimore Association of Consulting Psychologists and a charter member of the Maryland Society of Clinical Hypnosis. Dr. Citrenbaum may be contacted at 402 E. Quadrangle, Village of Cross Keys, Baltimore, MD 21210.

William I. Cohen, M.D., is currently Clinical Assistant Professor of Pediatrics at the University of Pittsburgh School of Medicine and also maintains a private practice in developmental and behavioral pediatrics, specializing in the evaluation and management of developmental disorders of children and families. Dr. Cohen may be contacted at 315 Melwood Avenue, Pittsburgh, PA 15213.

Mark E. King, Ph.D., is currently an Associate Professor in the School of Health Related Professions, University of Pittsburgh, and also maintains a private practice, specializing in clinical hypnosis. He is the senior author of IRRESISTIBLE COMMUNICATION, on which this contribution is based, and has also written two other books. Dr. King may be reached at the School of Health Related Professions, Pennsylvania Hall, University of Pittsburgh, Pittsburgh, PA 15261.

RESOURCE

Haley, Jay. UNCOMMON THERAPY: THE PSYCHIATRIC TECHNIQUES OF MILTON H. ERICKSON, M.D.. New York: W. W. Norton & Co., 1973.

ADVANCES IN BIOFEEDBACK: A BEHAVIORAL MEDICINE APPROACH TO TREATMENT OF STRESS RELATED DISORDERS

George Fuller-von Bozzay

New treatments have been developed to combat stress effectively without resorting to drugs and their often harmful side effects, and at the same time allow the person to learn behavioral and physiological self-control. The emerging specialty of behavioral medicine integrates behavioral self-management and medical approaches to treatment. Biofeedback is its primary modality. This contribution will discuss the basic applications of biofeedback and then consider the professional issues related to clinical practice. A list of recommended resources for the biofeedback clinician is also provided.

The early definition of biofeedback was "the use of instrumentation to mirror psychophysiological processes of which the individual is not normally aware, but which may be brought under voluntary control" (Fuller, 1977, p. 3). After many refinements, a more precise definition has emerged: "Biofeedback is a learning procedure in which sophisticated electronic instrumentation aids the individual in controlling physiological variables. With practice and integration into daily life this learning has lasting health benefits" (Fuller, 1980, pp. 1.18-1).

Biofeedback instruments provide an electronic mirror of one's physiology and allow a person to become aware of his or her bodily changes. The individual then develops greater self-control over aspects of the physiology which had formerly been thought of as not under voluntary control. The person begins to take responsibility for his or her own health maintenance. As a learning procedure, information must be received as to whether the responses are correct or incorrect.

Just as in learning to play darts, the person must receive sufficient feedback to make the minor corrections necessary to come closer and closer to the bull's eye. Even though the individual may not be able to identify exactly what tiny muscular changes were made to hit the bull's eye, he or she is able to improve. It would be difficult, if not impossible, for the person to learn to hit the bull's eye if blindfolded. And yet, we are generally blindfolded in our ability to detect and control significant aspects of our physiologies, such as brain waves and blood pressure. The instruments allow a means for feedback so that appropriate corrections can be made. Once the control is achieved, the instruments are no longer needed. However, as with any other skill, this requires practice.

THE CURRENT STATUS OF THE MAJOR INSTRUMENTS

The electronic instrumentation used in biofeedback training is a product of our modern technology. The formerly cumbersome and large laboratory equipment has now been reduced to small microminiaturized units. Electrodes or sensors receive information from the body, amplify, filter, transform, and display the information in a meaningful form back to the person. This biofeedback loop provides the person with accurate information as to changes in bodily functioning.

With the addition of the therapist or facilitator to motivate and suggest methods of change and integrate this information with psychological issues, learning becomes meaningful for day-to-day use in deepening relaxation and reducing stress, as well as reversing the process of many stress related medical disorders. Relaxation, meditation, autogenic training, and other procedures are used in conjunction with biofeedback, which no longer requires the awesome and imposing tangle of wires and equipment most people expect to find in a research laboratory. Most clinical applications of biofeedback are done within a very comfortable setting and homelike atmosphere so that what is learned there transfers readily to the person's daily life. The instruments are vitally important for learning to take place, but are no longer necessary once the person has attained physiologic control.

There are four instruments that are most commonly used in biofeedback. I will describe each one, indicating what they are, what they do, the basic physiology of the system, how and where training is done, and the applications of each device.

ELECTROMYOGRAPHIC FEEDBACK

EMG, or Electromyographic Feedback, measures muscle tension. The electrical firing of the muscle fibers gives information about muscle contraction and relaxation. The instrument feedback, whether visual or auditory, is usually proportional to changes in muscle tension. It has perhaps the most general application of the four major instruments. The muscles of the face, neck, and shoulders are particularly important, as these muscles seem to reflect total body tension and are often chronically contracted, as in the case of muscle contraction headache.

Electrical impulses from the brain and spinal cord travel through motor nerves which terminate in muscle fibers and, with sufficient stimulation, produce muscle contraction. The EMG, measured from electrodes on the surface of the skin, receives the electrical activity, and the microvoltage is directly proportional to the mechanical muscle contraction. The lower the microvoltage level of EMG activity, the more relaxed is the muscle that is being measured.

The electrical discharge of the muscle is translated into auditory and visual displays. The person typically hears the raw EMG (a click rate or tone), or watches a meter (digital readout or lightbar display), either of which is proportional to the muscle activity such that, in a sense, the person can "hear" or "see" the muscle under the skin. Becoming aware of the difference between contraction and relaxation, the individual can gain control over the muscle activity which was previously impossible to do.

While the major placement of the EMG electrodes has been on the forehead to measure frontalis and nearby muscles, other muscles such as the trapezius in the upper back and shoulders, the forearm, or a total upper body placement measured from ankle to ankle are all used. Precise placements for neuromuscular re-education can reflect specific muscle activity. It is generally impractical and inconvenient to use dozens of electrodes over the entire body for accurate overall muscle tension assessment, since the frontalis may represent a reasonable reflection of the total body tension.

Major Applications of EMG. The major applications of EMG include general relaxation and lowered arousal training, phobic desensitization and anxiety reduction, and tension or muscle contraction headaches. It is also used for neck and back pain, essential hypertension, bruxism and temporomandibular joint syndrome, and neuromuscular re-education (e.g., stroke and cerebral palsy). In addition, EMG has been used in cases of insomnia, spasmodic torticollis, and spinal cord injuries.

Illustrative Case Example. Mr. T, a 28 year old unemployed college teacher, had had tension headaches since the age of 20. For the previous 3-1/2 years these headaches had occurred daily, producing severe pain for which he took a variety of pain killers. Mr. T had taken 25 milligrams of valium a day for the last 5 years, which he wanted to discontinue, but felt unable to do. During the headache episodes he found himself not interested in things around him, becoming irritable, preoccupied with thought of the headache, and experiencing tension across the top of the head and forehead, bilaterally.

During the first session, a complete social and medical history was obtained and discussion of his chronic anxiety explored. At the end of the first session a baseline hand temperature and a galvanic skin response (GSR) was obtained; hand temperature was relatively nonsignificant (being in the low 90's); GSR, while high, did not show dramatic shifts during imagery of anxiety-producing situations, although his pattern showed a GSR response before he felt any sensation of change. (Typically, patients have an image "in mind" and are aware of it slightly before the GSR responds on the display unit.)

The most important feature in the diagnostic exploration using biofeedback instrumentation was his extremely high trapezius EMG (minimum resting level of 25 microvolts), which he was unable to lower through his own efforts at relaxation. During the second session, Mr. T was trained in progressive relaxation, during which time his trapezius EMG reduced from 25 mv. to 16 mv. (a marked reduction but still relatively high compared to normal populations). He was instructed to practice relaxation for two 15-minute periods daily; in the third session he carried out the relaxation procedure without instruction from the therapist, with EMG showing a similar (marked) reduction in muscle tension. In the third session, the patient received EMG feedback with a tone proportional to muscle tension, and a meter showing the microvoltage activity of the muscle (in microvolts). Mr. T was instructed to relax himself as deeply as possible, and then to relax more deeply by lowering the tone. With this procedure, he was able to achieve 4.5 mv.

In the succeeding 15 sessions, Mr. T continued with EMG training, plateauing at a level of .75 mv. The focus of the training in later sessions was to maintain low EMG levels, not to necessarily reduce the microvoltage further. His headache frequently dropped to a mild occurrence each week, which he was able to relate to specific tension-producing events. His need for valium gradually diminished and his feelings of dependence on its effects dissipated. Mr. T was seen on two occasions at 4-month intervals following treatment. He reported occasional mild tension headaches after a hectic day of teaching. He had, however, discontinued all medications and relied on his successful ability to reduce the tension by relaxation.

This illustration describes the typical case in which the most significant drop in microvoltage of EMG is at the beginning of training, with decreasing reductions in later sessions. The object of continuing training is to enable the patient to differentiate and maintain the tension reduction rather than returning to previous levels.

THERMAL FEEDBACK

Thermal Feedback of skin surface temperature is a convenient, though indirect, measure of blood flow. The flow is determined by the constriction and dilation of the peripheral vessels, regulated by smooth muscles which are controlled by the sympathetic branch of the autonomic nervous system. One way for an individual to become immediately aware of the effect of stress upon the body is to take note of the drop in hand temperature in a stressful situation. Activity of the vascular system is very responsive to stress. Sympathetic nervous system activation uses vasoconstriction, especially in the periphery as the smooth muscles contract around the blood vessels, thus reducing their diameter. Given constant conditions, skin temperature is directly related to peripheral circulation. An increase in skin temperature can reflect a relaxation of the sympathetic nervous system. The intra- and extra-cranial vessels are specifically involved in producing the pain of a migraine headache.

A small thermistor is typically placed on the surface of the skin, often on the hands, to monitor skin temperature. There is a close relationship between autonomic nervous system activity and skin temperature variation in the hands. The fingertip is usually the most responsive to stress stimuli. The person receives feedback on changes in skin surface temperature (sometimes with as much accuracy as 1/100th of a degree) by watching a meter or lights or listening to a tone. Progress can be enhanced by visualizing handwarming images. The person may be able to change hand temperature dramatically, sometimes by as much as 20 degrees, demonstrating volitional control of the sympathetic nervous system. It should be borne in mind that skin temperature is not necessarily correlated with internal core body temperature.

Major Applications of Thermal Feedback. The major applications of thermal biofeedback include peripheral vascular disorders such as Raynaud's Disease, in which the extremities become painfully cold because of inadequate blood supply, migraine headaches, in which the contraction and then dilation of the cranial vessels produce stretching and pain, and hypertension and other stress-related disorders in which low arousal training is useful. Thermal biofeedback has also been found useful in psychotherapy to track changes in psychological resistance.

Illustrative Case Example. Mrs. K is a 23 year old married housewife who was referred by her physician for biofeedback treatment of her resistive hyperhydrosis. Her hands and feet sweated profusely and had done so for as long as she could remember. Frequency of the symptom was estimated at 50% of the day. Previous treatment included tranquilizers (Robinal with phenobarbitol) and diuretics. One physician's prescribed treatment was that the patient wash her hands with formaldehyde and fasten plastic bags to her hands and feet before bed. She commented that this made sleep very uncomfortable.

The patient, a cosmetologist, was particularly affected by her symptoms in that she had to apply make-up and handle the customers' hair. Her hobbies, including knitting, were also greatly affected (she could drench a ball of yarn).

The treatment included the use of temperature feedback, GSR/moisture detector (having both a baseline measure and feedback of surface moisture of the hands), homework (including a history of the hyperhydrosis, some of which was obtained from other family members), and a daily record of sweating. In addition, a deep muscle relaxation training was initiated.

The patient was seen for a total of eight visits. She learned hand cooling quickly; she could volitionally cool her hand temperature (skin surface) from 86 degrees to 74 degrees Fahrenheit in 5 minutes by the third training session. It was explained that the purpose of the training was not to cool her hands but to be able to influence hand moisture by cooling them when they were hot, and warming them when they were cold.

The GSR was used in conjunction with visualization of stressful scenes, and habituation of GSR responses to these scenes was obtained. Within the first three sessions the patient was able to readily cool her hand temperature (both hands tracked with 0.5 degree), and she was able to stabilize GSR. Mrs. K learned to raise and lower GSR (at a very gross setting so that it operated as a moisture detector), which thus indicated the amount of moisture on her hands. She thereby became readily aware of the parameters of turning "on and off" palm sweating. Her hand sweating record for the first 4 weeks showed dramatic decrease in the symptom each week. By the 6th week her hands were sweating only once or twice a day for no longer than 15 minutes. In the final session, the patient could literally turn her hand moisture on and off by alternately warming and cooling her hands. She asked to continue treatment for a different problem, a moderate overweight condition. She no longer experienced the hyperhydrosis severely as of the eighth session, nor at subsequent follow-ups.

ELECTRODERMAL FEEDBACK

EDR or Electrodermal Feedback includes a number of different measures such as GSR (Galvanic Skin Response), SPR (Skin Potential Response), and SCL (Skin Conductance Level). The EDR is a particularly good index of general activation of the physiologic system and is mediated by the sympathetic nervous system. It describes the electrical conductance across the skin secondary to changes in the sweat gland activity.

The activity of the sweat glands in response to increased sympathetic activation results in an increase in the level of conductance. There is a relationship between sympathetic activity and emotional arousal, although the specific emotion cannot be specified. Fear, anger, startle response, and sensual feelings are among emotions which can produce electrodermal changes. When there is a stressful stimulus, the perspiration in the sweat gland ducts rises as a result of sweat gland secretion. The electrical resistance decreases, resulting in an increased skin conductance. With relaxation, there is a concurrent decrease in skin conductance level.

Electrodermal instruments, whether called GSR's or skin conductance dermographs, are usually quite convenient and easy to use. The instruments range from tiny devices which can be held in the palm of the hand and have metal fingerplate contacts which give a sound feedback proportional to arousal, to instruments which measure many different electrodermal activities and have a full complement of meter, tone, and light feedback. The electrodes or sensors are typically silver-impregnated cloth pads placed on the fingertips. While watching the meter or listening to the tone, the person can see quite dramatically the arousal response to a hand clap startle stimulus, an upsetting thought, or the attempt at relaxation of the system.

Major Applications of Electrodermal Feedback. Applications of electrodermal feedback are typically more general than specific and include many applications in which decreased sympathetic activity and low arousal training is desired (e.g., in systematic desensitization for phobias, anxiety states in guided imagery, or exploration of feelings as in psychotherapy). In the case of cyclical arousal episodes, as in stuttering and asthma, this type of biofeedback training has shown usefulness.

Illustrative Case Example. A 32 year old male junior executive was a phone stutterer who, when he answered the phone, stuttered for as long as a minute before saying "Hello." Bright and effective as a person, he found the stuttering interfered greatly with his life. He reported some stuttering since childhood.

After relaxation training facilitated with EMG and some exploration of the variables of the problem, GSR training was done. When some control had been achieved, the phone desensitization process began. He was to maintain a low arousal, taking about 15 minutes to have the GSR at a low level of conductance, then call someone. An alternative was to have the secretary call in for him to maintain a low arousal while on the phone. If he began to get an increase in arousal as he was dialing the phone, he was to stop, reduce the GSR, and continue only if below a predetermined criterion. This continued until he could perform an activity such as talking on the phone while keeping low GSR. He finished dialing the phone and attempted to maintain low arousal while the phone was ringing. If there was an increase, he would bring it down while the phone was ringing. Fortunately, on his first attempt, the phone rang several times and he was able to bring the GSR back down. In one case, he called a girlfriend (whose name he had never been able to say on the phone) and was successful in saying "Cathy" without a stuttering episode. This was a rewarding experience for him and allowed an "on-line" way of using the instruments.

ELECTROENCEPHALOGRAPHIC FEEDBACK

EEG or Electroencephalographic Feedback is a measure of the synchronous firing neurons of the cortex. Small microvoltages of brain wave activity can be amplified, and a signal fed back to the person, who can then attempt to modify certain frequencies as they are correlated with subjective psychological states.

Brain waves have been categorized into four basic groups. Although the frequencies are somewhat arbitrary and are in combination with other frequencies, there is typically a psychological correlate which can be identified. Beta, which is a relatively fast (12-20 Hz) frequency, has been associated with concentration and attention, arousal, and even stress and anxiety. Alpha, a slower (8-12 Hz) frequency, has been associated with relaxation, calmness, and a meditative, nonfocused blank mind. Theta, an even slower (4-8 Hz) frequency, has been associated with hypnogogic and hypnopompic imagery – the pictures which passively pass through the mind just upon falling asleep and waking up. Some have suggested that this twilight state is one of greater creativity. Finally, Delta, which is the slowest (below 4 Hz) frequency, is associated with deep sleep and very low mental arousal.

Small sponge or silver electrodes are typically placed on the surface of the scalp for EEG readings of various cortical areas. Occipital-parietal placements on one hemisphere are quite common in EEG training for enhancing Alpha-wave frequencies. More precise placements are used with equipment specifically designed for subdominant frequencies, such as the neuroanalyzers used in biofeedback for seizure disorders. Power spectrum analysis, which involves a complex three-dimensional representation of the impulses emitted at different frequencies in a given period of time, will bring even more advanced approaches to the clinician.

Major Applications of Electroencephalographic Feedback. EEG applications have focused on general relaxation training, especially when the person would benefit from the quieting of mental activity (as in obsessive/compulsive neurosis and ruminative depression), concentration and reading disorders (for the person to learn how to shift focus and to prevent drifting into Alpha frequencies), insomnia and pain reduction, and, with special equipment, major motor seizures in epileptics.

Illustrative Case Example. The patient was a 36 year old male physician with a busy group practice, happy home and marriage, no clear sign of depression or complicating mental distress, but a 10-year history of sleep onset (45 minutes to 1-1/2 hours corroborated by his wife) and sleep duration (3 to 4 hours uninterrupted with inability to return to sleep) insomnia. He exercised sufficiently, ate well, and received little relief from Dalamane. The symptoms had worsened in the last 3 years. The patient was trained in Jacobson's progressive deep muscle relaxation (alternate tension/relaxation) and baseline EEG's were obtained. He was instructed to practice relaxation training twice daily, and returned for weekly appointments. Each week his EEG (occipital left hemisphere) frequency was shaped (reinforcement given for below average frequency production). He began at 16 Hz. By the third session, he was obtaining a 9 Hz average, reporting a floating-in-space sensation and blank mind, which was pleasant for him. By the 12th week he was obtaining 6 Hz averages, reporting hypnogogic imagery, and falling asleep in the office within 15 minutes. His sleep records showed 20-minute onset and 6 to 7 hour duration. By the 14th session, he was no longer taking medication, sleeping 7 to 8 hours uninterrupted, relaxing in the office, and falling asleep in 10 to 15 minutes. (Note: One weekly appointment was missed, which regressed him to levels of 2 weeks prior.) He was terminated after 18 sessions. Follow-up at 6 months showed a stable sleep pattern of 7 to 8 hours.

OTHER INSTRUMENTATION

Other instruments for the biofeedback of blood pressure, pulse wave velocity, heart rate, penile erection feedback, vaginal feedback, and gastrointestinal feedback are in use. In addition, sophisticated computer systems which can be used to train several individuals with different feedback modalities simultaneously (perhaps being controlled from a central console), are currently available. Videotape feedback and television color graphic displays that show progress and training as well as give incentives and motivation during the training process are now a part of the biofeedback system.

STEPS IN THE TREATMENT PROGRAM

A typical treatment program would include intake, treatment session, termination, and follow-up. While there will be variation, most treatments go through the following steps: (a) Referral (either by a hospital, professional, or self-referral), (b) an intake appointment in which information, forms, symptom checklists, psychological tests, and medication history is obtained, (c) development and agreement by the patient on the treatment plan (done at the conclusion of the intake), and (d) at the end of the biofeedback treatment, post-treatment physiological and psychological measures to determine the degree of change as well as a provision for follow-up in order to help the patient maintain his or her learning and the benefits achieved. This may be as simple as one visit or phone contact after 6 months and 1 year.

TREATMENT OVERVIEW CHART		
INTAKE PROCEDURES	TREATMENT SESSIONS	FINAL VISIT
Referrals	Progress Review	Transfer of Training
Telephone Screening	Counseling/Psychotherapy	Learning Internalization
Initial Visit	Home Practice Record	Post-Treatment Profile
Clinical Information	Relaxation Training	Future Recommendations
Psychological Evaluation	Biofeedback	
(MMPI; Locus of Control, Life Change Inventory)	Concurrent Therapy	FOLLOW-UP
Medical/Psychological History	Physical Therapy	Refresher Training
Psychophysiological Profile	Exercise Program	Progress Check
Baseline, Stress, Recovery	Relaxation Group	6-Month 12-Month

Figure 1.

Upon arrival, the patient is given information forms and symptom checklists, as well as a psychological evaluation. An intake interview includes a medical-psychological history specific to the symptom, and a psychophysiologic profile.

The psychophysiologic profile is a type of stress test which allows the therapist and patient to see the present level of functioning for several systems simultaneously. This may include the neuromuscular, cardiovascular, and sympathetic nervous systems. These measurements determine the baseline, the reaction to stressors, the recovery from stress, the ability to relax, and frequently, a measurement of stress management techniques and biofeedback in enhancing the relaxation process. It is with this psychophysiologic profile in combination with the history, interview, and psychological evaluation results that a treatment plan is developed. The number of visits per week, the type of instruments to be used, and perhaps even the approximate length of treatment can be determined.

PROCEDURE FOR FULLER PSYCHOPHYSIOLOGIC PROFILE

Five vital questions:

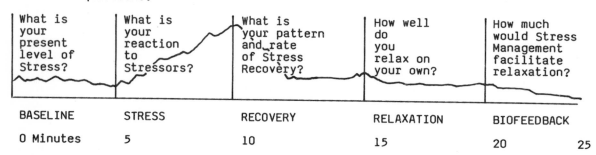

| What is your present level of Stress? | What is your reaction to Stressors? | What is your pattern and rate of Stress Recovery? | How well do you relax on your own? | How much would Stress Management facilitate relaxation? |

BASELINE	STRESS	RECOVERY	RELAXATION	BIOFEEDBACK	
0 Minutes	5	10	15	20	25

BASELINE   Sequence of Stressors:
Quiet sitting, no activity

STRESS
1. Hand clap
2. Serial sevens backwards from 1,000
3. Unpleasant thought
4. Breath holding
5. Ice water hand immersion, rubber band on finger pinch or arm constriction (1 min. each). (Optional)

RECOVERY   Quiet sitting, no activity

RELAXATION   May use one or both:
1. Own - using some present method
2. Standardized - using Progressive Relaxation training method of Autogenic Phrases (2-1/2 min. each).

BIOFEEDBACK   May use one or both:
1. With instrument showing best recovery in **RECOVERY** phase.
2. With instrument showing most response in **STRESS** phase (2-1/2 min. each).

Figure 2.

In difficult cases there may be consultation or a staff meeting in order to determine the best therapist and treatment plan for a patient's needs. The treatment is then begun, often on a once or twice weekly basis, frequently with home practice assignments including record keeping of the frequency and intensity of the symptom, relaxation practice, medication use, and possibly even home practice with portable training instruments.

In a typical course of treatment, the patient is seen in a setting which is comfortable and relaxing so that there is an adequate transfer of training from the office to everyday life.

Biofeedback training is only one part of the total treatment session. The therapist may discuss the results of the home pratice exercises, the events and stressors of that week, and attempt to facilitate and integrate what is being learned with the person's current life issues and goals. A record of progress is maintained as well as training records of the session, and typically when the goals have been achieved, there is a conclusion or termination session which is compared with the intake session, and a follow-up for maintenance of learning and continuation of symptom-free behavior.

During the treatment, portable home trainers may be worn to develop awareness of the occurrence of the symptoms or for home practice training in between sessions. In order to increase motivation, special instruments are also used in the office setting which allow different kinds of feedback displays and heighten interest and awareness.

With children, this increased motivation for learning is especially important. The biofeedback process of learning to control the system can become part of an exciting game. Behavioral medicine procedures and biofeedback techniques can be integrated into a powerfully effective stress management program. It is frequently an eye-opening experience for individuals to learn that they can develop control over a system that they never thought was possible, and to be able to maintain that control without the use of drugs but through a process of internal self-awareness.

PROFESSIONAL ISSUES

Using the Biofeedback Institute in San Francisco as an example of a multidisciplinary, behaviorally oriented clinic which treats a variety of disorders, the following description would apply to clinics attempting to integrate the various approaches used in behavioral medicine.

REFERRALS

Referrals are made by physician and other professionals in community health and rehabilitation agencies, former or current clients, and others. Additionally, some clients learn of the biofeedback clinic as a result of lectures to professional groups, classes, articles and television programs, and listings in the telephone directory. Although no advertising is done, a fact sheet on the functions and services can be provided upon request. At the outset, most referrals come from professionals (primarily physicians). However, each year an increasing percentage come from former clients who recommend the Biofeedback Institute to friends.

FEES AND BILLING

The Institute's sessions are time based at a 50-minute hour. This time unit is used for three reasons: It has precedence as a customary unit, it allows enough time for most biofeedback training protocols, and it also allows time to discuss relevant psychological issues, as well as to complete the billing and appointment setting. This allows maximum utilization of equipment and space. It has been our experience that 30-minute appointments tend to last 40-50 minutes in actuality, since 30 minutes is rarely enough time to complete the biofeedback process and allows little "talk time."

There is a base fee for the 50-minute session, applicable to all clients, unless a reduction is made by the therapist for special financial reasons. Groups have a separate flat rate, dependent on the nature of the group.

Billing is done by a single-entry system. The client typically pays the fee at the end of each session. The therapist (not an administrative person) usually completes the statement stub, which also shows receipt (credits), service provided and charge, and the next appointment time. We have found that collection of fees is better maintained when payments are made at the time of the visit, and when the client deals directly with the therapist who established the fee contract, rather than a secretary. Payments are made directly to The Biofeedback Institute. Statements are sent monthly for outstanding accounts. Difficulties in billing are also recognized in presenting treatment issues. Clients understand that they are responsible for the fee. If third party payers are involved, the client handles the fee in full and is reimbursed by the insurance carrier.

THERAPIST REIMBURSEMENT

Therapists are reimbursed on a client-hour basis in accordance with a matrix. This matrix bases reimbursement for contract services on the number of accumulated client hours, years of affiliation with the Institute, and average fee obtained. This has been found to be an effective reinforcing structure.

The concept of a mixed professional group has presented some problems in terms of billing, health insurance, and legal considerations. Frequently, a heterogeneous professional group has difficulty incorporating under the same umbrella. It is required, however, to obtain different types of liability insurance for individual staff members. Moreover, in terms of health insurance, the process of billing patients becomes somewhat complicated. For example, all therapists are reimbursed by the Institute on the same matrix, regardless of discipline. But a third-party carrier will often have a different rate of reimbursement for EMG training administered by a physical therapist than it would for the same kind of work done by a psychotherapist.

INSURANCE COVERAGE FOR BIOFEEDBACK

In the past three to four years, considerable progress has been made in educating insurance carriers about biofeedback and its efficacy as a treatment procedure. However, there is considerable work left undone.

More and more, insurance carriers are reimbursing for biofeedback by specifying the conditions for which biofeedback treatment may be used, by offering guidelines as to the number of sessions and charges they will cover, and by informing their field officers of their stance, either as written policy or unwritten.

It is generally true that the major carriers are more likely to cover biofeedback services, although there are three notable exceptions which are technically not insurance companies. Blue Cross and Blue Shield (which have separate policies on a district-by-district or state-by-state basis) in some cases reimburse and in others do not, dependent upon the individual jurisdiction. Medicare and Medicaid tend not to cover biofeedback services. Finally, CHAMPUS, after considerable pressure and lobbying effort by the Biofeedback Society of America, has only recently changed its stance to include biofeedback services. However, this has not been formalized through Congress.

Private carriers that have generally reimbursed for biofeedback, although not in every case, are as follows: Aetna, Allstate, Bankers Life, Connecticut General, Equitable, Great West Life, Hancock, Hartford, Lincoln National, Metropolitan Life, Pacific Mutual, Prudential, and Travelers. It should be added that carriers covering Worker's Compensation have generally covered biofeedback.

These insurance companies have by and large developed guidelines based on input from various sources, including the insurance committee of the Biofeedback Society of America, practitioners who have sent information along with claim forms and correspondence, and the company's own psychological and medical consultants. The guidelines typically explain the type of treatments provided, the learning process involved, the conditions for which biofeedback has been considered effective treatment, and the course of treatment that will be considered customary. Many of the carriers also attempt to educate their field offices by describing biofeedback as a process in which the patient is taught through visual or auditory aids to control autonomic bodily functions such as body temperature, heart rate, and muscle tension. Further, they expand on the learning process by explaining that an increased awareness of bodily functions is developed, that there is an attempt to gain control over those functions, and that there is a transfer of this control to everyday life without the use of biofeedback equipment. The more knowledgeable companies further recognize that a clinical specialist plays a major role in the first stage of this process, but the major responsibility lies with the participant who must be motivated to help himself or herself.

While there are discrepancies among the various companies as to the conditions for which biofeedback is considered effective, the following conditions are most often mentioned: migraine and tension headaches, muscle spasms (including torticollis), hypertension, chronic pain, insomnia, facial tic, bruxism, temporomandibular joint pain, and anxiety. While this list is not exhaustive, it is certainly reasonable in covering the major conditions for which biofeedback has been found to be effective. Conditions not on the carriers' lists may be submitted for review. For example, the treatment of fecal incontinence which has been clearly supported by the data as effective, may well be considered reasonable for coverage.

The most difficult and misinformed part of the guideline generally has to do with the number of treatments that are considered essential. Too often the carriers place a limit on the number of treatment sessions, such as five to seven visits, and may allow a maximum of ten visits if the doctor indicates that this would complete the treatment. While many practitioners in biofeedback consider this number too low, it is easy to see how this misunderstanding could have arisen. Numerous research articles use a small number of treatments in the research paradigm and many clinicians have been quoted as having an average of under ten sessions for biofeedback treatment, even though this could include drop outs and single session consultations.

Finally, the carriers typically do not pay for expenses having to do with the purchase of biofeedback equipment or even lease or rental of portable equipment for patients. Some even limit the charge which may be made for biofeedback treatment, at times, to as little as $20 to $25. It is not yet clear whether this fee is set because it is assumed that the treatments are only 30 minutes in length (although many practitioners are seeing the patient for 50 minutes to an hour), or whether it is felt that the services are delivered by a technician under the clinician's supervision, even though many (if not most) clinicians supply the services directly.

The Health Insurance Association of America, in discussion with industry representatives on various biofeedback reimbursement practices, has taken the following position:

1. "That there are no existing written policies or guidelines regarding payment or nonpayment of biofeedback treatment."

2. That, as with "other medical technologies and therapeutic interventions, reimbursable services are those used in conjunction with specific illness (e.g., a person given treatment to alleviate pain secondary to a specific illness or condition would be reimbursed up to a given maximum for total treatment rendered, with the maximum being determined by the insurance contract and guidelines regarding reasonable and customary rates for the region)." This implies that chronic pain associated with certain terminal cancer conditions may be reimbursed but that a person being treated for "pain control" would not.

3. While carriers usually respond with automatic payment for treatment of generally recognizable conditions at biofeedback centers, including management of such conditions as migraine and hypertension, "reimbursement for stress management and other nondiagnostically related interventions are more selective and depend more heavily on the specifics of the insurance contracts and the facts of the particular case."

4. The determination of which cases will be covered is inevitably made with the assistance of the carrier's medical department.

5. It is doubtful whether there will be a unilateral industry position on biofeedback as long as federal payors and certain medical societies regard biofeedback as experimental.

(Summarized from correspondence by Carol Cole-Posner, Assistant Director, Health Insurance Association of America, March 7, 1980.)

In summary, reimbursement for biofeedback is currently a matter of educating the insurance carriers and providing them with information so that guidelines and policy can be developed. There is still inconsistency in the carriers' guidelines, but more and more of them are covering biofeedback services. Finally, there is a widespread feeling that biofeedback practitioners are "barking up the wrong tree" in attempting to deal only with insurance carriers as the determiners of policy. Instead, it is felt by some that practitioners should seek to educate their local medical and psychological societies so that biofeedback treatment will become accepted as usual and customary practice. When this occurs, insurance carriers will have no choice but to cover such services. Thus, it is important for professionals using biofeedback to educate others within their own professions so that they become more knowledgeable about the efficacy of biofeedback treatment.

TRAINING

A critical issue in the development and success of biofeedback in the treatment of psychophysiological and other disorders lies in the training of the professional or assistant who administers the services. It has been only very recently that any formal programs were developed for providing basic training in the use of biofeedback.

The California Society approved several training programs in California which provide the following:

Didactic Instruction: Basic information on biofeedback, including theory, use of instruments, research, clinical applications and procedures, relaxation techniques, and so on (40 hours required).

Case Studies: Focus on syndromes and clinical cases. Procedures, problems, contraindications, homework, ethics, placebo effects, and so forth (10 hours).

Personal Training: Personal biofeedback experience with instruments of at least four different types (10 hours with certified trainer; 15 hours additional).

Clinical Experience: Experience working with others in a clinical setting. Sessions are discussed with supervisor (30 hours).

Supervision: Supervision of clinical experience and other matters of concern to program participants (15 hours).

CERTIFICATION

Several states have formulated or are developing standards for certification. Certification is not to be confused with licensure by the State. The intent of certification is to find a minimal level of competence that could be measured and recognized. It is not a license, and certification should not be regarded as a "pseudo-license" to be misused (autonomous practice on a fee-for-service basis) by currently nonlicensed individuals without extensive professional training.

As an example, the Biofeedback Society of California (BSC) certification program presently evaluates the person's ability to apply biofeedback in some responsible and meaningful way within his or her professional area, or under the supervision of a professional in the case of a biofeedback assistant. The intent is not to test someone's ability in physical therapy or medicine or psychology, but to test basic understanding of the use of biofeedback as a modality.

BSC has established an oral and written examination which may be taken separately. There is a simple pass/fail system for each portion of the examination. Application to take the examinations is accepted when the applicant demonstrates that he or she has met the training requirements, either through a formal program or by other experience (equivalent training). In addition to protection of the public, the purpose of developing certification procedures is to provide adequate and effective standards for anticipated State regulation of biofeedback.

The Biofeedback Certification Institute of America (BCIA) has recently developed a national certification program which employs a multiple-choice, written examination.

LEGISLATION

There are typically no laws governing the use of biofeedback in and of itself. Most states do, however, license various professions (medicine, psychology, physical therapy). Some professions have moved to have biofeedback included in their current licensure laws. For example, in California, as of January 1, 1977, the Psychology Licensure Act includes the use of biofeedback. One important effect of this amendment is that most national legislation, including the Medical Devices Act, defines a user as a licensed provider, thus leaving the states to determine which professions are covered. In order to clarify whether or not a professional is able, under the law, to incorporate the use of biofeedback devices into his or her practice, it would appear that each profession, in each state, must include biofeedback in the current licensure laws.

If the use of biofeedback is seen by the state to be part of the practice of various professions, use of biofeedback by a nonlicensed individual in the treatment of a disorder could make that individual subject to legal action for practicing (medicine, psychology) without a license. As a hypothetical example of the legal difficulties that could be forthcoming with the nonlicensed use of biofeedback, consider the situation I describe below.

Joe Brown, after attending seminars in biofeedback and doing extensive reading, buys an EMG instrument. He sets up a small office and accepts a fee for doing EMG biofeedback. Mr. Smith comes to him with colitis, and Joe Brown suggests that biofeedback would be helpful in that colitis is a tension-related disorder. Mr. Smith subsequently dies of colon obstruction. The family brings charges against Joe Brown. A determination is made that Mr. Brown was treating Mr. Smith's colitis, accepting a fee for the service, and practicing medicine without a license. He is punished as prescribed by law.

When the states move to regulate the use of biofeedback instrumentation, they will, in all likelihood, look toward guidelines currently enforced by those who are most involved in the field (i.e., the membership of state biofeedback societies). One very positive outcome of this manner of approach is that those most knowledgeable in biofeedback practice will have the responsibility for formulating the procedures, not legislators or administrators who may not fully understand the implications of arbitrary decisions regarding biofeedback use.

George Fuller-Von Bozzay, Ph.D., is currently Director of the Biofeedback Institute and Associate Clinical Professor in the Department of Biological Dysfunction , U.C. Medical Center, San Francisco. In addition, he is on the faculties of San Francisco State University and U.C. Berkeley Extension, and is a consultant to the California School of Professional Psychology and several hospitals. He is the author of numerous publications in the field of biofeedback and has also co-authored several introductory psychology texts. Dr. Fuller-Von Bozzay may be contacted at The Biofeedback Institute of San Francisco, 3428 Sacramento Street, San Francisco, CA 94118.

RESOURCES

PUBLICATIONS

Autogenic Systems, Inc., THE HANDBOOK OF PHYSIOLOGICAL FEEDBACK (4 vols.). Berkeley, CA: ASI, 1976.

Barber, T. X., DiCara, L. V., Kamiya, J., Miller, N. E., Shapiro, D., & Stoyva, J. (Eds.). BIOFEEDBACK AND SELF-CONTROL, 1970: AN ALDINE ANNUAL ON THE REGULATION OF BODILY PROCESSES AND CONSCIOUSNESS. Chicago: Aldine Publishing Co., 1971.

Birk, L. (Ed.). BIOFEEDBACK: BEHAVIORAL MEDICINE. New York: Grune & Stratton, 1974.

Basmajian, J. R. (Ed.). BIOFEEDBACK: PRINCIPLES AND PRACTICE FOR CLINICIANS. Baltimore, MD: Williams & Wilkins Co., 1979.

Blanchard, E. B. & Epstein, L. H. A BIOFEEDBACK PRIMER. Reading, MS: Addison-Wesley, 1978.

Bongar, B. & Taylor, L. P. CLINICAL APPLICATIONS IN BIOFEEDBACK THERAPY. Los Angeles, CA: Psychology Press, 1976.

Beatty, J. & Legewie, H. (Eds.). BIOFEEDBACK: PRINCIPLES AND PRACTICE FOR CLINICIANS. Baltimore: Williams & Wilkins Co., 1979.

Brown, B. B. NEW MIND, NEW BODY: BIO-FEEDBACK; NEW DIRECTIONS FOR THE MIND. New York: Harper & Rowe, 1974.

Brown, B. B. STRESS AND THE ART OF BIOFEEDBACK. New York: Harper & Rowe, 1977.

Butler, F. A SURVEY OF THE LITERATURE. New York: Plenum, 1978.

Fuller, G. D. BEHAVIORAL MEDICINE, STRESS MANAGEMENT AND BIOFEEDBACK: A CLINICIAN'S DESK REFERENCE. San Francisco: Biofeedback Press, 1980.

Fuller, G. D. BIOFEEDBACK: METHODS AND PROCEDURES IN CLINICAL PRACTICE. San Francisco: Biofeedback Press, 1977.

Fuller, G. D. PROJECTS IN BIOFEEDBACK. San Francisco: Biofeedback Press, 1980.

Gaarder, K. R. & Montgomery, P. S. CLINICAL BIOFEEDBACK: A PROCEDURAL MANUAL. Baltimore, MD: Williams & Wilkins Co., 1977.

Gatchel, R. J. & Price, K. P. (Eds.). CLINICAL APPLICATIONS OF BIOFEEDBACK: APPRAISAL AND STATUS. New York: Permagon Press, 1979.

Hume, W. I. BIOFEEDBACK: RESEARCH AND THERAPY. Montreal: Eden Press, 1976.

Kamiya, J., Barber, T. X., DiCara, L. V., Miller, N. E., Shapiro, D., & Stoyva, J. (Eds.). BIOFEEDBACK AND SELF-CONTROL, 1976-77: AN ALDINE ANNUAL ON THE REGULATION OF BODILY PROCESSES AND CONSCIOUSNESS. Chicago: Aldine Publishing Co., 1977.

Karlins, M. & Andrews, L. M. BIOFEEDBACK: TURNING ON THE POWER OF YOUR MIND. Philadelphia: Lippincott, 1972.

Lamott, K. ESCAPE FROM STRESS. New York: G. P. Putnam's Sons, 1974.

Lawrence, J. ALPHA BRAIN WAVES. New York: Nash, 1972.

McCrady, R. E. & McCrady, J. B. BIOFEEDBACK: AN ANNOTATED BIBLIOGRAPHY OF PUBLISHED RESEARCH WITH HUMAN SUBJECTS SINCE 1960. Pomona, CA: Behavioral Instrument Co., 1975.

Owen, S., Toomim, H., & Taylor, L. P. BIOFEEDBACK IN NEUROMUSCULAR RE-EDUCATION. Los Angeles: Biofeedback Research Institute, 1975.

Payne, B. & Reitano, C. T. BIOMEDITATION. Brookline, MA: BFI, Inc., 1977.

Peper, E., Ancoli, S., & Quinn, M. MIND/BODY INTEGRATION. New York: Plenum Press, 1979.

Schwartz, G. E. & Beatty, J. (Eds.). BIOFEEDBACK: THEORY AND RESEARCH. New York: Academic Press, 1977.

Schwartz, G. E. & Shapiro, D. (Eds.). CONSCIOUSNESS AND SELF-REGULATION. New York: Plenum Press, 1976.

Stern, R. & Ray, W. J. BIOFEEDBACK. Homewood, IL: Dow Jones-Irwin, 1977.

Whatmore, G. & Kohli, D. R. THE PSYCHOPHYSIOLOGY AND TREATMENT OF FUNCTIONAL DISORDERS. New York: Grune & Stratton, 1974.

Wickramasekera, I. BIOFEEDBACK, BEHAVIORAL THERAPY AND HYPNOSIS. Chicago: Nelson-Hall, Inc., 1976.

PROFESSIONAL SOCIETIES

There are four major national societies as well as state societies whose membership are engaged in biofeedback treatment:

The **Biofeedback Society of America (BSA)**, Francine Butler, Ph.D., Executive Director, 4301 Owens Street, Wheat Ridge, CO 80033.

The **American Association of Biofeedback Clinicians**, Kathleen Kilkenny, Executive Secretary, 2424 Dempster, Des Plaines, IL 60016.

The **Society of Behavioral Medicine**, Redford B. Williams, Jr., M.D., President, Box 85330, University Station, Knoxville, TN 37996.

The **American Academy of Behavioral Medicine**, 8616 Northwest Plaza Drive, Suite 210, Dallas, TX 75225.

SUICIDE PREVENTION PROCEDURES

Calvin J. Frederick

Suicidal behavior is a perennial problem which has existed since the dawn of history, and probably even before that. It has been listed as one of the ten leading causes of death in the United States for most of the twentieth century. While it is not likely to ever disappear completely, such behavior and its effects upon others can be mitigated by research, training, and effective clinical practice.

The rate for suicidal deaths per 100,000 population annually, a figure which applies to all ages, races, and both sexes, reached an all time high of 17.4 in 1932, during the last phase of the Depression. Although the suicide rate declined during the 1940's and 1950's, it still remained among the first ten causes of death for all ages. Suicide began to climb again in the late 1960's and has now reached alarming proportions, in particular among younger age groups. There has recently been an increase of more than 200% in males 10-15 years of age and among both sexes in the 15-24 year age range. When accompanied by stressful situations, an apparent absence of interpersonal resources, and doubtful coping skills, young persons can be considered very high risks. The elderly can be viewed as high risk individuals as well, since they often lack these same resources and coping mechanisms, and frequently feel they are merely a burden to those around them. It should be emphasized that persons of any age, race, socioeconomic group, religion, or sex can be at risk for suicidal death when stressful situations are present which are seen as being beyond the capabilities of the person to manage (Frederick, 1978).

In responding to the suicidal client, it is necessary for a clinician to be innovative, sensitive, and affirmative. The suicidal person must view the intervenor as an individual who is stable, competent, knowledgeable, understanding, perceptive, and strong. The last thing a person in crisis wants or needs is someone who is, in their view, ambivalent, easily manipulated, and lacking in aplomb. Having faith and trust in the clinician in an emergency situation can mean the difference between life and death, since the suicidal person otherwise may feel let down and assume that all meaningful resources have been exhausted (Frederick, 1978, 1980, 1981; Frederick & Resnik, 1970; Frederick, Resnik, & Wittlin, 1973).

THE SUICIDAL EQUATION

There are a number of general factors which seem to set the stage for suicidal behavior.

STRESS

When any stressful situation is present which lasts more than two weeks without readily foreseeable resolution it does not augur well for sound emotional well being. Stress may result from any number of sources, including loss of a significant other through death, divorce, or separation, loss of job, failure in school, humiliation, or loss of self-esteem.

HISTORY OF SUICIDAL BEHAVIOR

Such behavior may be direct in the form of an actual overt act or indirect as indicated by reckless driving, heavy drinking of alcohol, heavy drug usage, prolonged improper eating, or lack of attention to medical infirmities.

EVIDENCE OF AN AFFECTIVE DISORDER

Affective disturbances, particularly clinical depression, should alert any clinician to the possibility of suicide. Depression is not an essential condition for a suicidal act, but it is highly correlated with life threatening behavior. Such symptoms as early morning awakening, fitful sleep, loss of appetite, loss of sex drive, moodiness, fatigue, or expressions of helplessness and loss of hope herald an acute state as a precursor to suicide. Among younger age groups, especially those in the lower teens, depression will often not show itself in such classical form; rather, it may manifest itself in conduct disturbances such as poor school work, rebellion, nonconformity, and withdrawal from friends.

PLAN FOR SUICIDE

In nearly all cases, a concrete plan for the act has developed when suicide is imminent. If the plan is general and not specifically defined, it is less likely to be of acute concern than when a specific plan has been formed. For example, if the potential victim has purchased a gun, rope, poison, knife, or other lethal object, a more acute situation is apt to exist than when definitive items are not present. If pills have been accumulated or if there is talk of jumping from a high place, such conditions would be of the same serious proportions as those where lethal objects exist. If the talk is more general, such as, "I haven't really thought of how I might kill myself yet, but I feel as though I might just end it all," the acute quality which calls for urgency of action as in a clearly defined plan, is not present. The lethal quality of the method to be used is of particular concern (e.g., a gun is more lethal than a handful of aspirin tablets).

RESOURCES

If close friends or family are available for use as adjuncts to intervention, this is important to know. When the person is relatively alone, the prognosis is more guarded, other things being equal. Feelings of rejection by important others should be explored to evaluate their effect upon the person at any given point in time.

MOOD

When the person has been morose and depressed and then becomes agitated, a critically serious situation exists which often culminates in suicide. The depths of depression can be so incapacitating that there is literally not enough energy available for the potential victim to take his or her own life. However, when the depression abates, as it inevitably will, energy for movement which is used to commit suicide becomes accessible. The person should not be left alone during this period. Comments about self-blame for some real or imagined event should be noted and assessed when treating the individual in crisis.

MEDICAL STATUS

The general health of the person experiencing a stress-laden crisis can help or hinder intervention and treatment. Healthy persons will frequently respond to the use of physical activity as a way of reducing tension and avoiding the insidiousness of depression. In the case of certain physically infirmed or debilitated persons, different procedures, such as promoting interaction with others, are employed.

TYPICAL PATTERNS

Traditionally, males have been regarded as committers of suicide, while females have been viewed as attempters. While this is still true statistically, females appear to be employing more violent methods in recent years and, hence, the probability of lethal first attempts has increased. Both sexes engage in suicidal acts for a number of reasons (e.g., feelings of defeat, loss of hope, feelings of personal rejection, hurt and anger, the desire to get back at others by making them sorry, misguided martyrdom, loss of face, fear of disgrace, self-defeat).

In one actual case, a 17 year old was found in his car early one morning in the high school parking lot, a victim of carbon monoxide, which was piped through a vacuum cleaner hose attached to the exhaust pipe. Although basically quite bright intellectually, his grades had dropped noticeably after rejection by a girlfriend and temporary suspension from an athletic team resulting from his breaking of some training rules. The rejection and loss of face was more than he could bear.

Another actual case, in which this author was called to testify in court, was that of a 56 year old woman who was found hanging in the bathroom of a large city hospital six days after admission for "suicidal ideation" and thoughts. A close relative had committed suicide in a mental hospital during the victim's early youth, and she had become increasingly fearful that a similar fate would befall her. She had been given an antidepressant, but her pleas for help one hour prior to her death were ignored by the admitting physician with no instructions for the ward staff. (Charges of negligence and malpractice against the hospital resulted.)

While suicides affect all ages, some rather typical profiles among young persons who are at high risk may be helpful. A typical profile for the young suicidal male would be one where the father has died or been separated before the boy is 16 years old. Especially among whites, the father is often a successful professional or businessman. There has been a characteristic lack of a solid father-son relationship, which results in feelings of rejection, anxiety, sleeplessness, substance abuse, or heavy smoking due to the tension experienced.

A young suicidal female is frequently the offspring of a narcissistic mother and an ineffectual father. After feeling rejection by parental figures, and often a boyfriend, she may attempt to take her life. Fathers are more important figures with both sexes than is commonly recognized. Traditionally, mothers have been viewed as the prime parent of the child and have sometimes been the recipient of most of the blame for childhood misbehavior and the subsequent emotional and mental disturbances. While both parents are important, the root of many serious emotional problems, particularly those with males, can be placed with the father.

TYPES OF SELF—ANNIHILATING BEHAVIOR

Three behavioral terms are used to characterize acts of a self-annihilating or destructive nature.

SELF-ASSAULTIVE BEHAVIOR

Self-assaultive behavior suggests an attack or assault upon the self. An act of this kind may not be clearly suicidal. It is not uncommon, for instance, for children to threaten injury to themselves or others. They may verbalize the fact by warning a parent or parental surrogate that they intend to hurt themselves. People experiencing repeated injuries are termed "accident prone." Such acts are often aimed at obtaining love and sympathy not gained through other avenues. This type of behavior can develop out of sibling rivalry in an effort to draw attention away from the rival at virtually all costs.

SELF-DESTROYING BEHAVIOR

Self-destroying behavior ordinarily connotes more seriously distressed cases than those in the self-assaultive range. There are varying degrees of intensity, and clearly self-destroying acts blend unmistakably with overt suicide. Psychological equivalents of suicide or self-destruction can be difficult to recognize, since they can be beneath the level of consciousness. For instance, there is the case of a person with severe insulin-dependent diabetes who fails to take insulin properly, even after having been carefully instructed about the importance of the procedure. Persons with serious cardiac problems or other medical disorders, which require vigilant personal monitoring and care, fall into this category if they neglect themselves repeatedly, especially with knowledge of the potentially dire consequences.

Different degrees of understanding may exist regarding death, even among adults. Some people live in a virtual dream world and feel as though they will be saved at the last moment, that nothing will happen to them no matter what they do. On the other hand, young persons may feel the risk is worth taking just one time, especially if there is a need to acquire peer-group approval. There is doubt about the exact age at which children really comprehend the concept of death, particularly suicidal death. Youngsters rarely understand suicidal death prior to the age of seven or eight years. Some authors believe the concept of suicide is not fully comprehensible before the age of nine or ten. In the author's experience, the youngest age at which suicide appeared to be clearly understood occurred in a very bright five year old boy. After a thorough examination of both child and parent, it became unmistakably clear that he was engaged in overt suicidal attempts which were rooted in conflict with his mother because he wanted to be with his divorced father. The age at which youngsters can comprehend the nature and quality of their actions about death often vary with cultural background, relationship to parents, presence of older siblings, intelligence, and exposure to violence, both within and outside the home setting.

SUICIDAL BEHAVIOR

Suicidal behavior can be viewed as less equivocal than the other two categories. It may be defined as any willful act designed to result in one's own death. People can injure and destroy parts of themselves without actually taking their own lives, of course. This is the reason why self-assaultive or self-destructive behaviors are useful dimensions on this continuum of behaviors. A finality is present in suicide which sets it apart, in concept and principle, from the other behaviors, even though the difference can be only a matter of degree.

TRADITIONAL SUICIDAL SIGNS

A number of contributing factors appear in suicidal behavior in general, but the experience of personal loss seems to be a pervasive theme. Such losses include those which are internal (e.g., loss of self-esteem, loss of confidence, or loss of face, resulting in humiliation) and external (loss of standing in society or school, loss of job, loss of a loved friend or relative). Many precipitating events, which may seem unimportant and insignificant to others, are viewed as overwhelming to the persons affected. Shneidman, Farberow, and Litman (1970), from the Los Angeles Suicide Prevention Center, have done much to develop the principles set forth here. Shneidman, in particular, has articulated the importance of signs such as these, some of which have been expanded or refined by this author.

Clues that can aid in suicidal identification will be both **overt** and **covert**. Overt behavioral clues include actions such as purchasing a rope, guns, or pills. Covert behavioral clues are revealed in the behavior patterns already noted for both young persons and adults. Signs of deterioration are often revealed by a sudden change of behavior, which may not be flagrantly rebellious enough to include rule breaking and legal violations. Verbal clues can be open or masked as well. A person in crisis may speak openly of suicide, or cover it by talking of wills, legal matters, death or dying, and problems supposedly occurring to a third person.

Marked symptoms of clinical depression are not always strikingly apparent, especially among younger persons. Even when signs are manifest, young persons below 18 years of age may not show all the classical signs, such as loss of appetite and weight, apathy, loss of libido, and insomnia. It is a mistake to believe that an individual will not commit unless clinically depressed. In point of fact, adult depression and youthful depression may not be synonymous.

SUICIDAL BEHAVIOR PATTERNS AMONG YOUTH

1. The young person may experience difficulty communicating with parents. In fact, this is part of the disturbance. They are more likely to communicate with a peer or another interested individual in whom they have some faith and trust. Thus, if it is apparent that a

youth cannot talk to his or her parents, one should be alert to the possibility of a serious problem.

2. The youth may give away a prized possession with the comment that it will not be needed any longer.

3. The youth is apt to be more morose and isolated than usual.

4. A young male may experience the loss of a father or a close male figure through death or divorce.

5. A young female is apt to reveal difficulty with her mother, especially in the presence of an inadequate father figure.

6. An adolescent is likely to smoke heavily, as an indication of severe tension or anxiety.

7. General efficiency and school performance may decline markedly.

8. An increase in substance abuse, accompanied by anxiety, isolation, or irritability, may occur.

9. The youth may have a history of self-poisoning. Even though apparently "accidental," one should be alert to instances of prior self-poisoning behavior. The person who tries to commit suicide frequently has a history of self-poisoning, often requiring medical treatment. Ultimately, this behavior will result in self-destruction.

10. The youth may have been an abused child. Children from homes in which the professional suspects child abuse or finds the so-called "battered child" syndrome should be given serious concern, since there is mounting clinical evidence to suggest that future violence, including suicide, can develop from abuse in childhood. Any feelings of rejection by parents should be noted, even if severe physical punishment is absent.

11. Youths exhibit behavioral or verbal signs which suggest a desire to get back at parents. A common component in suicidal behavior is to wish to make those left behind sorry that they did not treat the victim better while still alive.

12. Psychosis may be present in a young child (particularly less than 12).

SUICIDAL BEHAVIOR PATTERNS AMONG ADULTS

1. A past history of suicidal behavior is often present and should be explored at an appropriate point.

2. A past or recent loss of an important person in the individual's life may continue to plague the potential victim.

3. A loss of interest in activities (e.g., bowling or playing cards) which are usually important may occur.

4. Depressive symptoms are likely to become manifest, including the classical ones (e.g., early morning awakening which gets progressively worse, fitful sleep, anorexia, apathy, isolation and withdrawal to bed, chronic complaints, irritability, and fatigue).

5. Any of the major disorders may be manifest.

6. Paranoid suspicions and hostility may be present, but mental disorders are not a necessary component.

7. Expressions of guilt may occur which cannot be expatiated.

8. The person may suffer loss of libido.

9. Feelings of helplessness are openly expressed.

10. The person experiences a loss of hope for the future.

Some behaviors, such as giving away a valued object or possession, inquiring about the hereafter and legal matters relating to insurance, may appear in younger persons as well as adults, depending upon the age and life situation.

PSYCHOLOGICAL FIRST AID

I believe that the following procedural steps for dealing with persons in a suicidal crisis are basic and essential.

PROCEDURAL STEPS

Step 1: Listen And Hear. Of vital importance to a person in an emotional crisis is to have available someone who will listen and really hear what the person in crisis is saying. Every effort should be made to establish a connection with the feelings beneath the words spoken.

Step 2: Be Sensitive To The Relative Seriousness Of The Thoughts And Feelings Being Expressed. When the person speaks of clear-cut self-destructive plans, the situation is usually much more acute than when plans to die and thoughts of dying are less definitely stated.

Step 3: Determine The Intensity And Severity Of The Emotional Disturbance. It is possible for an individual to be extremely upset but not suicidal. When a person has been markedly depressed but then becomes agitated and moves about restlessly, it is usually cause for alarm. It is possible that the psychomotor aspects of retarded activity in depression may have lifted, and the resultant agitation is a precursor to the suicidal act.

Step 4: Take Any Suicidal Complaint Seriously. Do not undervalue or dismiss what the person is saying. In some instances, the person in crisis may express feelings in a low key, but behind this apparent calm may be profoundly distressed feelings. All allusions to suicide must be taken seriously. It is far better to err on the side of being overly cautious than not cautious enough.

Step 5:   Inquire Directly About Thoughts Of Suicide.   Suicide may be suggested but not overtly addressed in the crisis period by a potential victim. Experience discloses that harm is rarely done by inquiring directly into such thoughts at an appropriate time. In fact, the individual frequently responds to the query and is glad to have the opportunity to bring the issue out into the open.

Step 6:   Do Not Be Misled By Comments That The Emotional Crisis Is Past.   The person may feel initial relief after talking of suicide, but the same stressful crisis will recur later. Follow-up is a critical safeguard.

Step 7:   Be Affirmative And Supportive.   Strong, stable resources are essential in the life of a distressed individual. Provide emotional strength by conveying the impression of competence, and that everything possible will be done to prevent the person from taking his or her life. Problems will work out with the cooperation of the person in crisis.

Step 8:   Evaluate The Resources Available.   The individual may have both inner psychological resources (e.g., ego defenses such as rationalization and intellectualization) which can be strengthened and supported, and outer resources in the environment, such as ministers, relatives, and friends who can be contacted. When these are absent, substitutions for them must be found. Continuing observation and support may become vital.

Step 9:   Act Definitively.   Do something tangible, such as arranging for a subsequent contact with yourself or another professional expert. Nothing is more frustrating to an individual in crisis than to feel as if nothing has been received from a meeting with a professional person and it may enhance the notion that a last hope is gone. A future appointment gives the person something to hang onto.

Step 10:   Do Not Avoid Asking For Assistance And Consultation.   Call upon whomever is needed, depending upon the severity of the case. Do not try to handle everything alone. Convey an attitude of firmness and composure so that the person can believe that something realistic and appropriate is being done to help.

Step 11:   Never Demean Or Respond Pejoratively To Suicidal Expressions.   Accept the person as he or she is while emphasizing the existence of more positive qualities. The last thing a person in stress needs is negativism.

Step 12:   Make A Contract Where Appropriate.   Many suicidal persons in severe crisis will welcome making a contract not to kill themselves for a certain period of time. While it should not be relied upon entirely, it may take them off the spot and reduce tension.

There are a number of other specific steps which may be taken and behaviors adopted by the clinician in the intervention process.

It is wise to arrange for a receptive individual to stay with the person during the acute crisis. He or she should not be left isolated, alone, or unobserved for an appreciable time when acutely distressed. Also, the environment should be as safe and provocation-free as possible. Family and friends should be called in to maintain personal connections, if possible. The individual should not be challenged in an attempt to shock away the suicidal ideas, nor should there be any attempt to argue about suicide. The individual should be given emotional support for living and reassurance that the depressed feelings are temporary and will pass. An emphasis can be placed on the fact that there are options available as long as there is life, but absolutely no options once the person has died. The permanence of death can also be stressed. It is sometimes helpful to mention the stigma that may be placed on innocent and personally valued survivor victims, if the potential suicide is resultant from some cause other than anger or hostility toward family or friends. Further, the clinician can help the person to ventilate feelings necessary to reduce tension.

If an acutely suicidal person does not appear to show some positive change during an interview, hospitalization may be a necessary step. This procedure will run much more smoothly if the individual is cooperative and agreeable to hospitalization and he or she should be consulted on this option.

The goal of these procedures is to restore feelings of personal worth and dignity, which are equally important to basic ego strength. By so doing, the intervenor can make the difference between life and death and a future potentially productive citizen will survive.

RESPONSES TO REPRESENTATIVE COMMENTS OF SUICIDAL PERSONS

These comments and responses represent characteristic dialogues between the person in suicidal crisis and a trained intervenor. The ideas noted are what is of importance; the remarks are not necessarily a verbatim script. They are not listed in any special sequence.

1. Suicidal Person: I don't know how I can go on.

    Intervenor: Things are not hopeless. Feelings of sadness and depression will pass. Depressions are self-limiting. As long as there is hope, there is a good chance that things will get better. Matters can change. As long as you are alive, changes can occur. Once dead – the decision is irreversible. Altered and improved situations cannot be enjoyed once you are gone. No major decision should be made in the throes of an emotional crisis or conflict. Solid choices with which one can be comfortable can be made only after conflict resolution has occurred. Give yourself time to permit new events to occur.

2. S: I have a right to take my own life if I choose, don't I?

    I: Yes, but others in your life have a right to live unmarred lives of their own, too. Your friends and family should be able to walk with heads high, with feelings of pride and dignity in having you as a friend or close family member. (Many times there are siblings and parents who are innocent victims of suicidal death, quite apart from any conflict or resentment which may have been present with a spouse or lover.)

3. S: People would be better off without me.

    I: Do you not think it would be best to let the others make that judgment for themselves? It is likely that you mean more to some people than you think. You may be laying an emotional burden on them which they cannot handle, and which will cause them unmeasurable distress in the future.

4.   S: I seem to mess up everything I do. Nothing turns out right.

     I: What are the best and worst things you have ever done? Let's look at and talk about best things you have ever done first. Think about how good you felt about it and tell me more about what happened. You see, you are capable of doing something worthwhile. Now, what is the worst thing you have ever done? How did other people feel about it? Perhaps it was not as bad as you thought. You do not need to continue doing anything that you really believe to be bad. You can change it by the way you think or act.

5.   S: Life isn't worth living. I can end it all and stop the tormented feelings.

     I: Maybe you are looking at life with blinders on - employing tunnel vision. You must widen your view, see other options. Let's look at what you feel is so troubling to you now. Tell me what the worst aspect of your life is as you now view it. Another person in the same situation might react quite differently; this is only your perception at the moment.

6.   S: I have thought of killing myself before. It has been something I have felt at other periods. It comes back. It doesn't seem to go away for good.

     I: I wonder what has kept you from taking your life before now. What thoughts and feelings have kept you together and helped at other times? Clearly, you have strengths and resources to call upon which have served you in the past or you would not be here today. Moreover, it is apparent that you want to find a way out or you would not be talking with me now. Let the positive, constructive forces within you begin to take over. Every time you dwell on the destructive, suicidal part of yourself, it reinforces the weak, negative side of you. The strong, healthy part of you must be permitted to grow.

7.   S: I feel so down, so low a lot of the time, but at others I become so agitated I don't think I can stand it.

     I: The feelings tend to overwhelm you but they will pass. The ache and despair of depression will lift. Such feelings will not continue indefinitely, although you may find that hard to believe the way you feel right now.

8.   S: Maybe so, but one solution is to just end it all. That would end it and relieve me of the ache and the pressure.

     I: (The patient is crying for help, testing the intervenor here.) Is that the solution you really want? (The patient is talking as if he or she will still be alive later with the words "relieve me of the ache and the pressure." At some point such as this, if appropriate, hope can be given by making a contract with the patient to maintain life for a given period of time.) I know things can get better for you and I am willing to work with you, but I want you to agree not to kill yourself for the next three months, and at the end of that time we will renegotiate our contract.

The kind of agreement indicated in the last exchange provides an anchor, takes off some of the pressure from the patient, and conveys that idea that hope is real and that he or she is worth helping. Hospitalization should always be explored with an acutely suicidal person who does not seem to improve or worsens during interviews, but confinement, itself, is simply a maintenance arrangement until active treatment can begin.

It will be of value to the reader to underscore the fact that the remarks and responses by the suicidal person in crisis and the clinician cited above are not to be necessarily seen as literal expressions, although some of them may be on certain occasions. The philosophy of the approach to such problem behavior is the significant feature. The reader will observe that the responses are neither psychoanalytic nor nondirective in nature. Both of these classical approaches are not only unsuitable but can be damaging to the individual in a suicidal crisis. Such a person does not possess the inner resources or verbal skills needed to comprehend psychoanalytic interpretations, supply associative material, or be verbally facile enough to deal with client centered reflections of feeling. What the suicidal person needs is support in abundance, direction in thought and feeling, guidance to effective action, reassurance, and advice when indicated. The notion that people will not grow and gain insights on their own with direct advice and guidance, I believe, is sheer folly. The person in a suicidal crisis needs immediate help. Innovative and perceptive direction can restore distraught lives to healthy productivity in a way which is often unique and creative. More traditional, dynamic psychotherapy may be helpful following the crisis period, however, after careful examination.

FRONT LINE INTERVENTION

It is important to keep in mind that skilled clinicians are typically not the first to become aware of serious personal crises. A number of persons who come in contact regularly with people in crisis may provide front line intervention, both in terms of spotting the difficulty during its incipiency and in rendering initial "psychological first aid." Such persons may be club leaders, clergymen, teachers, and physicians. Youngsters who are in difficulty emotionally are apt to talk to another adult, rather than to their own parents. It is important for a youngster to have a leader or counselor who can establish the image of a stable and trustworthy friend. Due to the lack of such a relationship with adults, young people often turn to peers, many of whom are not capable of providing support or may be harmful influences. Persons at any age can and do take their own lives and the signs should be understood by all of us. Skilled suicidologists (persons trained in suicide prevention) can contact such front line intervenors to offer training and to enlist them as sources of referrals. Suicidal persons frequently do not contact psychologists or psychiatrists directly at the onset of their disturbances and need to be referred for treatment.

LEGAL CAVEATS

Since malpractice is a possibility when treating suicidal persons, I believe it is prudent to be aware of basic precautions involved in such interactions.

BASIC PRECAUTIONS

Suicide Must Be Proven. Legally, suicide is presumed not to have occurred as an essential premise of life. When doubtful or equivocal suicides are at issue, a psychological autopsy is often done to determine the actual cause of death. This is an extensive reassessment of the events preceding and surrounding the death, with all factors taken into account, and with extensive interviews of important persons who knew or were associated with the victim for at least six months prior to death.

Proximate Cause Must Exist. In legal terms **proximate** cause and **remote** cause are elements for evaluation in ascertaining negligence or malpractice. Proximate cause means that, due to a clear error of omission or commission on the part of the professional, the victim was so influenced that suicide followed. Without such influence suicide would not have occurred. Remote cause is that which exerts some influence on the subject but which is not so directly impactful that death would ensue. Remote cause is insufficient for proof of malpractice; proximate cause is necessary for conviction.

The Average Man Or Person Standard Enters. This standard states that the professional intervenor or therapist behaved in a manner, at all times, consonant with what would be expected and provided by another person with equal training, under the same conditions at that particular time. In essence, the suicide prevention professional intervenor would do well to constantly ask himself or herself if what is being done is likely to be the same thing that another colleague would do under those circumstances. For example, one might question lack of direction and guidance for the patient or lack of consideration of the possibility of hospitalization in acute cases where there is nobody to observe the patient in crisis.

Never Delay Or Avoid Consultation. No professional can do everything under all conditions. Be ready to ask for assistance or suggestions from another responsible party. If a legal action should follow, the professional is better off demonstrating that a single opinion or judgment was not all that entered into decision-making or disposition of the case.

Hospital Patients Should Be Monitored Assiduously. With seriously suicidal persons, the possibility of loss of life increases when the subject is not constantly observed during acute periods. During the night, the subject should be checked every 10 to 15 minutes. At time of discharge, the decision should be a team effort and risk of suicide carefully evaluated. Risks must be taken to promote self-confidence, ego strength, and responsibility, but only after the most thorough-going input from all available sources.

If these procedures are followed, the professional should have little fear of being found culpable in a lawsuit surrounding a suicidal death. Family members can be helpful adjuncts in treatment, and their involvement may also help guard against possible repercussions after a tragic event has occurred.

Calvin J. Frederick, Ph.D., is currently Chief of the Psychology Service at the VA Medical Center in West Los Angeles, Brentwood Division and is a Professor in the Department of Psychiatry and Biobehavioral Sciences at the University of California at Los Angeles. Formerly, he served as Chief of Disaster Assistance and Emergency Mental Health at the National Institute of Mental Health and was a Professor at the George Washington University School of Medicine. His articles on suicide have appeared in numerous publications. Dr. Frederick may be contacted at the Veteran's Administration Medical Center, Brentwood Building 258, 11301 Wilshire Boulevard, Los Angeles CA 90037, 691/B116 B.

RESOURCES

Beck, A. T., Resnik, H. L. P., & Lettieri, D. J. THE PREDICTION OF SUICIDE. Bowie, MD: Charles Press, 1974.

Frederick, C. J. Current trends in suicidal behavior in the United States. AMERICAN JOURNAL OF PSYCHOTHERAPY, 1978, 32, 172-200.

Frederick, C. J. Drug abuse as indirect self-destructive behavior. In N. L. Farberow (Ed.), THE MANY FACES OF SUICIDE. New York: McGraw-Hill, 1980.

Frederick C. J. Suicide prevention and crisis intervention in mental health emergencies. In C. E. Walker (Ed.), CLINICAL PRACTICE OF PSYCHOLOGY. New York: Pergamon, 1981.

Frederick, C. J. & Resnik, H. L. P. Interventions with suicidal patients. JOURNAL OF CONTEMPORARY PSYCHOTHERAPY, 1970, 2, 103-109.

Frederick, C. J., Resnik, H. L. P., & Wittlin, B. J. Self-destructive aspects of hard-core addiction. ARCHIVES OF GENERAL PSYCHIATRY, 1973, 28, 579-585.

Shneidman, E., Farberow, N. L., & Litman, R. E. THE PSYCHOLOGY OF SUICIDE. New York: Science House, 1970.

ANTIDEPRESSANT MEDICATION IN THE OUTPATIENT TREATMENT OF DEPRESSION: GUIDE FOR NONMEDICAL PSYCHOTHERAPISTS

Kenneth Byrne and Stephen L. Stern

Depression is probably the presenting complaint most frequently encountered by practitioners of outpatient psychotherapy. Although psychotherapy alone may be helpful to many depressed patients, others may more readily respond to therapy in combination with antidepressant medication. As a group, clinical psychologists receive little training about the nature of these drugs and the kind of patients likely to benefit from them. This article is intended as an introduction to the role of this group of medications in clinical practice.

EVALUATION OF THE DEPRESSED PATIENT

There are many factors to consider in the complete evaluation of a depressed patient. This article focuses on those aspects directly relevant to determining the appropriateness of antidepressant drug therapy.

SYMPTOMS OF DEPRESSION

One important criterion in determining whether a patient is a candidate for antidepressant medication is the presence of biological symptoms, which include disorders of sleep, appetite, sexual functioning, and psychomotor activity. It is important to question the patient specifically about these symptoms, since many patients will not spontaneously mention them.

The most characteristic sleep disturbances in depression are early morning awakening and middle-of-the-night insomnia, in which patients awaken in the early morning hours or the middle of the night and have difficulty returning to sleep. Difficulty falling asleep, though common in depression, is nonspecific, since it can also be seen in patients with anxiety. Some depressed patients may experience hypersomnia, that is, sleeping significantly longer than usual. Both patients with insomnia and hypersomnia complain of fatigue and low energy during the day.

---

*This contribution is reprinted from Vol. 12(3) of PROFESSIONAL PSYCHOLOGY, copyright 1981 by the American Psychological Association. Reprinted/Adapted by permission of the publisher and authors.

Decreased appetite and weight loss are common in depression. However, some depressed patients may eat more than usual and gain weight.

Both men and women may complain of decreased interest in and satisfaction from sex, and men may complain of impotence. Women may experience menstrual irregularity.

Disorders of psychomotor activity consist of retardation and agitation. The patient with psychomotor retardation speaks and moves slowly, whereas the agitated patient constantly fidgets and may pace up and down.

Patients with biological symptoms often report a decreased interest in their usual activities. They may also experience anhedonia, a loss of ability to experience pleasure. Their mood may not be reactive to environmental changes but may vary according to the time of day. Classically, it is worst in the morning.

Some patients may initially describe problems other than depression, such as anxiety or a generalized boredom with life and difficulty experiencing pleasure. They may describe their life-style as "grey" and limited or may talk of "existential woes" and the meaninglessness of human existence. Most patients with these "masked depressions" (Lesse, 1974) will admit to a feeling of sadness if questioned **directly**, though some may not. The diagnosis of depression is difficult in these cases, but may be suggested by the presence of biological symptoms, a history of a recent loss, or a personal or family history of depression or mania. It is extremely important that these patients be properly diagnosed and treated for the underlying depressive disorder.

PSYCHIATRIC HISTORY

In evaluating the current complaints, it is important to ask in detail about previous periods of depression, including precipitating events, symptoms, and treatment. It is also essential to inquire about possible prior episodes of mania or hypomania. These periods are typically characterized by a euphoric mood, though in some cases irritability may be present. The patient is very active and talkative, requiring less sleep than usual, with unrealistically inflated self-esteem and poor judgment. Impulsive spending or sexual escapades are typical of these episodes. During periods of severe depression, the patient's view may be so distorted that these "high" periods are forgotten. Thus, it is helpful to question a spouse or other family member, as part of taking the history. It is also worth asking the patient about this again, after the severe depression has lifted. Patients with a past history of mania are considered to have a bipolar depression. Those without such a history are said to have a unipolar depression.

FAMILY HISTORY

It is essential to determine if there is a family history of depression or mania, since the existence of these disorders in family members may increase the likelihood that this patient will benefit from antidepressant medication. Include parents, grandparents, aunts, uncles, cousins, siblings, and children. Also remember to ask about alcoholism, since this is very often associated with an underlying depression. If there has been a family history of depression, it is useful to know what treatment was instituted, if any, and with what results. If a family member responded positively to medication, there is a good chance that this patient may also respond well.

MEDICAL STATUS

The examiner should also inquire about the patient's current and past medical status. This should include questions about what medication the patient takes and what other doctors have been consulted. One should specifically inquire about the presence of heart problems, high blood pressure, chest pains, and memory difficulties. If the patient is on other medications or has some physical illness, such as heart disease, it will be useful to alert the prescribing physician, since such issues play an important role in decisions about the type and dosage of medication. It is possible that either a medical illness or a medication (in particular, medication for high blood pressure) might be the cause of the patient's depression. Do not overlook asking about use of alcohol or illicit drugs. Many depressed patients essentially medicate themselves by frequent use of alcohol, "uppers," or marijuana. Finally, depressed patients should also have a physical examination to rule out organic illness that might produce a depression. This can usually be arranged in consultation with the consulting psychiatrist.

SELECTION OF PATIENTS LIKELY TO BENEFIT FROM ANTIDEPRESSANT MEDICATION

The decision to refer a patient for medication evaluation is based primarily on the symptoms of the depression and its severity. Most patients with moderate to severe depression accompanied by biological symptoms should be referred. A family history of depression will also indicate a likely candidate, particularly if a relative had a positive response to medication. A patient who was helped by drug treatment in the past is likely to benefit again. If a depression is mild, particularly if it has been of brief duration, it is reasonable to treat the patient with psychotherapy alone for a few weeks and re-evaluate. For a moderate depression **without** biological signs, it is reasonable to try psychotherapy alone for a few weeks and then re-evaluate. All patients with severe depression should be referred for evaluation regarding medication or psychiatric hospitalization.

A group of depressed patients has been identified and diagnosed as "atypical depressions" (Bielski & Friedel, 1977). These individuals tend to experience few biological symptoms and have a depressed mood that is reactive to the environment. This is often accompanied by fatigue, anxiety, irritability, initial insomnia, and phobic and hypochondriacal symptoms. These patients can usually also be treated with medication with favorable results.

MEDICATIONS USED IN TREATING DEPRESSION*

There are three principal groups of medications used in treating depression. They are discussed in the following material and summarized in Table 1.

---

*Three new antidepressant medications have recently become available for clinical use. They are amoxapine (Asendin), maprotiline (Ludiomil), and trazodone (Desyrel). Although they are structurally different from standard tricyclics, it is not yet clear whether they offer a significant clinical advantage.

TRICYCLIC ANTIDEPRESSANTS

Tricyclics are the most widely used and generally the most effective antidepressant medications. There are seven tricyclic drugs in current use in this country: amitriptyline (Elavil, Endep), imipramine (Tofranil, SK-Pramine), doxepin (Sinequan, Adapin), nortriptyline (Pamelor, Aventyl), desipramine (Norpramin, Pertrofrane), protriptyline (Vivactil), and trimipramine (Surmontil). Although all these drugs are, in general, equally effective, certain patients may be helped by one but not by another. There is no proven way of predicting which drug will be best for a particular patient. Psychiatrists often choose tricyclics on the basis of their sedative properties. Amitriptyline, doxepin, and trimipramine are the most sedating, with protriptyline and desipramine least sedating, and imipramine and nortriptyline in an intermediate range. More sedating medications are often prescribed for anxious, agitated patients or for those with insomnia; less sedating or activating drugs are used when psychomotor retardation is present.

TABLE 1: ANTIDEPRESSANT MEDICATIONS

Category	Generic Name	Trade Name	Approximate dosage range[a] (mg/day)
Tricyclic antidepressants	Amitriptyline	Elavil Endep	75-300
	Desipramine	Norpramin Pertofrane	75-200
	Doxepin	Adapin Sinequan	75-300
	Imipramine	Imavate SK-Pramine Tofranil	75-300
	Nortriptyline	Aventyl HCl Pamelor	50-100
	Protriptyline	Vivactil	15-60
	Trimipramine	Surmontil	75-300
Monoamine oxidase (MAO) inhibitors	Isocarboxazid	Marplan	10-50
	Phenelzine	Nardil	45-90
	Tranylcypromine	Parnate	20-40
Lithium carbonate	Lithium carbonate	Eskalith Lithane Lithobid Lithonate	900-1800

[a]Some patients, particularly the elderly, adolescents, and those with medical illnesses, may require lower dosages. Others may require higher dosages. For the new antidepressants, the approximate dosage ranges are: amoxapine (Asendin) 150-600 mg/day, maprotiline (Ludiomil) 75-300 mg/day, and trazodone (Desyrel) 150-600 mg/day.

Some depressed patients may begin to feel better a few days after starting medication, whereas others may feel better after 2 or 3 weeks. Such a delay is also common with monoamine oxidase (MAO) inhibitors and lithium. Many patients who respond rapidly to antidepressants may do so because of a placebo effect; that is, their belief in the medication leads to their rapid improvement. About half the patients who ultimately respond to a tricyclic would also respond to a placebo. There is, however, no reliable way of determining in advance who would be a placebo responder.

Common side effects of the tricyclics include dry mouth, blurred vision, lightheadedness, rapid heart beat, and sedation. Most side effects tend to decrease with time. They can also be reduced, if necessary, by decreasing the dosage or switching to another medication. Occasionally, these drugs may affect cardiac functioning in elderly patients or those with heart disease. For physically healthy patients, a single daily dose at bedtime usually minimizes side effects during waking hours, improves sleep (if it is a sedating tricyclic), and is also easier to remember. To be effective, it is extremely important that the medication be taken in a regular daily dosage, not on an "as needed" basis. Since these drugs can be very dangerous in overdose, they should be used with particular caution with potentially suicidal patients.

MONOAMINE OXIDASE (MAO) INHIBITORS

Although the MAO inhibitors are probably not so broadly effective as the tricyclics, they appear to be effective in certain patients with "atypical" depression and with hypersomnia and weight gain. Patients with bipolar depression may also do well on these agents, used in combination with lithium to avoid precipitating a manic episode. Other patients who do not respond to tricyclics may also benefit from MAO inhibitors. There are three MAO inhibitors in current use in this country: phenelzine (Nardil), tranylcypromine (Parnate), and isocarboxazid (Marplan).

Patients receiving MAO inhibitors must adhere rigorously to a diet that excludes certain foods such as cheese, chocolate, raisins, beer, and wine; otherwise, they may experience a reaction in which their blood pressure rises markedly. These drugs are quite safe when taken with the necessary precautions. Like tricyclics, they are very dangerous in overdose.

The MAO inhibitors produce some of the same side effects as the tricyclic drugs, including dry mouth and lightheadedness. Irritability and agitation occasionally occur, and insomnia is fairly common. To minimize insomnia, they are usually taken early in the day.

LITHIUM CARBONATE

This simple chemical salt dramatically relieves the symptoms of mania in most patients with manic-depressive illness (bipolar affective disorder). It has also been shown to be effective in preventing future episodes of mania and depression and in the treatment of selected cases of acute depression. Patients with bipolar depression are the most likely to show an antidepressant response to lithium.

Many psychiatrists consider lithium to be the initial drug of choice for bipolar depressed patients because it appears to be as effective as tricyclics but will not precipitate a manic episode, as tricyclics may. Others recommend using a tricyclic alone or in combination with lithium. Lithium may also be helpful in some unipolar depressed patients who do not respond to tricyclic drugs, perhaps particularly those with a family history of mania.

Lithium is a safe drug when prescribed by a physician familiar with its use and when necessary precautions are observed. The level of lithium in the patient's blood must be closely monitored to maintain it within the therapeutic range. Lithium is less likely to be effective in doses below the therapeutic range and is potentially quite dangerous above that range. It is usually prescribed in divided doses throughout the day. Common side effects of lithium at therapeutic levels include tremor, weight gain, and increased urine volume, with a compensatory increase in thirst.

OTHER MEDICATIONS

Neuroleptics or antipsychotics, such as thioridazine (Mellaril), benzodiazepines, such as diazepam (Valium), and stimulants, such as methylphenidate (Ritalin), are sometimes prescribed as the primary medication for depressed outpatients. The evidence for their effectiveness in this population is limited. Their use poses risks of neurologic side effects for the neuroleptics and of dependency for the other drugs. Thus, their use as the primary drug for depressed outpatients is not recommended.

MAKING THE REFERRAL

For psychotherapists who have not been medically trained, the question of drug treatment can bring up a variety of feelings. Perhaps most common are professional rivalries and remaining insecurities about one's competence. These can sometimes underlie seemingly plausible reasons for not making medication referrals. Among these are the idea that if depressive symptoms are relieved through medication, the patient will lose motivation for further psychotherapy. For some patients this will be true and probably indicates that they were poor candidates for insight psychotherapy to begin with. In many other cases, the relief of painful depressive symptoms enables the patient to participate much more fruitfully in the psychotherapeutic process. Medical consultation may also be avoided because of the idea that medication will gratify the patient's "dependency needs." If there is a reasonable chance that painful symptoms will be helped by medication, the patient will gain more than he or she might lose by this "gratification." There will also be many other opportunities to explore this area.

It is preferable to make the referral to a psychiatrist, although if this is not feasible, a nonpsychiatric physician may also be helpful, provided that he or she is experienced in the use of antidepressant medications. It is essential that the psychologist have a good working relationship with the physician, based on mutual respect and open communication. Anything less than this is likely to stir up unnecessary anxieties in the therapist and is bound to affect the overall treatment. We suggest the therapist be familiar with the psychiatrist's typical practice regarding appointment times, length of sessions, and fees. It is also helpful to have someone who can be available to the patient and psychologist by phone.

In making the recommendation for a consultation, the psychologist should not state that the patient will be placed on medication, since the psychiatrist may feel that it is not indicated. It is usually best to talk with the psychiatrist beforehand to give a brief description of the patient's problem, the course of therapy thus far, a brief history of previous treatment, and the diagnostic impression.

It is not uncommon for depressed patients to respond negatively to the idea of drug treatment, perhaps especially those who refer themselves directly to a psychologist, since they may have made this choice partly because of an aversion to medication. The therapist needs to explore the reasons for this reluctance. One common reason is a concern that medication will be habit forming. The patient should be reassured that this is not the case for any of the antidepressants. Some patients may be insistent on wanting to overcome the problem "by myself, without medication." In this case it is helpful to explain that medication can often relieve unpleasant symptoms and facilitate the psychological changes that are part of the psychotherapy process. After there has been improvement, the medication can be gradually decreased and eventually withdrawn entirely without the person becoming depressed again. (However, some patients with frequently recurring depression may need to stay on medication indefinitely.)

The psychologist can also inquire whether the patient has had a negative experience with medication, such as unpleasant side effects or a failure to be helped. Patients can be reassured that there are many antidepressants available, so that they are quite likely to be helped, even if they did not have a positive outcome before.

If a patient still refuses to consider drug treatment, it is reasonable to continue psychotherapy and bring the matter up again if necessary.

How patients respond to medication, as to any other therapeutic modality, will be influenced considerably by their own character structure and the dynamics of the psychotherapeutic relationship. The use of medication must be integrated into the overall psychotherapy. Some of the theoretical and clinical aspects of this integration are discussed in a recent paper by Radomisli (1979).

Appropriate usage of antidepressant medications can be an extremely useful complement to psychotherapy. It can provide rapid relief from painful depressive symptoms, allowing the patient and therapist to move on toward other goals.

Kenneth Byrne, Ph.D., is currently with the Management consulting firm of Hay Associates in Philadelphia. He holds a doctorate in clinical psychology from Hahnemann Medical College. Dr. Byrne can be reached at 7903 Winston Road, Philadelphia, PA 19118.

Stephen L. Stern, M.D., is currently director of the Affective Disorders Clinic and Associate Professor of Psychiatry, The Ohio State University College of Medicine, and Staff Psychiatrist, VA Outpatient Clinic, in Columbus, Ohio. He received his medical degree from New York University. Dr. Stern may be contacted at 473 W. 12th Avenue, Columbus, OH 43210.

RESOURCES

Bielski, R. J. & Friedel, R. O. Subtypes of depression - diagnosis and medical management. WESTERN JOURNAL OF MEDICINE, 1977, **126**, 347-352.

Lesse, S. (Ed.). MASKED DEPRESSION. New York: Jason Aronson, 1974.

Radomisli, M. The use of antidepressant medication as an adjunct to psychoanalytic therapy. In D. S. Milman & G. D. Goldman (Eds.), PARAMETERS IN PSYCHOANALYTIC PSYCHOTHERAPY. Dubuque, IA: Kendall Hunt, 1979.

STRESS INOCULATION THERAPY FOR ANGER CONTROL

Raymond W. Novaco

Disorders of anger and aggression have been insufficiently understood by clinicians and can pose special problems for treatment. Anger has received scant attention in the psychological literature, certainly far less than anxiety and depression. Behavioristic traditions favored the study of aggressive actions over the examination of anger, but the extensive attention to aggression in psychological research was largely confined to the area of personality and social psychology and was lacking in clinical relevance. Prior to Novaco (1975) no treatment procedure existed for anger problems, although some efforts were being made to utilize systematic desensitization. The classical conditioning models, however, offered neither an adequate conception of anger disorders nor a sufficient therapeutic method for their modification.

Therapeutic modification of anger and aggression is complicated by difficulties associated with treating persons who are prone to provocation. Angry clients can elicit anxiety in therapists, as the potential of danger is sensed. Descriptions and expressions of anger, rage, and hostile impulses may unduly alarm therapists who may then intentionally or inadvertently curtail the client's disclosures and thereby undermine the helping process. Moreover, persons who have angry, antagonistic dispositions or response styles are inclined to become frustrated and impatient, which can interfere with the treatment process itself. When desired treatment effects are not quickly forthcoming, the client may become inclined to disengage from therapy. In this regard, it is advantageous for the treatment program to be clearly defined, structured, and time-limited, so as to minimize ambiguity and frustration that might result from vague expectations regarding treatment.

This contribution describes the application of a cognitive-behavioral approach to the treatment of anger problems. The treatment procedure, although uniquely conceptualized, incorporates a variety of methods developed in the field of behavior therapy, including methods referred to as self-control, semantic therapies, cognitive therapies, and problem solving therapies. Extensive accounts of these various approaches and the developing area of cognitive-behavioral interventions can be found in Beck, Rush, Shaw, and Emery (1979); Kendall and Hollon (1979); Mahoney and Arnkoff (1977); and Meichenbaum (1977).

The treatment approach to anger disorders, or what I have called "chronic anger problems" and "proneness to provocation," was rooted in the belief that enough was known about aggressive behavior and about how to intervene clinically with maladaptive thoughts and emotions to formulate a therapeutic procedure that could be systematically applied to the management of anger.

From the aggression and the behavior therapy literature, a set of propositions regarding anger management was generated, from which a treatment procedure was constructed that incorporated cognitive coping and relaxation training components (Novaco, 1975). The cognitive coping procedures were based on the work of Meichenbaum (1974, 1975a) on self-instructional methods. The relaxation training procedures followed from the techniques developed by Jacobsen (1938), and formulated as a self-control procedure by Goldfried (1971).

No previous work of an experimental sort existed with regard to the effect of cognitive interventions on anger regulation. The experimental investigation reported in Novaco (1975, 1976b) was the first such study. However, desensitization by relaxation counter-conditioning had been shown to be effective in reducing anger in several experimental investigations (Evans & Hearn, 1973; Hearn & Evans, 1972; O'Donnell & Worell, 1973; Rimm, deGroot, Boord, Reiman, & Dillow, 1971), as well as in case studies (Evans, 1971; Herrell, 1971). I found that the cognitive treatment interventions were an effective means of reducing anger and facilitating constructive coping in response to provocation (Novaco, 1975; 1976b). Furthermore, the cognitive therapy component was more effective than the relaxation therapy component.

The treatment approach to anger subsequently was reconceptualized in terms of a concept called **stress inoculation** that was first proposed by Meichenbaum and Cameron (1973) and later by Meichenbaum (1975b). This reformulation was prompted not only by the attractiveness of the stress inoculation model, but also by my growing interest in the area of human stress and adaptation. The stress inoculation approach was first developed for anger problems as applied to the training of law enforcement officers who routinely must manage an assortment of provocation and conflict situations (Novaco, 1977a) and was then applied clinically in a case study of a hospitalized patient with severe anger problems (Novaco, 1977b). Meichenbaum and Novaco (1978) have described the development of this treatment approach and its usefulness as a preventive intervention.

My growing interest and experimental work in the area of stress led to a greater emphasis on environmental determinants of anger. Contextual conditions and life circumstances were seen to activate physiological arousal and shape anger-engendering cognitions. Therefore, an effort was made to articulate the treatment model and the conception of anger in a way that incorporated what was known about human stress, as well as human aggression. These concepts are developed below.

ANGER, AGGRESSION, AND STRESS

Provocation to anger has salient manifestations. Anger arousal is marked by physiological activation in the cardiovascular and endocrine systems, tension in the skeletal musculature, antagonistic thought patterns, and, at times, aggressive behavior. The view of anger taken here is that it is an emotional state defined by the presence of physiological arousal and cognitive labeling (Konecni, 1975b; Novaco, 1975). The cognitive label need not be precisely that of "anger" but may be something semantically proximate, such as "annoyed," "irritated," "enraged," "provoked," and so on. The cognitive labeling dimension may be otherwise viewed as the "subjective affect" dimension of the emotional state.

Implicit in the cognitive labeling is some impulse to action. That is, the cognitive labeling process inherently involves an inclination on the part of the person to act in an antagonistic or confrontative manner towards the source of provocation. These action impulses, in part, define the emotional state and are incorporated in the cognitive labeling process. This is to say that people are "angry," rather than described otherwise, precisely because they are antagonistically inclined. The urge to attack, injure, or destroy by real or symbolic actions is part of what differentiates the emotional state as anger, as opposed to something else, like "being upset" or "tense."

From this perspective, certain quandaries are resolved by definition. A common question one encounters among clinicians, particularly those who favor psychodynamic models, is: What about the person who is angry but does not know it (repressed anger)? Assuming that the clinician is getting reliable and valid information from the client, a person who does not "know" that he or she is angry (or something semantically approximate) is not angry. The clinician or someone else may judge that the client should be angry, in view of the prevailing circumstances, but observer judgments must not be confused with the subject's own emotional state. Additionally, the therapist may successfully persuade or induce clients to reconstrue their feelings as anger, and, upon doing so, clients then behave in angry ways which may have some instrumental value for problem resolution. The clinician might then come to the erroneous conclusion that this proves the individuals were indeed angry all along. The point is that once a person actually becomes angry, he or she then begins to think, feel, and act in a different manner (i.e., the person thought, acted, and felt the way people do when they are angry, as opposed to something else). For these reasons and obvious theoretical axioms, the concept of repressed anger is not meaningful in the present system.

The general model of anger is that of a cognitively mediated emotional state that is reciprocally related to cognitions and to behavior. The theoretical foundation of this model and its relationship to a larger conceptual framework for human stress have been developed in Novaco (1979). A central proposition is that there is no direct relationship between external events and anger. The arousal of anger is a cognitively mediated process. Expectations and appraisals are designated as the principal classes of cognitions that determine the occurrence of anger (Figure 1).

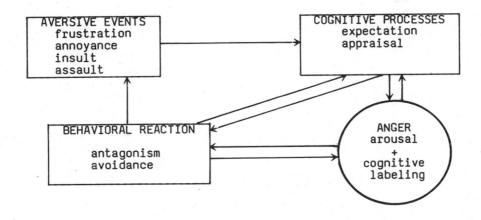

Figure 1.

Another proposition is that anger is neither necessary nor sufficient for aggression, yet it is a significant antecedent of aggression and has a mutually influenced relationship with aggression. This bidirectional causality postulate (Konecni, 1975a) means that the level of anger influences the level of aggression and vice versa. Whether or not aggression occurs following provocation is thought to be a function of various social learning factors other than anger, such as reinforcement contingencies, expected outcomes, and modeling influences. These same social learning factors can also influence the occurrence of aggression independent of anger arousal. Thus, it is possible for someone to aggress without becoming angry, as when the infliction of injury or damage is expected to produce personal gain or when the aggressive act is a well-learned behavior. Anger is viewed as an affective stress reaction (Novaco, 1979). That is, anger arousal is one kind of response that occurs in conjunction with exposure to environmental demands.

Stress is understood as a hypothetical state defined by the functional relationships between environmental demands (stressors) and adverse health and behavior consequences (stress reactions). The demands or stressors are elements of various environmental fields (i.e., physical, biological, psychological, social) which exert pressure on the organism to adapt. The routine exposure to environmental demands, in the absence of commensurate coping resources, induces stress reactions that represent impairments to psychological functioning and physical health.

The reasons for the stress perspective are threefold: (a) the range of conditions that function as determinants of anger, (b) the range of consequences linked with repeated occurrences of anger, and (c) the involvement of anger in behavior styles of coping with stress. Each of these points has direct relevance to the therapeutic intervention approach. Because of their importance to the treatment procedure, I will elaborate on them when presenting the intervention method.

The stress inoculation procedures are a coping skills therapy. That is, they attempt to develop the client's competence to adapt to stressful events in such a way that stress is reduced and personal goals are achieved. The term "inoculation" is a medical metaphor. The therapeutic process hypothetically works by first developing coping skills and then exposing the client to manageable doses of a stressor that arouse, but do not overwhelm, his or her defenses. The client thereby learns to cope with the stressful events that have a high probability of occurrence in his or her life. Additionally, by learning how to regulate thoughts, emotions, and behavior and to optimize environmental conditions so as to reduce exposure to stressors, anger management is achieved by preventive means, as well as by coping activities.

As a cognitive-behavioral intervention, the treatment is based on theoretical ideas of cognitive mediation. The anger management procedures are based on the conviction that emotional arousal and the course of action that such arousal instigates are determined by one's cognitive structuring of the situation - specifically, by one's **expectations** and **appraisals**. This emphasis on cognitive determinants reflects the influence of the personality theories of George Kelly (1955) and Julian Rotter (1954), as well as the impetus provided by Albert Ellis (1962), who in turn refers us to the Stoic philosophers and the teachings of Buddhism. Secondly, the procedures are predicted on the proposition that how one acts in a situation influences how one feels. This follows from the James-Lange theory of emotion (James, 1890).

The Konecni (1975a) bidirectional causality model also assumes that there is a continuous feedback loop between behavior and internal emotional state.

The treatment approach consists of three basic phases: (a) cognitive preparation, (b) skill acquisition, and (c) application training. Each of these phases will be described in detail below, along with a recommended format for conducting each therapeutic session. First, some things must be said about how to understand anger problems.

THE ASSESSMENT OF ANGER PROBLEMS

As an emotional state, anger has adaptive as well as maladaptive functions. It may energize coping activity, act as a discriminative cue for problem-solving efforts, or serve as a vehicle for communicating negative sentiment. On the other hand, it can disrupt information processing, defeat the opportunity for self-scrutiny, and instigate aggressive behavior. Analysis of the functional properties of anger (Novaco, 1976a) indicates that it should not automatically be viewed as a negative or undesirable condition of the organism. The determination of anger as a clinical problem is a matter to be evaluated in terms of various response parameters (frequency, intensity, duration, and mode of expression) by which we can gauge the severity of anger reactions with regard to effects on performance, health, interpersonal relationships, and lawful behavior. Ultimately, the determination that someone "has a problem with anger" is the result of a cost analysis. That is, what are the psychological, social, and medical costs associated with the person's anger reactions, and to what extent is the client willing to absorb those costs.

The assessment process begins with an understanding of anger functions. That is, in order to determine whether the person has an anger problem, one should first recognize the variety of ways that anger affects behavior. This functional analysis of anger is elaborated in Novaco (1976a). The basic ideas are that anger has the following functions, which are not mutually exclusive: (a) it **energizes** behavior by increasing the vigor of our responses; (b) it **disrupts** information processing and task performance; (c) it is an **expressive** communication of negative sentiment; (d) it serves as a **defensive** reaction to ego-threat; (e) it acts as a **discriminative** cue for coping; (f) it **instigates** aggressive activity; (g) it **potentiates** a sense of control; and (h) it **promotes** an image of the self, in the sense of impression management. Recognizing the multiple functions of anger, one can see that anger affects us in both positive and negative ways as judged from the outcomes of the psychological process. The therapeutic approach is designed to help the client maximize the positive functions and minimize the negative or maladaptive functions.

Bearing in mind these general concepts, the assessment of anger should address the **dimensions** of anger reactions. That is, anger responses to provocation events can be examined with respect to several parameters: (a) frequency, (b) intensity, (c) duration, and (d) mode of expression. Information on these parameters, obtained in the clinical interview, should be derived from a situational analysis whereby the client's anger reactions are examined according to the settings, persons, and triggering stimuli that evoke them. A person's anger patterns may vary considerably across settings. For example, someone may get angry infrequently at work, but when anger does arise in that setting, the anger is suppressed and remains at a high level for long periods of time. In contrast, that same person may become angry frequently at home, but not at high levels of arousal, and may express it directly, thereby getting over it quickly. Although little is known empirically about these parameters of anger reactions, the treatment should be geared to what is learned in their regard. This will be discussed in the presentation of the treatment procedure. At this time, I am gathering parametric data on anger in conjunction with a large epidemiological project.

With regard to the "cost analysis" mentioned above, the **consequences** of anger reactions can be examined in relation to (a) effects on performance, (b) effect on relationships, and (c) effects on health. When anger has become chronic, it is part of a style of dealing with life demands and challenges. The client, as well as the therapist, must recognize the degree to which anger can impair work performance and other task-driven activities, sour relationships with loved ones and associates, and contribute to health jeopardizing conditions. By identifying the dimensions and consequences of anger reactions in conjunction with their situational correlates, the focus of treatment can be sharpened.

A thorough assessment is obviously important for any therapeutic method, but the situational and dimensional analysis is of particular importance for the stress inoculation approach. First, the therapeutic procedures are self-control methods, which require that clients become astute observers of their own behavior. Second, the stress inoculation approach utilizes a technique whereby the person learns to prepare for a provocation experience and to engage in self-instructions to guide captions and behavior in responding to aversive events. Careful attention must therefore be given to the social circumstances of anger reactions, identifying the settings of anger episodes, the events and persons that trigger the anger reactions, and the form of the anger reaction as distinguished by the parameters given above. This information is directly relevant to the construction of the provocation hierarchy to be used in the "application training" phase of the treatment.

In order to determine the range of situations in which a client's anger is aroused, the type of situation most likely to arouse anger, and the overall magnitude of a respondent's proneness to provocation, an inventory of provocation circumstances, the Novaco Provocation Inventory (NPI) has been developed. An early version of this inventory was reported in Novaco (1975). The current instrument consists of 80 items for which the respondent rates the degree of anger on a 5-point scale. Extensive data have been collected on the inventory for clinical and nonclinical samples, and a report is in preparation. The inventory has a high internal consistency (r=.93 or above for various samples) and a satisfactory test-retest reliability (r=.82). Descriptive statistics and the inventory itself can be obtained by contacting me.

The total score for the inventory is the principal measure of anger, although subscales have been found to have differential predictive value. In the clinical interview, the client's ratings across the range of items on the NPI provide an avenue of inquiry into the anger problem. By sequentially reviewing with the client those items for which high anger ratings were obtained (i.e., given ratings of 5), a structured interview on anger patterns can be conducted. Respondents often discover common denominators for their anger reactions when their responses to the inventory are reviewed. For example, clients have commented, "I found that I am mostly bothered by things people say to me," or, "It seems that I get upset most when I'm not treated fairly," or, "It's all these little annoyances that shouldn't really bother me." In addition to the pre-treatment assessment, the inventory serves as a useful instrument to gauge the progress of treatment.

The situational analysis begun in the clinical interview and the inventory assessment proceeds further with the client's self-monitored tabulation of anger reactions. This self-monitored assessment should be conducted throughout treatment, but it is of key importance at the start of therapy. By means of a structured diary, the client records anger incidents (thus tabulating frequency) and is instructed to rate the degree of anger experienced when the event occurred. It is also useful to have them evaluate how effectively they handled the provocation. This self-monitoring procedure was used in Novaco (1975, 1977b), and it is integral to the "cognitive preparation" phase of the treatment, as is the entire assessment sequence.

Beyond the interview, inventory, and self-monitoring assessments, the use of physiological and behavioral test procedures might be considered. Because of the ease of measuring blood pressure and heart rate, and because of the relevance of cardiovascular arousal to anger, these physiological measures should be obtained and utilized in the treatment process and evaluation (cf. Novaco, 1975). Behavioral tests which gauge the client's coping skills can also be constructed, most easily in role play interactions. If videotape equipment is available, role play performance can be recorded and given as feedback to the client.

DETERMINANTS OF ANGER

An anger problem is not an anger problem. That is to say, the kinds of psychological deficits that result in the inability to manage anger are not homogeneous across individuals or clinical populations. The anger-related deficits of hypertensives, child abusing parents, time-urgent corporate executives, hospitalized depressives, juvenile delinquents, paranoids, combat veterans, and impulsive youngsters are likely to be quite different. Nor should these category labels be understood to imply homogeneity with respect to anger determinants.

Clients' anger experiences can be examined in terms of the events that happen in their lives, how they interpret and experience those events, and how they behave when and after these events occur. The factors will be referred to as **external circumstances, internal processes,** and **behavioral reactions.**

EXTERNAL CIRCUMSTANCES

The NPI facilitates the identification of anger-eliciting events. The cluster of events that routinely provoke anger for the client may be similar in nature (frustrations, annoyances, insults, inequities) or they may vary widely. To be sure, events are not provocative in themselves, nor do particular provocations have universal meaning or effect. The impact of an aversive event will depend upon a number of factors internal to the client.

The external determinants of anger, however, should not be understood to pertain only to discrete events. I have become increasingly persuaded that anger is very often a result of contextual influences that prime the individual to experience anger at some subsequent occurrence. My research on traffic congestion and long distance commuting (cf. Stokols & Novaco, 1981) and on conditions associated with military recruit training (cf. Novaco, Cook, & Sarason, 1983) indicates that cumulative exposure to aversive environmental elements progressively shapes a disposition for anger. While we are inclined to identify proximate events as the source of, or reason for, an anger reaction, it may well be the case that the anger was in large measure due to ambient, distal circumstances, rather than an acute, proximate event.

INTERNAL PROCESSES

Cognitive theorists have been fond of quoting the Stoic philosopher, Epictetus, who once said, "Men are not troubled by things themselves but by their thoughts about them." Two basic cognitive processes are thought to influence anger arousal: expectations and appraisals. Appraisal, which has been a prominent concept in the literature on psychological stress, pertains to the interpretation or meaning analysis of present and past events, as well as to the person's judgment about his or her ability to cope with the threat or demand. Expectations are the subjective probabilities that a person has concerning future events. These pertain both to the anticipated event and to one's behavior in response to the event. The theoretical development of these concepts of the cognitive mediation of anger and stress can be found in Novaco (1979).

Private speech is thought to reflect appraisals and expectations and to influence arousal and action. Private speech can act as a self-arousal mechanism. Antagonistic self-statements inflame anger. Ruminations about aversive experiences can prolong anger beyond the point that it would otherwise have dissipated. When we selectively remind ourselves about the noxious aspects of some experience, private speech serves to reinstigate the provocation. The content of the client's private speech thus should be examined for its anger instigative qualities, and it will provide information about the client's cognitive structuring of the situations of provocation. For angry clients, it is very important to short-circuit the preoccupation with provocation episodes. An extensive account of the development and function of private speech can be found in Meichenbaum (1977).

Somatic and affective factors also influence the occurrence of anger. Tension and agitation can prime anger reactions. High tension levels reflect a lowered ability of the person to cope with external demands. Consequently, provocation experiences have a magnified impact, and composed, conciliatory reactions are less likely to be available. Temperament or prevailing mood also influences anger. A person whose affective tone is characterized by ill humor is emotionally inclined to become angry or annoyed. In addition, anger can result from a failure to understand and appreciate the feelings of others. Lack of empathy has thwarted the resolution of many conflicts.

Sources of arousal summate. Arousal level is a function of aversive external circumstances, which successively add in their contribution, but internal conditions, such as the ingestion of stimulants and lowered blood sugar, also affect arousal state. Whatever the sources, physiological activation is a predisposing factor for anger. The regulation of anger must give attention to arousal reduction objectives.

Antagonistic responses to aversive events result in the definition of one's emotional state as anger. Anger is inferred from our behavior, as well as from other internal and external cues. According to the James-Lange theory of emotion, we derive knowledge about our emotion from observations of our own reactions in particular contexts. Furthermore, aggressive behavior in an interpersonal context is likely to incite others to behave aversively, which increases the probability for anger in the subject. Provocation sequences have been shown by Toch (1969) to escalate from minor annoyances to serious injury as each party in the interaction responds antagonistically.

For some clients, avoidance is the predominant response to provocation incidents. Here the anger is deliberately unexpressed at the time of provocation and may subsequently result in displaced aggression towards another target. The avoidance, withdrawal, or denial strategy may be adopted in one behavior setting (e.g., at the office) but, in another setting where inhibitory influences are absent (e.g., at home), the accumulated anger may be vented. Such avoidance response styles are likely to prolong physiological arousal (e.g., a longer recovery time for blood pressure to return to resting levels) and engender hostile attitudes, because the instigation to anger is left unchanged.

The factors that cause anger are transactionally related. Environmental circumstances, cognitions, arousal, and behavior operate in a reciprocally causal manner. It is oversimplified to view anger as caused by factors in any one of these domains (e.g., as being due to irrational belief systems) (Ellis, 1977). It is not a matter of thoughts causing emotions, or emotions causing behavior, or environmental contingencies causing everything else. Transactionality means that there exist processes of mutual influence between elements in the system. For angry clients, there are several aspects of the transactionality axiom that merit particular attention: (a) we are not the passive victim of life events but in fact have an active role in shaping the physical and social settings in which we function; (b) antagonistic thinking styles can prompt arousal and behavior which perpetuate the cognitive patterns; (c) arousal reduction promotes a balanced cognitive perspective, problem-solving, and adaptive action strategies; and (d) effective anger management in resolving conflicts enhances personal relationships and can elicit social reinforcement that supports a positive self-image.

Having introduced these ideas about anger and its determinants, the stress inoculation approach to treatment will be presented. Although the therapeutic method is not logically derived from the theoretical model of anger, the procedures do follow from the conceptual model and are logically consistent with it.

THE STRESS INOCULATION APPROACH

The therapeutic approach aims to impart anger control skills that are of three basic kinds: (a) preventive, (b) regulatory, and (c) executional. The general goals are to prevent anger from occurring when it is maladaptive, to enable the client to regulate arousal when it occurs, and to provide the performance skills needed to manage the provocation experience. Given the analysis of anger determinants just presented, it can be seen that anger control is not only a matter of what to do about anger when it is aroused, but preventing anger from occurring in the first place. The stress framework lends itself to these therapeutic goals.

Anger is incorporated into the larger theoretical framework of human stress for several reasons. First, one defining property of anger is physiological arousal, and it is unquestionably the case that arousal is activated by exposure to stressors, such as noise, heat, traffic congestion, crowding, difficult tasks, and high pressure job environments. The importance of this is that acute and prolonged exposure to such conditions may induce arousal that is experienced by the individual in conjunction with other events that pull for the cognitive label "anger." Exposure to certain stressors may produce arousal or excitation that decays slowly, leaving a residual excitation that can subsequently transfer to other experiences (Zillman, 1971). This residual excitation then adds in a nontrivial way to the arousal induced by subsequent events appraised in terms of anger. Thus, anger should be understood in terms of contextual conditions as well as the more immediate and identifiable provoking events. The stress framework provides theoretical guidelines for the disaggregation and analysis of contextual factors (environmental demands and moderators) that may act as determinants of anger and aggression.

Additionally, the routine exposure to stressors in the absence of commensurate coping resources has a cumulative adverse effect over time. With regard to anger, it is asserted that persons who are prone to provocation and are without the psychological resources for coping are thereby susceptible to health impairments (e.g., cardiovascular disorders), to diminished work efficiency, and to disruption of personal relationships. The point here is that chronic anger can have extensive consequences that go far beyond the simple experience of a perhaps unpleasant emotional state. Concepts of stress and adaptation can be useful for understanding the enduring or long-term effects of anger. The extended and unanticipated costs of anger proneness can easily go unrecognized.

Thus, the stress framework can improve our identification of the range of circumstances that engender anger and the varied impacts that anger can have on well-being. Furthermore, it is here suggested that among persons who are prone to provocation the anger response represents a learned coping style. That is, chronic anger reactions can be understood as a way of coping with life demands.

The anger management procedures intervene at the cognitive and behavioral levels to promote adaptive coping with provocation. The stress inoculation approach involves three basic steps or phases: cognitive preparation, skill acquisition, and application training. The theoretical developments of these phases of the treatment method can be found in Novaco (1979) and Meichenbaum (1977).

COGNITIVE PREPARATION

The cognitive preparation phase is designed to educate clients about the functions of anger and about their personal anger patterns, to provide a shared language system between client and therapist, and to introduce the rationale of treatment. An instructional manual for clients is used to facilitate these tasks. Clients are asked to keep a diary which serves as a data base for discussion of the treatment concepts.

The anger control components of the cognitive preparation phase consist of (a) identifying the persons and situations that trigger anger, (b) distinguishing anger from aggression, (c) understanding the multiple determinants of anger, (d) understanding provocation in terms of interaction sequences, and (e) introducing the anger management techniques as coping strategies to handle conflict and stress.

This phase is implemented during the pre-treatment assessment and the first two treatment sessions. The activities of the treatment sessions are described in detail below.

SKILL ACQUISITION

The intervention attempts to promote cognitive, arousal reduction, and behavioral coping skills, consistent with the analysis of anger determinants. At the cognitive level, the client is taught to alternatively view provocation events (Kelly, 1955) and to modify the exaggerated importance often attached to events (Ellis, 1973). A basic goal is to promote flexibility in one's cognitive structuring of situations. In this regard, expectations and appraisals linked with anger arousal are targets for modification. Particular attention is paid to inordinately high expectations of others' behavior and to the appraisal of events as personal affronts or ego threats. The ability to "not take things personally" is a fundamental skill. This is accomplished by fostering a task orientation to provocation, which involves a focus on desired outcomes and the implementation of a behavioral strategy to produce those outcomes.

A central cognitive intervention technique consists of the use of self-instructions (Meichenbaum, 1974). The cognitive control of anger by means of private speech is accomplished by first dissecting a provocation experience into a sequence of stages: (a) preparing for a provocation, (b) impact and confrontation, (c) coping with arousal, and (d) subsequent reflection (conflict unresolved, or conflict resolved). Stages (c) and (d) provide for the possible failure of self-regulation and for the mitigation of additional self-arousal by ruminations. The self-regulated private speech functions as an instructional cue that guides the client's thoughts, feelings, and behavior in the direction of effective coping.

It is of the utmost importance that the self-instructional package be individualized and generated by the client with regard to particular situations of provocation. I am not proposing that simply making "positive thinking" utterances to oneself will necessarily have anger control effects. Coping self-statements must follow from altered expectations and appraisals. Examples of coping self-statements are contained in Table 1. These are to be offered to clients as examples, but the client should be encouraged to generate his or her own self-statement package.

For arousal reduction, the client is taught relaxation skills and is also encouraged to begin a program of exercise or aesthetic enjoyment that is explicitly directed at reducing arousal monitored by the client and therapist. Relaxation training is used as a counterconditioning process (Wolpe & Lazarus, 1966), incorporating Goldfried's (1971) self-control concepts. Clients are

TABLE 1: EXAMPLES OF ANGER MANAGEMENT SELF-STATEMENTS REHEARSED IN STRESS INOCULATION TRAINING

Preparing for a Provocation

This could be a rough situation, but I know how to deal with it.
I can work out a plan to handle this. Easy does it.
Remember, stick to the issues and don't take it personally.
There won't be any need for an argument. I know what to do.

Impact and Confrontation

As long as I keep my cool, I'm in control of the situation.
You don't need to prove yourself. Don't make more out of this than you
    have to.
There is no point in getting mad. Think of what you have to do.
Look for the positives and don't jump to conclusions.

Coping with Arousal

Muscles are getting tight. Relax and slow things down.
Time to take a deep breath. Let's take the issue point by point.
My anger is a signal of what I need to do. Time for problem solving.
He probably wants me to get angry, but I'm going to deal with it
    constructively.

Subsequent Reflection

---

1. Conflict unresolved

    Forget about the aggravation. Thinking about it only makes you
        upset.
    Try to shake it off. Don't let it interfere with your job.
    Remember relaxation. It's a lot better than anger.
    Don't take it personally. It's probably not so serious.

2. Conflict resolved

    I handled that one pretty well. That's doing a good job.
    I could have gotten more upset than it was worth.
    My pride can get me into trouble, but I'm doing better at this all
        the time.
    I actually got through that without getting angry.

---

also encouraged to cultivate their sense of humor. Humor has been found to reduce aggression-related arousal (Singer, 1968; Smith, 1973), and its use in the present procedure pertains to not taking oneself and one's predicaments too seriously. The relaxation procedures are introduced in Session 2. Of course, other procedures aimed at the same arousal reduction goals, such as hypnosis, meditation, biofeedback, yoga, or Tai Chi can be substituted, particularly if they are better suited to the client's needs and interests.

The behavioral coping skills concern the effective communication of feelings, assertiveness, and the implementation of task-oriented, problem-solving action. The client is helped to maximize the adaptive functions of anger and to minimize its maladaptive functions. When arousal is activated, the client is taught to recognize anger on the basis of internal and external cues, and to then either communicate that anger in a nonhostile form, or use it to energize problem-solving action, keeping the arousal at moderate levels of intensity.

Establishing a task-oriented response set facilitates problem-solving behavior. It is emphasized that anger is an emotional response to stressful demands, signaling that problem-solving strategies are to be implemented. Anger management behavior involves a strategic confrontation whereby the client learns to focus on issues and objectives, as well as the behaviors instrumental to achieving them. This prevents the accumulation of anger and prevents an aggressive over-reaction by imposing thought between impulse and action.

APPLICATION TRAINING

The value of application has been emphasized by a variety of skills-training approaches (D'Zurilla & Goldfried, 1971; Meichenbaum, 1975b; Suinn & Richardson, 1971). The anger management principles are essentially aimed at building personal competence, and therefore involve augmenting the client's ability to manage provocative situations and testing his or her proficiency.

The practice is conducted by means of imaginal and role playing inductions of anger. The content of these provocation simulations is presented sequentially in hierarchical form. That is, a hierarchy of anger situations **that the client is likely to encounter in real life** is constructed with the client (Sessions 2 and 3), and the coping skills that have been rehearsed with the therapist then are applied to these scenarios beginning with the mildest, and progressing to the most anger arousing. This process continues throughout the course of treatment and enables both client and therapist to gauge the client's proficiency.

TREATMENT PROCEDURE

The procedural sequence described here is intended to be flexible. Individual differences of clients and of therapists will require modifications in timing and emphasis. In addition, the therapeutic mode, whether individual or group, will necessitate adjustments in procedure. In general, the sessions are designed to be 1 hour in length for individual therapy and 1-1/2 hours if conducted in groups. In an experimental study involving probation counselors, it was found that counselors trained in these procedures performed significantly better in assessing and treating anger than did control counselors, and these training effects were strongly maintained on follow-up measurements (Novaco, 1980).

SESSION I

The first session follows the completion of pre-treatment tests, such as the anger scales or other behavioral measures (cf. Novaco, 1975). Test performance is reviewed with clients, using the high anger responses as points for discussion. Following a brief review of these test materials, the clients' problems with anger are assessed more fully through an interview process. The interview analysis should follow these steps:

    1. Obtain a statement by the clients regarding (a) the degree to which they
        believe there is a problem with anger; (b) the greatest concern they have

about their anger; and (c) how working on this problem will make their life different.

2. Conduct a "situation x person x mode of expression" analysis of the anger problem. That is, examine the range of **settings** in which the clients function (i.e., home, work, school, commerce, recreational, driving), the **persons** involved in those settings (i.e., parents, mates, siblings, friends, fellow workers, strangers), and **how** anger is **expressed** when aroused under these various circumstances (i.e., verbal antagonism, physical antagonism, passive aggression, avoidance, self-degradation, constructive action).

3. Try to assess the clients' deficits in anger control by examining the determinants of anger arousal. That is, examine the external events, internal processes, and behavioral reactions that are predominantly involved for the clients.

   a. **External Events** (frustration, annoyance, insult, inequity, abuse, etc.)

   What particular aspects of situations trigger anger arousal? Are there any particular forms of provocation that are most often encountered and which easily arouse anger? How reasonable is it to be angry when these events occur?

   b. **Internal Factors**

   1. **Cognitive** (appraisals, expectations, self-statements)

   Try to help the clients become aware of the many ways in which their thoughts influence feelings. What do these provocation events mean to the clients? How do they interpret the behavior of others? Does their anger come from how they expect others to behave? Are these expectations unreasonable? What kinds of things do they say to themselves when provocations occur? This can all be facilitated by having the clients close their eyes and "run a movie" of the anger experience or relive their thoughts and feelings.

   2. **Affective** (tension, temperament, empathy)

   Are the clients tense or agitated? Look for nonverbal cues as indicators. Do they feel "on edge," "wound-up," "up-tight?" Any problems with sleeping? Any physical problems related to tension like headache, chest pains, nervous stomach, high blood pressure? How capable are they at laughing at themselves or seeing the less serious side of life? Are they sensitive to the feelings of others?

   c. **Behavioral Factors** (antagonism, hostility, avoidance)

   How do the clients customarily respond when provoked in a given situation? How does their behavior influence how they feel? How do others respond to their reactions? How capable are they at communicating their feelings to others? Are there any signs of positive assertiveness?

4. The rationale for treatment should be presented to clients in accord with the material presented here. That is, clients should be given an overview of what will be done and the theory behind the procedure.

(**Note:** Assessment is a process that is not completed in a single session, and it is inevitable that what is presented above as material for Session 1 will carry over to Session 2. Remember, these are guidelines.)

Homework. At the end of the first session, clients are asked to maintain a diary of anger experiences. The diary should provide three pieces of information: (a) the frequency of anger experiences (obtained by an account of each incident), (b) the degree of anger experienced, as rated by the clients for each incident, and (c) the degree of proficiency demonstrated by the clients in managing anger in that situation, also as rated by the clients (cf. Novaco, 1977b).

Clients are given a set of index cards on which to record hierarchy incidents. They should be instructed to write down a set of anger experiences that they have had and are likely to experience again, ranging from minor annoyances to infuriating events. They will invariably need help with this task in the next session.

Following from the cognitive analysis, instruct the clients to "listen to yourself with a third ear" so as to tune in to anger instigating private speech. Have them try to notice the kinds of self-statements they emit when anger is experienced.

SESSION II

The second session begins with a review of homework assignments from the initial session. These consist of (a) anger diary ratings, (b) index cards for hierarchy scenarios, and (c) reports on internal dialogue ("listen to yourself with a third ear").

1. Using the clients' diary statements about recent anger experiences, continue to obtain assessment of the anger problems. That is, get a more refined view of the situations, persons, and mode of expression involved with anger arousal.

2. Establish a hierarchy. Order index cards containing anger scenarios so that a graduated series of seven situations are produced. Set these aside until the end of the session when the lowest anger situation will be used.

3. Introduce relaxation training. Begin by doing deep breathing exercises and emphasize the importance of breathing control in achieving relaxation. Go through the full set of muscle exercises. Pay particular attention to breathing rate and to any part of the body that clients have difficulty relaxing.

   The Jacobsen (1938) procedure of alternative tensing and relaxing muscles is recommended, since angry people are inclined to tense their muscles and this procedure tells them to do what they are already doing, thus minimizing resistance to relaxation induction.

4. While the clients are still relaxing have them imagine a quiet, mellow, tranquil scene. After having them imagine that scene for 30 seconds, present the first anger hierarchy scene, which should be a mild annoyance:

   "Just continue relaxing like that. Now I want you to imagine the following scene: (Present the scene as described on the card.) See it as clearly and vividly as you can. If you feel the least bit angry as you imagine it, signal me by raising the index finger of your right hand."

   If the clients do not signal anger for 15 seconds, then instruct them to "shut it off and just continue to relax. You are doing very well."

   If the anger is signaled, instruct them as follows: "You have signaled anger, now see yourself coping with the situation. See yourself staying composed, relaxing, settling down. Continue to imagine the scene but see yourself handling it effectively." (15 seconds)

   Bring the clients back to the tranquil scene for another 30 seconds of imagination and continued relaxation. Then have them take a deep breath before opening their eyes.

5. Review how the procedure went. Obtain information on how they experienced the anger scene. Explain the strategy of successive approximations to the top of the hierarchy. Instruct them to practice the relaxation exercises at home and to continue to "listen to themselves with a third ear," to tune in to anger eliciting private speech.

SESSION III

At this point the clients have hopefully begun to tune in to our view of the anger process and share in our language system. This is not a small matter. Like looking through a special lens, it helps to sharpen their observations and gives them a new handle on the things that trouble them.

This session will introduce the important staging strategy and continue work on the hierarchy using both cognitive and relaxation coping.

1. Review the diary and continue to refine your assessment of the clients' problems. Examine the timing and impact of anger-facilitating self-statements using a diary example. Try to specify at this point what the clients' predominant styles of coping are. Praise them for working on homework tasks. Check on the accuracy and usefulness of the hierarchy.

2. Begin the cognitive interventions by first explaining that our feelings are caused not by events themselves but by our thoughts or beliefs about those events. How we think determines how we feel. Mention the Ellis concept of A-B-C in further making this point. Then,

   a. Select example provocations from the clients' lives and identify the **A**ntecedent events, **B**eliefs, and **C**onsequent behaviors.

   b. Make an attempt to alter B. That is, try to help clients alternatively view the situation. Modify their appraisal of its significance, the intentions of others, and so forth, or alter any maladaptive expectations of the behavior of others, themselves, or the consequences of the situation.

   Determine how they construed the situation (preconceptions of the event, how they interpreted others' behavior, how they justified their own actions) and give particular attention to their internal dialogue before, during, and after the incident.

3. Using information from the diary, have the clients sort out the situations for which anger is justified versus those for which it is less justified or even counterproductive. Mention the varied functions of anger and state that our objective is to maximize the positive functions and minimize the negative. As they become better at recognizing when it is okay to be angry and when it is not okay, they will be more able to use their anger in positive ways.

4. Induce relaxation. Follow the same steps as the last session. This time also add some relaxing imagery.

5. Present the next hierarchy scene. First have them imagine themselves being in a tranquil, peaceful place. Then have them see themselves in the provocation situation. **In addition to the relaxation in coping with the anger experience, have them see themselves coping cognitively with the provocation.**

6. Review their experience of the relaxation and cognitive coping process. Remind them to practice the relaxation at home.

SESSION IV

1. Review anger diary and ask if any progress has been made on hierarchy situations in real life. That is, inquire how the clients have done on those situations you have practiced under relaxation. Check again on appropriateness of hierarchy.

2. Select an example incident. Try to **modify thoughts** about the anger situation such as intolerance for mistakes, unreasonable expectations of self and others, impatience, or the felt necessity for retaliation. Try to sharpen the clients' discrimination of when anger is justified.

3. Arrive at a sharp understanding of the clients' feelings of anger in those situations to as complete an extent as possible. Try to make them become fully aware of the signs of anger physiologically and behaviorally. Have them tune in to the bodily cues of anger and the effects it has on their behavior.

4. Help them understand the feelings of others in that situation. What is it like to be the other guy? Role play will usually help with this. Have them take the role of the other person and you take their part. Encourage empathy for the other person's point of view.

5. Introduce the staging idea of breaking down an anger experience into chunks. Indicate that trying to handle something all at once is difficult, so we will instead attack it part by part. Use an example to illustrate the various stages.

    a. **preparing** for a provocation (when possible)
    b. **impact** and confrontation
    c. **coping** with arousal and agitation
    d. **reflecting** or thinking back when conflict unresolved or conflict resolved

    This will require that you model explicitly how to view an anger experience and cope with it using these stages. Therefore, you will have to "think out loud" how to handle the situation cognitively. Use self-statements as the means to express constructive appraisals and expectations. Give clients a handout describing the examples of self-statements for the various stages. Emphasize the personal control aspects.

6. Have the clients rehearse these strategies. Have them try out the steps in the coping sequence for the same incident.

    Ask them to "say out loud" how they are thinking their way through the situation. Have them generate a set of self-statements that suits them for this situation.

7. Induce relaxation and work on next two hierarchy items. Remember to use relaxation imagery and instruct them to see themselves coping cognitively.

SESSION V - X

1. Review diary incidents and evaluate progress on treatment objectives. Sharpen assessment of particular difficulties in managing anger. Be sure to praise any accomplishments.

2. Emphasize how anger can be used as a **signal** to cue us in to what to do in a situation. State that, to use anger in positive ways, arousal must be kept at moderate levels. This leads to **impulse control** or thinking before acting. Once again, review the material on staging and self-statements for managing provocation.

3. Begin behavioral interventions. This is intended to gear the clients to a **problem-solving** approach to conflict. These can be made in three important areas:

   a. **Communication of feelings:** Effective provocation management requires that the clients **know what to say.** Take an example and, in role play, demonstrate or model how to express anger constructively. Have clients rehearse the recognition and expression of anger in role play.

   b. **Assertion:** Help clients understand that confrontation does not mean hostility. One way to accomplish this is by setting up a role play in which you instruct them to be as hostile as they can, then examine their behavior and search for more constructive forms of expression. This is particularly effective if you first have them play a very passive, submissive role.

      In coaching their assertive behavior, have them become more proficient in being direct, firm, and explicit in making requests for change in another person's behavior.

   c. **Staying task oriented:** Help them stay focused on the desired outcomes of anger situations. This means not taking things personally, knowing what one wants to get out of a situation and working toward that goal. Anger situations should be seen as **problems** that need a solution. Help them discover strategies that will achieve constructive resolution.

4. Work on the next hierarchy item, first imaginally, then in role play. Use abbreviated relaxation procedures prior to the imaginal presentation. Emphasize the task oriented concept in role play.

SUMMARY

Stress inoculation is a particular kind of cognitive-behavioral therapy that emphasizes coping skills so as to develop competence in response to stressful events and to regulate disturbing emotions. The stress inoculation approach differs from other cognitive-behavioral therapies with regard to the explicit attention given to environmental/contextual determinants of problem conditions and the explicit exposure to graduated dosages of problem-relevant stimuli. Through a process of paced mastery, the client develops cognitive and behavioral proficiencies for coping with stress.

The cognitive and behavioral skills are designed to control negative, self-defeating ideation, to divert attention from anger engendering stimulation, to promote alternative constructions of provocation events, to regulate physiological arousal, and to implement problem-solving behavior. Special attention is given to the client's self-statements in order to guide thoughts, emotions, and actions toward effective coping. This aggregate of coping strategies is modeled by the therapist and rehearsed by the client and then systematically practiced in conjunction with simulated provocations.

As a self-control therapy, the effectiveness of the treatment depends upon the active participation of the client; consequently, this approach is not suited to those who are highly resistant to change or who lack internal motivation for treatment. Quite obviously, the cognitively-based interventions require adequate cognitive functioning and would not have value for psychotic or mentally retarded populations.

The stress inoculation approach, in the areas of anxiety and pain, as well as anger, has received encouraging experimental confirmation (cf. Meichenbaum & Novaco, 1983) and holds considerable promise for advances in therapeutic interventions.

Raymond W. Novaco, Ph.D., is currently an Associate Professor in the Program in Social Ecology at the University of California, Irvine. He received his training in clinical and community psychology at Indiana University. He has published a number of books and articles in the area of stress inoculation and is currently involved in research on the environmental determinants of human stress and processes of adaptation, particularly with regard to cognition and emotion. Dr. Novaco may be contacted through the Program in Social Ecology, University of California, Irvine, Irvine, CA 92717.

RESOURCES

Beck, A. T., Rush, A. J., Shaw, B. F., & Emery, G. COGNITIVE THERAPY OF DEPRESSION. New York: Guilford Press, 1979.

D'Zurilla, T. & Goldfried, M. Problem solving and behavior modification. JOURNAL OF ABNORMAL PSYCHOLOGY, 1971, **78**, 107-126.

Ellis, A. HOW TO LIVE WITH AND WITHOUT ANGER. New York: Readers Digest Press, 1977.

Ellis, A. HUMANISTIC PSYCHOLOGY: THE RATIONAL-EMOTIVE APPROACH. New York: Julian Press, 1973.

Ellis, A. REASON AND EMOTION IN PSYCHOTHERAPY. New York: John Stuart & Co., 1962.

Evans, D. Specific aggression, arousal, and reciprocal inhibition therapy. WESTERN PSYCHOLOGIST, 1971, **1**, 125-130.

Evans, D. & Hearn, M. Anger and systematic desensitization: A following. PSYCHOLOGICAL REPORT, 1973, **32**, 569-570.

Goldfried, M. Systematic desensitization as training in self-control. JOURNAL OF CONSULTING AND CLINICAL PSYCHOLOGY, 1971, **37**, 228-234.

Hearn, M. & Evans, D. Anger and reciprocal inhibition therapy. PSYCHOLOGICAL REPORTS, 1972, **30**, 943-948.

Herrell, J. M. Use of systematic desensitization to eliminate inappropriate anger. PROCEEDINGS OF THE 79TH ANNUAL CONVENTION OF THE AMERICAN PSYCHOLOGICAL ASSOCIATION. Washington, DC: American Psychological Association, 1971.

Jacobsen, E. PROGRESSIVE RELAXATION. Chicago: University of Chicago Press, 1938.

James, W. PRINCIPLES OF PSYCHOLOGY (Vol. 2). New York: Holt, 1890.

Kelly, G. A. THE PSYCHOLOGY OF PERSONAL CONSTRUCTS (Vol. 1 & 2). New York: Norton, 1955.

Kendall, P. & Hollon, S. COGNITIVE BEHAVIORAL INTERVENTIONS. New York: Academic Press, 1979.

Konecni, V. J. Annoyance, type and duration of postannoyance activity, and aggression: The "Cathartic Effect." JOURNAL OF EXPERIMENTAL PSYCHOLOGY: GENERAL, 1975, **104**, 76-104. (a)

Konecni, V. J. The mediation of aggressive behavior: Arousal level vs. anger and cognitive labeling. JOURNAL OF PERSONALITY AND SOCIAL PSYCHOLOGY, 1975, **32**, 706-712. (b)

Mahoney, M. & Arnkoff, D. Cognitive and self-control therapies. In S. L. Garfield & A. E. Bergin (Eds.), HANDBOOK OF PSYCHOTHERAPY AND BEHAVIOR CHANGES (2nd ed.). New York: Wiley, 1977.

Meichenbaum, D. COGNITIVE BEHAVIOR MODIFICATION. Morristown, NJ: General Learning Press, 1974.

Meichenbaum, D. COGNITIVE BEHAVIOR MODIFICATION. New York: Plenum Press, 1977.

Meichenbaum, D. A self-instructional approach to stress management: A proposal for stress inoculation training. In C. Spielberger & I. Saranson (Eds.), STRESS AND ANXIETY (Vol. 2). New York: Wiley, 1975. (b)

Meichenbaum, D. Self-instructional methods. In F. H. Kanfer & A. P. Goldstein (Eds.), HELPING PEOPLE CHANGE. New York: Pergamon Press, 1975. (a)

Meichenbaum, D. & Cameron, R. STRESS INOCULATION: A SKILLS TRAINING APPROACH TO ANXIETY MANAGEMENT. Unpublished manuscript, University of Waterloo, 1973.

Meichenbaum, D. & Novaco, R. W. Postscript-stress inoculation: A preventative approach. In C. Spielberger & I. Sarason (Eds.), STRESS AND ANXIETY (Vol. 10). Washington, DC: Hemisphere Publishing Corp., 1983.

Meichenbaum, D. & Novaco, R. W. Stress inoculation: A preventive approach. In C. Spielberger & I. Sarason (Eds.), STRESS AND ANXIETY (Vol. 5). New York: Halstead Press, 1978.

Novaco, R. W. Anger and coping with stress. In J. Foreyt & D. Rathjen (Eds.), COGNITIVE BEHAVIOR THERAPY: RESEARCH AND APPLICATION. New York: Plenum Press, 1978.

Novaco, R. W. ANGER CONTROL: THE DEVELOPMENT AND EVALUATION OF AN EXPERIMENTAL TREATMENT. Lexington, MA: D. C. Heath, Lexington Books, 1975.

Novaco, R. W. The cognitive regulation of anger and stress. In P. Kendall & S. Hollon (Eds.), COGNITIVE-BEHAVIORAL INTERVENTIONS: THEORY, RESEARCH & PROCEDURES. New York: Academic Press, 1979.

Novaco, R. W. The functions and regulation of the arousal of anger. AMERICAN JOURNAL OF PSYCHOLOGY, 1976, **133**, 1124-1128. (a)

Novaco, R. W. A stress inoculation approach to anger management in the training of law enforcement officers. AMERICAN JOURNAL OF COMMUNITY PSYCHOLOGY, 1977, **5**, 327-346. (a)

Novaco, R. W. Stress inoculation: A cognitive therapy for anger and its application to a case of depression. JOURNAL OF CONSULTING CLINICAL PSYCHOLOGY, 1977, **45**, 600-608. (b)

Novaco, R. W. Training of probation counselors for anger problems. JOURNAL OF COUNSELING PSYCHOLOGY, 1980, **27**, 385-390.

Novaco, R. W. Treatment of chronic anger through cognitive and relaxation controls. JOURNAL OF CONSULTING AND CLINICAL PSYCHOLOGY, 1976, **44**, 681. (b)

Novaco, R. W., Cook, T., & Sarason, I. Military recruit training: An arena for stress coping skills. In D. Meichenbaum & M. Jaremko (Eds.), STRESS REDUCTION AND PREVENTION. New York: Plenum Press, 1983.

O'Donnell, C. & Worell, L. Motor and cognitive relaxation in the desensitization of anger. BEHAVIOR RESEARCH AND THERAPY, 1973, **11**, 473-481.

Rimm, D. C., de Groot, J. C., Boord, P., Reiman, J., & Dillow, P. V. Systematic desensitization of anger response. BEHAVIOR RESEARCH AND THERAPY, 1971, **9**, 273-280.

Rotter, J. B. SOCIAL LEARNING AND CLINICAL PSYCHOLOGY. Englewood Cliffs, NJ: Prentice-Hall, 1954.

Singer, D. L. Aggression arousal, hostile humor, and catharsis. JOURNAL OF PERSONALITY AND SOCIAL PSYCHOLOGY MONOGRAPH SUPPLEMENT, 1968, **8**(1, Pt. 2).

Smith, R. E. The use of humor in the counter-conditioning of anger response. BEHAVIOR THERAPY, 1973, **4**, 576-580.

Stokols, D. & Novaco, R. W. Transportation and well-being. In I. Altman, J.

Stokols, D. & Novaco, R. W.   Transportation and well-being.   In I. Altman, J. Wohlwill, & P. Everett (Eds.), TRANSPORTATION AND BEHAVIOR.   New York: Plenum Press, 1981.

Suinn, R. & Richardson, F.   Anxiety management training: A non-specific behavior therapy program for anxiety control. BEHAVIORAL THERAPY, 1971, **2**, 498–510.

Toch, H. VIOLENT MEN. Chicago: Aldine Publishing Co., 1969.

Wolpe, J. & Lazarus, A. BEHAVIOR THERAPY TECHNIQUES. Oxford: Pergamon Press, 1966.

Zillman, D. Excitation transfer in communication-mediated aggressive behavior. JOURNAL OF EXPERIMENTAL SOCIAL PSYCHOLOGY, 1971, **7**, 419–434.

INTRODUCTION TO SECTION II: PRACTICE MANAGEMENT AND PROFESSIONAL DEVELOPMENT

In this section of **INNOVATIONS,** we have included contributions which concentrate on the business and management aspects of clinical practice. Too often, a practice will either fail or not achieve its potential because the otherwise competent clinician has failed to pay attention to critical areas of practice management and professional development.

The section opens with Woody's discussion of ten fundamental steps to minimize the possibility of a malpractice suit, a subject of growing concern in today's litigious society. This author offers the unique perspective of an attorney-psychologist.

Weitz discusses the problem solving process and the solutions he developed when he made the decision to sell his practice. He has also included the contract he developed for this purpose.

Vincent's contribution concerns procedures for test analysis and report generation utilizing word processing equipment. He provides specific suggestions for automated analysis which could be adapted to your own practice.

The Editor of **PSYCHOTHERAPY FINANCES,** Herbert Klein, presents a business approach to the marketing of therapy services, with comments from experienced practitioners in the field. He offers specific suggestions for gaining broader exposure for your practice.

The **INNOVATION** editors offer a checklist of important areas that need to be considered by the practitioner considering private practice. Established practitioners can also use this checklist to evaluate their practices and identify potential problem areas. An annotated bibliography of current books on practice management is also included.

Kelley offers concise formulas for establishing fees for consulting services. He gives careful consideration to advantages and limitations of various approaches.

AVOIDING MALPRACTICE IN PSYCHOTHERAPY

Robert Henley Woody

The trainer or supervisor of psychotherapists frequently hears such statements as, "It's strange, I spend all day, everyday, in the most intimate of discussions, yet I feel so isolated from people - I'm starved for professional contacts." This type of comment captures the special vulnerability of psychotherapists, especially those in independent practice. The very nature of psychotherapy (i.e., the reasons for the relationship require centering on the client, and personal need fulfillment for the therapist is excluded) creates an often unacknowledged pressure to take actions that are not in the best interests of the client. Such actions are most likely to occur when therapists lack professional stimulation and colleagial monitoring of therapeutic activities. In the loneliness and isolation of the treatment office, there exists the potential for malpractice.

Every client receiving psychotherapy has a legal right to high quality treatment; this means that certain positive features must be present and certain negative features must not occur. Further, for a wide variety of reasons, society at present is particularly litigious regarding failure to meet the client's or patient's legal rights, and psychotherapists are in no way exempt from this trend. The result of a failure to honor the therapy client's rights is malpractice.

By its very definition, malpractice means that something bad has happened. The happening, as already alluded to, can be something that occurs (a commission), or something that should occur but does not (an omission).

In malpractice, the psychotherapist makes an unwarranted departure from accepted professional standards and a harm is inflicted upon the client, with the result being some sort of damage. The violation of the standard of care must be the cause of the harm that leads to the damages. I will elaborate on this point later in the chapter.

"Malpractice in psychotherapy," the topic of this contribution, encompasses all liability-producing conduct that arises in the provision of professional services by a psychotherapist (regardless of disciplinary identity). Thus, it includes negligence (the primary legal principle commonly associated with malpractice), intentional tortious misconduct (such as a physical assault), breach of contracts (such as promising a therapeutic result), defamation, invasion of privacy, and failure to prevent injury to the client's self or to third parties, to name but a few of the legal possibilities (King, 1977).

Opinions vary about what specific actions (or lack thereof) by a psychotherapist provoke a legal response such as malpractice. In considering malpractice in psychiatry, Trent (1978) analyzed relevant insurance data and posited the following 12 types of claims or cases: (1) improper hospital commitment; (2) death; (3) pressing for fee collection; (4) subpoena to testify; (5) sexual behavior with patients; (6) drug reactions; (7) unauthorized release of confidential information causing damage to the patient; (8) improper administrative handling; (10) electroconvulsive therapy (ECT); (11) improper treatment; and (12) injury to a nonpatient during professional services. These categories are medically oriented, and may not be applicable to all psychotherapists, such as those who are not physicians. At the same time, they do capture the breadth of legal problems. Wilkinson (1982) offers what may be a more meaningful set of liability areas for the psychotherapist. They include: (1) liability for client-inflicted injuries and suicide; (2) harm by the client to third persons; (3) errors in judgment (such as when making custodial accommodations or releasing information); (4) treatment methods; (5) drug-related liability; and (6) sexual misconduct. These categories of liability will provide the conceptual framework for this contribution.

My major objective here is to provide concrete ideas about how to avoid malpractice allegations. In so doing, an extensive legal analysis of critical cases will not be provided; this type of documentation can be obtained elsewhere (Knapp & Vandecreek, 1982; Wilkinson, 1982; Woody, in press). Rather, citations will be used sparingly, with deference being given to recommendations for practice.

RECOMMENDATION 1: WHEN A COMPLAINT ARISES, REVERT TO A DEFENSIVE POSTURE

This recommendation goes against the essence of psychotherapy. The entire set of psychotherapeutic processes are predicated upon the psychotherapist and the client being able to trust, confront, and communicate openly and undefensively. This litigious era, however, negates the tenet that the psychotherapist can resolve allegations about the quality of treatment. Wright (1981) acknowledges the psychologist's propensity for confrontation in this sort of situation, and points out that any confrontation or communication by the psychotherapist intended to "therapeutically resolve" the problem may well prove to be evidence used against the psychotherapist later on. Such self-implemented efforts by the psychotherapist, as opposed to turning to an attorney for defense, can well result in the infamous "foot-in-the-mouth" dilemma.

Along with Wright, Brodsky (1978), asserting that "mental health professionals overreact emotionally and underreact functionally to malpractice threats and concerns" (p. 121), warns:

> The fear of malpractice suits is part of mental health professionals' perception of lawyers and litigious clients as harmful and noxious. Lawyers are dangerous. Any client who hints at filing suit is dangerous. (p. 121)

While it is inappropriate to adopt an alarmist view or to consider all lawyers and complaining clients as "dangerous," concern about defending one's own rights is more than justified.

RECOMMENDATION 2: KNOW YOUR STANDARD OF CARE AND COMMUNICATE IT TO THE CLIENT

The fundamental upon which a malpractice suit is based is that there has been a violation of the standard of care. From a legal point of view, every person has a societally-imposed duty to not create an unreasonable risk of injury to another person. As unique relationships are formed (such as between employer-employee, innkeeper-guest, transporter-passenger, husband-wife, or, for our purposes, psychotherapist-client), social policy has created special duties. These duties are translated into a standard of care.

Regardless of the relationship, the question is, "What would the reasonable person (read: psychotherapist) do in this relationship?" For the psychotherapist, it is necessary to exercise reasonable and prudent care and to possess a minimum of professional knowledge and ability. As Prosser (1971), a noted tort law authority, interprets it, this means that the professional must maintain skill and learning that is commonly possessed by members of the profession in good standing. The skill may be thought of as being that of the "average" member of the profession, but obviously there is a range of competency that could be potentially acceptable.

Judgment need not be flawless in the manifestation of professional skills:

> An error in judgment is not actionable only where the psychiatrist was acting in good faith, had made sufficient inquiry and examination into the cause and nature of the patient's disturbance, had exercised the requisite care in making the diagnosis and prescribing treatment, and otherwise had not deviated from generally accepted standards and practices. If the psychiatrist is careless in any of the steps preliminary to making a bona fide judgment, then liability may be imposed for the error in judgment (Wilkinson, 1982, p. 75).

It is important to avoid entry into any professional situation for which there is any doubt about preparation or competency, and, once functioning has commenced, to exercise the precautionary steps, such as in diagnosis and treatment, that a comparable professional known for being reasonable and prudent would exercise.

When I conduct seminars on malpractice for psychotherapists, a frequently heard question is, "To whom will I be compared?" The answer will vary with the situation and with the jurisdiction. Historically, a parochial comparison would have been applied. For example, if you were a psychologist with a Ph.D., you would have been compared with other psychologists with a Ph.D. in your home area.

With the passage of time, the matter has become a bit more complex. As a guideline (which can have exceptions), you will typically be compared to a reasonable sample of professionals with comparable academic training and experience within the general locale (say within a geographical region) if you are a "general practitioner." However, if you hold yourself out as a "specialist" in any manner (say through a yellow pages listing or on your letterhead), your comparison will be national in scope, and will be with a reasonable sample of other specialists.

If you hold a special credential, you will likely have a standard of care imposed that is consonant with other professionals holding that same credential. For example, it would be logical to assert that a psychologist holding the status of Diplomate in Clinical Psychology from the American Board of Professional Psychology should be compared to other psychologists holding the same Diplomate status, as opposed to being compared to a parochial sample of psychologists. Likewise, even if the professional had not been granted Clinical Member status by the American Association for Marriage and Family Therapy but practiced marriage and family therapy, it is logical that a plaintiff's attorney would strive to hold the professional to the standards promulgated by that association; and it also seems likely that many courts would support such a comparison, even if the professional claimed no identity with the association.

Part of the standard of care, therefore, involves openly specifying one's qualifications. Even if a competency or qualification is not explicitly stated but the client had a reasonable basis for inferring a competency or qualification, the therapist may be forced legally to live up to that standard.

Keeping one's clients well informed about the treatment is a good defense against allegations of malpractice. Schwitzgebel (1975) and Brodsky (1978) endorse a contractual approach, whereby the entry into psychotherapy will be prefaced by a contract that specifies the procedures to be followed (the likely results, the risks, the fees, and the professional's responsibility) and the client signs the contract.

Informed consent is one thing, but waiver of rights for a questionable professional service is another matter. That is, any attempt by a psychotherapist to get a client to sign a blanket waiver of professional liability (a) would likely shock the conscience of the court, (b) would not be allowed to absolve the psychotherapist in the event of damage to the client, and (c) might create a punitive thrust to the judicial decision.

If the psychotherapist is in a group practice, it is wise to provide the client with a specific statement about his or her liability for treatment. This is because if a client were damaged by a psychotherapist, the plaintiff's attorney would appropriately name all members of the group as defendants. For example, when a female patient filed a malpractice suit alleging she had sexual relations during the therapy sessions with her psychotherapist, all practitioners in the same clinic were named as defendants.

Why should this liability by association be allowed? The idea is that a reasonable standard of care for a psychotherapeutic group practice would include, among other things, a colleagial duty to be familiar with the quality of services that are being provided therein and to supervise accordingly. Theoretically, the group members stand to benefit financially by their association, so the liabilities must be shared. Thus, damage done by one psychotherapist is damage done by all of the psychotherapists, unless the others properly exercised their duties to safeguard the client. Even then, there might be liability imposed on them, depending upon the nature of the case. By informing the client, however, that each psychotherapist is solely responsible for the treatment quality and by the client's implied acceptance of this through entering into treatment, it is possible that this would be a reasonable defense for the other psychotherapists in the group.

It should be obvious that no standard of care, whether by explicit contract or by implication through professional actions, should connote an assured outcome. It would be appropriate to indicate the therapeutic goals, but these should not be, in any way, guaranteed.

How does a standard of care get formed and disseminated? One clinical group has an "Introduction to the _____ Clinic." Their brochure (a) specifies, in global terms, the types of services that are provided (e.g., psychotherapy, marriage and family therapy, sex therapy, psychological testing), (b) provides a capsule vita for each professional (along with a photo), and (c) offers a summary of agency policies (such as for payments or missed sessions). This brochure is given to all new clients. This group also has a one-page statement covering (a) the fact that each of the professionals is an independent practitioner and is solely responsible for the quality of his or her services, and (b) a list of conditions that are not under the aegis of the clinical group (e.g., socializing with clients, entering into business ventures with clients, guaranteeing therapeutic outcomes). This document is left in ready evidence in the waiting room.

Even with these sorts of precautionary measures, the standard of care may be violated. Subsequent recommendations will focus on specific actions that can be taken to avoid an alleged breach of the standard of care.

RECOMMENDATION 3: MAINTAIN A SUPERVISORY RELATIONSHIP

As might be assumed from the comments about the standard of care being based on what other reasonable and prudent professionals would do, the psychotherapist who maintains some sort of supervisory relationship with another professional is establishing a critical defense against allegations of malpractice. It would be a helpful defense to be able to show that the psychotherapist had prudently and openly shared concerns about the treatment with a supervisor (who might be a colleague in the same practice) and had received endorsement for the way he or she had handled the case.

As reflected in the earlier comments about liability for one's colleagues in the same clinical group, by actively seeking supervision and serving as a supervisor for others in the group, a defense against failure to safeguard clients is created.

RECOMMENDATION 4: HAVE THE CLIENT ASSUME THE RESPONSIBILITY FOR ALL COMMUNICATIONS

It is prudent to keep the client informed fully about all written communications, whether they be in the form of case notes, reports, insurance documents, or whatever. For example, insurance forms, which contain what could be an impactful DSM-III diagnostic label, should always be given to and discussed with the client. From a legal point of view, it would be preferable for the client to mail the form to the insurance company, although the very fact that the client gave the psychotherapist the form would likely establish authorization for a release of confidential information.

There should certainly never be any substantive clinical communication made (such as to an insurance company in response to a request for a progress report and prediction of cure) that has not been shown to and discussed with the client. In those rare instances where the information must be communicated and the client would, in fact, be harmed by knowing the information, it is best to (a) obtain a release for the specific communication in question, along with a waiver of right to have access to the report, and (b) avoid using any language that might exacerbate the emotional tone for the client.

Brodsky (1978) posits a so-called Promethean model for communications of this type (in Greek literature, Prometheus risked the wrath of Zeus through sharing knowledge and power of fire with mankind, was punished, but was released from his chains by Hercules). He states:

> The Promethean model is one of sharing power and information fully with the client, in any professional setting. All files, all information are shared with the client. No closed files are maintained and all the decision making is participatory. (p. 130)

It is difficult to see how this kind of client involvement in the recording and communication systems could be viewed negatively by a psychotherapist, except perhaps by one who strives for a god-like stature.

RECOMMENDATION 5: ESTABLISH A DIAGNOSTIC SYSTEM

Many psychotherapists believe that diagnostics are unnecessary. Without digressing, suffice it to say that a substantive theoretical argument could be made that every therapeutic step is, in fact, diagnostic in nature and that greater reliance on formal diagnostic procedures would enhance the efficacy of the treatment.

Be that as it may, contemporary social policy has led the courts to hold that psychotherapists have a duty to warn others if a client is potentially dangerous to self or third parties. Knapp and Vandecreek (1982), Wilkinson (1982), and Woody (in press) have reviewed the duty-to-warn cases. For the purposes of this contribution, the discussion can be limited to how best to assess for a possible warning of dangerousness. The answer is found in psychodiagnostics.

To be sure, there is no fool-proof method for evaluating dangerousness. There are certain psychological test indices (summarized by Walters, 1980), but they will all potentially lead to false positives (i.e., identifying someone as dangerous when, in fact, they will not prove to be dangerous in the long run). Rightly or wrongly, the courts have interpreted public policy as requiring that this risk of error be allowed and that psychotherapists exercise their prediction-of-dangerousness skills as well as is possible.

For this discussion of malpractice, the conclusion is that the standard of care for predicting dangerousness to self or to third parties requires that the psychotherapist apply some sort of diagnostic measure. Perhaps it will be simply inquiring about thoughts of harming self or others. For example, liability was removed from one psychiatrist because he did a case history that was deemed adequate, even though his diagnosis proved to be incorrect (TIMMINS v. STATE, 1968). As Wilkinson (1982) describes it:

> A primary duty of the psychiatrist is to make a proper diagnosis of the patient's condition. To do this, the psychiatrist must make a thorough examination into the patient's history, and must interpret this data correctly. Failure to do so will result in liability. (p. 75)

A psychotherapist cannot hide behind the notion that since his or her theory of therapy does not rely on psychodiagnostics (such as a client-centered advocate who believes in a nondirective, humanistic approach), there is no reason for diagnostics. In the courtroom, it would be fruitless (perhaps even detrimental) to say, "I take the client wherever he or she is, and let the treatment evolve." Like it or not, the legal perspective necessitates reasonable diagnostic assessment.

There is no single procedure that automatically fulfills the requirement of diagnosis. As mentioned, it might be adequate (reasonable) to simply inquire about certain critical factors. Depending upon the context or the nature of the case, it might be necessary to employ a standardized psychological test, such as perhaps relying upon one of the research-based indices of dangerousness that can be derived from the Minnesota Multiphasic Personality Inventory (as noted by Walters, 1980). Further, the qualifications of the psychotherapist and the type of client would enter into the determination of what sort of diagnostics would be necessary. For example, it is unlikely that a clinical social worker would be expected to make use of psychological tests (unless, of course, he or she had a joint practice with a clinical psychologist), but likewise he or she would be expected to restrict professional services to those clients who could be assessed adequately through social work methodologies. On the other hand, it would be difficult to excuse a clinical psychologist from using a psychological test with a client who had the characteristics that would cause a comparable clinical psychologist to employ tests for assessment.

In meeting this legal mandate, the important message is to accept a reasonable assessment strategy. As reflected in the TIMMINS case, a reasonable effort, perhaps regardless of how accurate it proves to be, is a viable defense.

RECOMMENDATION 6: BASE ALL PSYCHOTHERAPEUTIC INTERVENTIONS ON A WELL-ESTABLISHED THEORY

Malpractice can be due to a failure to base the psychotherapy on an appropriate theory. Prosser (1971) states, "A 'school' must be a recognized one with definite principles, and it must be the line of thought of at least a respectable minority of the profession" (p. 163). As for a seemingly-discreet theoretical approach (and based on an analysis of legal cases involving nontraditional forms of psychotherapy), Glenn (1974) believes that the standard of care would be derived from the closest theoretical school of thought.

It seems possible that any nontraditional form of psychotherapy runs the risk of appearing to be a radical departure from the "tried and true," and it is likely that courts would move toward traditional ideas about what the appropriate standard of care should be, even if it is at the expense of innovation. Wilkinson (1982) summarizes, "A psychiatrist who utilizes a treatment that is supported by a respectable minority of psychiatrists is not ordinarily guilty of malpractice if the treatment ultimately fails, so long as the psychiatrist's conduct was in conformity with the acceptable practices as espoused by the minority" (p. 76).

Following a traditional approach for the sake of being traditional (and avoiding legal liability) can be an affront to the essence of professionalism. It is only through innovation in clinical practices that advances in theory and technique can be obtained. Wilkinson (1982) acknowledges this problem as follows:

> Difficulties arise when the psychiatrist wishes to pursue a new treatment, but at the same time does not want to risk exposure to potential liability should the treatment prove ineffective, or even harmful to the patient. In such a situation, one must balance the need to protect the patient by assuring that only proven treatments are used, with the need to develop new methods that may produce even better and more effective results...unless modern psychiatry is allowed to explore new methods of treatment, the future growth of the profession and discovery of new cures will be greatly inhibited. (p. 76)

The balancing test applied by the court (i.e., whether or not advancing knowledge was more societally useful than a conservative treatment), would likely receive weighting from the degree of professionalism (again, under traditional definition) that the psychotherapist achieved. For example, an innovative therapeutic procedure that had been researched to some extent, that was specified (such as in a scholarly journal), was considered by professionals other than the psychotherapist in question (such as a review board of peers or a supervisor) for its applicability to the type of client at issue, and was applied by a professional with strong credentials would probably lead to the court's straining to justify the professional usage. It is the instance where there is an element of dubious motive and by a professional of questionable repute that the court would decisively denounce innovation or nontraditional procedures.

By theory or context, certain "schools" of psychotherapy possess unique liabilities. For a clear-cut example, consider the psychotherapist who serves as a member of a "behavioral medicine" team. Knapp and Vandecreek (1981) point out that the psychologist within the behavioral medicine framework (a) runs the risk of "crossing the line into practicing medicine" (p. 677), (b) may get committed to treatments that his or her training cannot adequately fulfill (thus, there should be collaboration with a physician), (c) cannot rely on the close emotional bond that has been common to psychodynamic therapy and which serves to deter legal actions, and (d) must recognize that the stigma has been removed from receiving mental health treatments, thereby removing a historical reason that kept clients from "going public," as would be necessary if a lawsuit against a therapist were filed.

As should be evident, the safest route is a conservative path, one that has been often trod by other professionals. To take a side excursion into the unknown hinterlands will probably be branded a "frolic on one's own," and will be stripped of professional respectability. To lead a quest for a more direct and productive access to uncharted treatment realms, if done with the honor of the true scientist-practitioner, will be heralded.

RECOMMENDATION 7: SERVE STRICTLY AS A PSYCHOTHERAPIST TO YOUR CLIENTS

As the first paragraph of this contribution indicated, it is tempting to allow the client to salve the isolated psychotherapist's ego. The intimacy of the psychotherapeutic relationship can foster pseudoconnections. It must always be remembered and staunchly maintained that the client came to the psychotherapist for treatment; the connection did not occur to create social relations between the client and the psychotherapist.

Sexual relations between the client and the psychotherapist constitute an increasing source of legal action. Erotic contacts in psychotherapy are not as rare as professionalism would dictate (Holyroyd & Brodsky, 1977; Kardener, Fuller, & Mensh, 1973). However, frequency of occurrence does not, in any way, justify the sexual contact. It is well established legally that an entire profession can be in malpractice if there is damage being done to the clients by omission or commission, if a balancing of the benefits and liabilities supports that the profession should be conducting itself differently.

In the case of sexual relations between the client and the psychotherapist, only the most spurious of arguments could be framed to justify sexual acting out. On the contrary, the codes of ethics for professional associations are increasingly spelling out that sexual relations are, in point of fact, the basis for an ethical violation (note the codes of ethics for the American Psychological Association, the National Association of Social Workers, and the American Association for Sex Educators, Counselors, and Therapists, to name but a few). Moreover, state statutes may well recognize the code of ethics (such as in the licensing laws for psychologists) and thereby make it such that an ethical violation under the aegis of a professional organization (such as the American Psychological Association) could lead to being an unlawful act under the statutes of the state; both criminal and/or civil sanctions could potentially be imposed against the violator (Woody, 1983).

It is safe to say that any professional accused of malpractice who has been found to have engaged in conduct deemed unethical by his or her primary professional organization would have a difficult time gaining absolution from the allegations in a court of law.

True professionalism mandates that the psychotherapeutic relationship be restricted to professional service. It cannot be an invitation to other sorts of conflicting relations, be they business, social, sexual, or whatever. Avoiding conflicting relations is especially difficult for the practitioner in a rural area. Due to the small population within a fairly restricted area of service, it may well be that there will be contacts that could be avoided if the context were a metropolitan area. Within the rural framework, there may be chance "social" contacts, such as would result from competing in a bowling league or bumping into each other at a community festival. But even these contacts should not become self-serving nor negate the tenets of psychotherapy. If the psychotherapist is unable to function with the single purpose of professional service, albeit perhaps tempered or defined in part by the community context, he or she may be inadequately trained; and both professional and legal sanctions should be imposed to remedy the situation, such as by requiring that he or she (a) gain further training, (b) alter the type of services rendered, or (c) cease to be a psychotherapist.

RECOMMENDATION 8: DO NOT ALLOW CLIENTS TO ACCRUE A DEFICIT IN PAYMENTS

Supposedly in the name of "being reasonable about meeting the costs of treatment," some psychotherapists allow clients to accumulate debts to them. As a rule of thumb, the larger the amount owed to you by a client, the more likely it is that the client will become disenchanted with your therapeutic expertise and find reason to take a legal action against you (Wright, 1981). Moreover, the therapeutic benefits for the client decline as well.

It must be suspected that the presumably good intention that underlies extending credit to a client might be based on a less-than-healthy motive, namely greed! That is, perhaps psychotherapists realize that revenues may be lost if clients are required to pay as they go, and they want to reap all that is possible. This translates, purely and simply, into greed, one of the long-recognized "seven deadly sins." In this litigious era, greed can certainly be "deadly" in a malpractice sense of the word.

RECOMMENDATION 9: LEARN TO RELY UPON AN ATTORNEY

It is paradoxical, to say the least, that a psychotherapist, who does not hesitate to levy a fee for his or her professional services, hesitates to pay a fee to another professional. Wright (1981) has recognized this tendency, and personal experience supports that it may be stronger than with nonprofessionals; that is, it may well be (again, perhaps because of the humanistic nature of psychotherapy) that the psychotherapist is more resistant to paying a fee to an attorney (even when professional stature is at issue) than the average lay person would be.

What might at best be labeled "thrifty" might at worst be labeled "miserly." Whatever it may be called, failure to seek the counsel of an attorney whenever there is any doubt about the legalities of a situation is to court professional disaster; it is a price that can be ill-afforded, regardless of cost for the legal counsel.

RECOMMENDATION 10: CARRY MALPRACTICE INSURANCE

In selecting malpractice insurance, it is essential to be aware of whether it does or does not cover the legal expenses (e.g., attorney fees); some policies cover damages only. The cost for legal representation can be substantial. As

Wright (1981) points out, the majority of legal suits, whether they be actually filed or only threatened, require that a legal defense be formulated, and this can be costly. Premiums paid for insurance coverage are a small cost when placed against the possible amount of damages or legal fees that could amass, even in a frivolous or nuisance lawsuit.

RECOMMENDATION 11: IF YOU WORK FOR AN AGENCY OR INSTITUTION, HAVE A CONTRACT THAT SPECIFIES THE EMPLOYER'S LEGAL LIABILITY FOR YOUR PROFESSIONAL FUNCTIONING

Many times, it has been witnessed that when an employee is faced with a legal action, the employer suddenly finds a reason why the agency or institution should not be responsible for either the damages or legal fees. At the time that employment is accepted, the employer should be asked for a contractual obligation to provide insurance coverage for damages and legal representation for acts arising out of and in the course of employment. Obviously, it is feasible that a professional could engage in an activity that would not be sanctioned as being part of employment, such as allegedly having sexual relations with a client, and it is, therefore, essential to have the contract liability be well defined.

Similarly, the employee must require that the employer maintain reasonable conditions for the provision of professional services. For example, two psychologists in a mental hospital reported that their employer required them to sign insurance forms attesting that they supervised lay-level counselors, but that the employer refused to allow them the time to actually do the supervision. It seemed evident that they were being parties to fraud and that, potentially, if one of the counselors was found to be liable for malpractice, the psychologists could be held liable as well. This was most likely one of those "no-win situations." That is, the employer might well have refused to allow them the supervisory time, and the psychologists might have been faced with resigning or knowingly incurring legal liabilities. These are the kinds of dilemmas that must be solved through an idiosyncratic analysis of the alternatives. It is difficult and risky, but then that is part of being professional.

CONCLUSION

These recommendations are designed to promote reasonable and prudent psychotherapeutic services, yet allow the psychotherapist an opportunity to continue to seek advances and gain personal satisfaction. In regard to the latter, satisfaction means being able to function free from the crippling effects of unnecessary fear of legal actions for malpractice. As one psychiatrist recently lamented, "Now that malpractice suits are so common, it is just no fun being a psychotherapist any more." Hidden in the comment is a clue to one of the problem areas for psychotherapists: fun. Certainly we want our work to be pleasant, but contrary to romantic notions about professionalism, the rational view of psychotherapy is that it is the rendering of an expert service; it is not intended to yield "fun" or to satisfy personal needs beyond the recognized benefits of employment. As the recommendations herein should underscore, well-defined professional psychotherapy can be provided without the storm clouds of malpractice actions looming overhead.

Robert Henley Woody, Ph.D., Sc.D., J.D., is currently Professor of Psychology and Director of Clinical Psychology Training at Central Michigan University and maintains a private practice in clinical/forensic psychology. He is a Diplomate in Clinical Psychology, ABPP, and a Diplomate in Forensic Psychology, ABFP. He is the author of numerous books and articles relevant to clinical and forensic psychology. Dr. Woody may be contacted at the Department of Psychology, Central Michigan University, Mount Pleasant, MI 48859.

RESOURCES

Brodsky, S. L. Buffalo Bill's defunct now: Vulnerability of mental health professionals to malpractice. In W. E. Barton & C. L. Sanborn (Eds.), LAW AND THE MENTAL HEALTH PROFESSIONS. New York: International Universities Press, 1978.

Glenn, R. D. Standard of care in administering non-traditional psychotherapy. UNIVERSITY OF CALIFORNIA, DAVIS LAW REVIEW, 1974, **7**, 56-83.

Holyroyd, J. C. & Brodsky, A. M. Psychologists' attitudes and practices regarding erotic and nonerotic contact with patients. AMERICAN PSYCHOLOGIST, 1977, **32**, 843-849.

Kardener, S., Fuller, M., & Mensh, I. A survey of physicians' attitudes and practices regarding erotic and nonerotic contact with patients. AMERICAN JOURNAL OF PSYCHIATRY, 1973, **130**, 1077-1081.

King, J. H., Jr. THE LAW OF MEDICAL MALPRACTICE. St. Paul: West Publishing, 1977.

Knapp, S. & Vandecreek, L. Behavioral medicine: Its malpractice risks for psychologists. PROFESSIONAL PSYCHOLOGY, 1981, **12**, 677-683.

Knapp, S. & Vandecreek, L. Tarasoff: Five years later. PROFESSIONAL PSYCHOLOGY, 1982, **13**, 511-516.

Prosser, W. L. HANDBOOK OF THE LAWS OF TORTS (4th ed.). St. Paul: West Publishing, 1971.

Schwitzgebel, R. K. A contractual model for the protection of the rights of institutionalized mental patients. AMERICAN PSYCHOLOGIST, 1975, **30**, 815-820.

TIMMINS v. STATE, 58 MISC.2D 636, 296 N.Y.S.2D 429 (1968).

Trent, C. L. Psychiatric malpractice insurance and its problems: An overview. In W. E. Barton & C. J. Sanborn (Eds.), LAW AND THE MENTAL HEALTH PROFESSIONS. New York: International Universities Press, 1978.

Walters, H. A. Dangerous. In R. H. Woody (Ed.), THE ENCYCLOPEDIA OF CLINICAL ASSESSMENT (Vol. II). San Francisco: Jossey-Bass Publishers, 1980.

Wilkinson, A. P. Psychiatric malpractice: Identifying areas of liability. TRIAL, 1982, **18**, 10, 73-77, 89-90.

Woody, R. H. Ethical and legal aspects of sexual issues. In J. D. Woody & R. H. Woody (Eds.), SEXUAL ISSUES IN FAMILY THERAPY. Rockville, MD: Aspen Systems, 1983.

Woody, R. H. Legal dimensions of the human services relationship: Informed consent, privileged communication, duty to warn, and professional malpractice. In R. H. Woody (Ed.), HUMAN SERVICES LAW. San Francisco: Jossey-Bass, in press.

Wright, R. H. What to do until the malpractice lawyer comes: A survivor's manual. AMERICAN PSYCHOLOGIST, 1981, **36**, 1535-1541.

I SOLD MY PRIVATE PRACTICE

Robert D. Weitz

In 1971, following 31 years of private practice in clinical psychology, including 26 years on a full-time basis, I decided that it was time to think about closing out this phase of my career in favor of semiretirement. Five years later, my plan became a reality; I will relate here how it was done.

The initial idea of a career change came about during a winter vacation in Florida during December of 1971. I became intrigued with the idea of being able to swim, fish, play tennis, and so on, throughout the year. With my wife's concurrence, it was decided that we would plan to move to Florida in due course.

To insure our future security, my first step was to seek licensure in Florida. I took the examination and received my Florida license in July of 1972. At that point, I began to make known to my colleagues and others that I was interested in selling my practice. There was no doubt in my mind that the practice was salable by the very nature of its organization, pattern of referrals, and other factors. An underlying question of significance concerned the determination of its value were the practice to be sold. With this in mind, I began to research the matter by consulting with other professionals, including lawyers, dentists, physicians, and others, who previously had sold their practices. With the aid of my accountant, it was decided that the selling price would be fixed at the average of the gross annual income for the three years immediately prior to the anticipated date of sale.

Now what was there about my practice that caused me to believe it could be sold? To begin with, I was the first private practicing psychologist in the State of New Jersey, and among the first in the entire country. In addition to my own services, I maintained a staff of three part-time psychologists and a secretary. My work was primarily concerned with psychological testing and psychotherapy, but, further, I served as a consultant to a number of public and private agencies, including police departments, court systems, rehabilitation services, schools, adoption agencies, and mental health facilities. These relationships provided a steady stream of referrals. In addition, referrals were regularly forthcoming from professionals in other fields (physicians, dentists, lawyers, optometrists, podiatrists) with whom personal relationships were established over the years. Last, but by no means least, there were regular referrals from the hundreds of clients and patients who were known to the office from past years.

When it became known that my practice was for sale, inquiries began to come forth, but, for the most part, the individuals involved were not license eligible and generally without adequate qualifications. They apparently viewed the purchase of the practice as a means of obtaining professional credibility for themselves. Ultimately, a qualified psychologist sought to purchase the practice and plans for the sale were established - or nearly so. I decided not to sell to that party, as he and his attorney sought to change the financial arrangements of the purchase plan each time we met. Their uncertainties undermined my confidence relative to my future financial security were the sale consummated. I terminated these negotiations at my lawyer's office during the meeting scheduled for signing the purchase contracts.

Once again the search for a buyer was in effect. By pure chance, I met the right person, the ultimate buyer, when I attended a sex therapy workshop conducted under the auspices of the New Jersey College of Medicine and Dentistry during the spring of 1975. One presentation was by a young man who was listed on the program as Staff Psychologist with the Division of Obstetrics and Gynecology. I was intrigued by his command of the subject, his ability to lecture without notes, and by the obvious confidence that he had in himself. I immediately sensed that here was the type of person who could readily succeed in the private practice of clinical psychology, and the type of individual to whom I would like to sell my practice. Following his presentation, I introduced myself to the young psychologist and congratulated him on his performance. From the discussion which followed between us, I learned that, in addition to being on the faculty of the College of Medicine and Dentistry, he conducted a small private practice as a clinical psychologist in another part of the state, and that in the future he hoped to expand his private work. I thereupon advised him that I was seeking to sell my practice and it was my personal opinion that the opportunity would be ideal for him. He expressed interest, and we agreed to meet a few days later to discuss the matter in greater detail. This in turn led to a dinner meeting, with our respective wives attending also. It was mutually agreed at the conclusion of the evening that the matter would be pursued further. Subsequent discussions followed with the prospective buyer and his accountant, and 2 months later the terms of sale were agreed upon. I have included a facsimile of the contract, which we signed, at the end of this chapter.

This contract included the following details:

1. The sale price was established at the average level of the gross income covering the three prior years, 1972 to 1975.

2. The purchaser would make an initial payment of 10% of the purchase price with the balance to be paid in weekly installments without interest over a 10 year period beginning January 1, 1976.

3. The purchaser would be covered by life insurance with the seller as beneficiary up to the financial limit of the balance due on the sale price, the estate as beneficiary beyond that amount.

4. The partnership would be established for two years following the sale with financial arrangements as follows:

    a. For the first year the purchaser would work at the practice 3 days a week, whereas the seller would continue on a full-time basis. Both parties would share equally in the expenses and income.

    b. For the second year of the partnership, the seller would work at the practice for 2 days a week and the buyer would work on a full-time basis. Both parties would continue to share equally the expenses and income.

5. At the end of the second year, the partnership would automatically be dissolved with the buyer assuming full ownership and management of the practice.

6. It was the seller's responsibility to introduce the buyer to as many of his referral sources as possible and to introduce him to the community at large.

7. At the conclusion of the partnership, the seller's name would remain on the stationery as a consultant.

With the contract signed, the sales plan went into effect at the beginning of January, 1976. The arrangements have proven favorable to all concerned.

Let us now reflect upon the details of the contract relative to the significance to the buyer and seller.

Using the standard based upon the average income over a period of 3 years as a basis for the purchase price gave the buyer a picture of the potential for future earnings. There was no clear-cut rationale established arriving at the sale price but, based upon the information gathered, it appeared to be equitable.

Concerning the payment plan established, of major significance was the question of taxes related to the sale. By establishing an installment payment plan, I, as the seller, was able to save considerably compared with my tax responsibility had I been paid in full at the outset.

The life insurance policy on the buyer was a 10 year term policy. This assured me of full payment in the event of the death of the purchaser. With each installment payment by the purchaser, that amount accrued to his estate in the event of his demise.

The plan of having the purchaser work only 3 days a week at the office for the first year allowed him to continue his medical school position. Sharing half the net income provided him with considerable increment in his yearly income. In addition, his presence resulted in a significant increase in the gross income for the office. The provision allowing me, as the seller, to receive half of the net income over the second year, while being present only 2 days a week, allowed me an easier transition with respect to my move to Florida. It did, however, require weekly commuting between Florida and New Jersey during the second year of the partnership.

As part of our agreement in the contract, the purchaser was introduced to many professionals and other significant people in the community. He was immediately invited to join the local professional and businessmen's club and other local organizations. New referrals to the office were immediately directed to him. His acceptance by the referral sources proved to be no problem whatsoever.

CONCLUSION

It is my opinion that many psychology practices have a sale value. To find a qualified purchaser and make the smoothest possible transition, however, requires time and a significant amount of patience. Details should be carefully worked out, and ample time should be given to the transition faced by patients, referral sources, and others affected by the change. Care should also be given to the financial aspects of the sale to derive the most benefit to both buyer and seller. With these thoughts in mind, a successful transition can be made to the satisfaction of all involved.

CONTRACT

Re: Sale of private practice of Dr. Robert D. Weitz to Dr. John Smith

This Agreement made this 25th day of September, 1975, between Dr. Robert D. Weitz, hereinafter called "Weitz," and Dr. John Smith, hereinafter called "Smith."

WHEREAS, Weitz and Smith are duly licensed and qualified psychologists, and

WHEREAS, Weitz maintains and conducts the practice of psychology at 57 Cedar Lane, Teaneck, New Jersey, and

WHEREAS, Smith desires to purchase and Weitz desires to sell an interest in such practice and eventually all of said practice,

NOW, THEREFORE, in consideration of the mutual promises, it is hereby agreed as follows:

1.   Smith agrees to purchase and Weitz agrees to sell to Smith all his right, title, and interest in his practice of psychology for the sum of _____, payable as follows:

a. $_____ upon execution of this agreement.

b. $_____ a week commencing January 1, 1976 and until January 1, 1978 (Total $_____).

c. $_____ a week commencing January 1, 1978 and until January 1, 1980 (Total $_____).

d. $_____ a week commencing January 1, 1980 and until the entire balance of $_____ is paid.

All payments hereunder shall be made without interest.

In the event of the death of Smith and the payment of life insurance proceeds to Weitz in accordance with Paragraph 7 hereof the obligations of Smith contained in this Paragraph shall be deemed paid.

In the event of the death of Weitz and the payment of life insurance proceeds to Smith in accordance with Paragraph 7 hereof, Smith agrees to immediately pay the entire proceeds of such insurance to the widow of Weitz, if living or if not, to the estate in full discharge of his obligations hereunder.

2. It is agreed that commencing January 1, 1976 and until December 3, 1977, Smith and Weitz shall be equal partners in the practice and psychology presently being conducted by Weitz under the following terms and conditions:

a. Smith shall devote 3 days per week during the first 12 months and full time for the second 12-month period.

b. Weitz shall devote his full time and effort to the partnership during the first 12 months. During the second 12-month period Weitz shall be required to devote only 2 days per week to the partnership.

c. Both parties shall share profits and losses equally.

d. In the event Weitz is maintaining a home in Florida during the second 12-month period his weekly costs of travel, not exceeding $200.00 per week, shall be borne as an expense of the partnership prior to any distribution of our accounting for profits.

3. It is further agreed that from and after January 1, 1978 the partnership shall be dissolved and Smith shall become the owner of all partnership assets including the right to continue to use the name of Weitz and that the interest of Weitz and his right to any of the former partnership assets shall immediately cease and terminate subject, however, to the provisions of Paragraph 4 hereof.

4. As security for the payment of the purchase price by Smith, Weitz shall receive a security interest in any interest transferred to Smith and in the assets of the partnership including but not limited to accounts receivable, good will, and furniture and equipment.

5. It is understood that Weitz is a Tenant under a lease dated November 1, 1974 covering premises at 57 Cedar Lane, Teaneck, New Jersey which term expires on October 31, 1976 and which lease contains an option to renew for an additional term of 2 years to October 31, 1978. Weitz agrees to use his best effort to have the lease assigned to Smith and Weitz jointly. In the event such an assignment is not permitted by the Landlord, Weitz agrees to exercise the option to renew said lease upon written request of Smith. In such event Smith shall be obligated to pay one-half of all rents and charges under said lease until January 1, 1978. Thereafter and until the termination of said lease and any renewal term, Smith shall be obligated for the payment of all rents and charges under said lease and he agrees to indemnify and hold Weitz harmless from any and all claims by the Landlord pursuant to the terms of said lease.

6. Upon termination of the partnership on December 31, 1977, and for a period of 10 years thereafter, Weitz will not, within the Counties of Hudson, Bergen, Passaic, and Essex, directly or indirectly, own, manage, operate, control, be employed by, participate in, or be connected in any manner with any profession similar to the type of profession conducted by Smith at the time of the termination of the partnership.

7. The parties agree to obtain life insurance on each others life under the terms and conditions set forth in Schedule A annexed hereto.

8. Upon the termination of the partnership, Smith agrees that so long as he continues to use Weitz's name he shall obtain and keep in full force and effect malpractice insurance with Weitz as a named insured in an amount not less than $1,000,000.00.

9. This agreement shall be binding upon the parties hereto, their heirs, personal representatives, and assigns.

IN WITNESS WHEREOF, the parties hereto have hereunto set their hands and seals the day and year first above written.

_____
ROBERT D. WEITZ

_____
JOHN SMITH

Robert D. Weitz, Ph.D., currently maintains a limited practice, specializing in the hypnotic therapy of stress related physical disorders. He is also Chair of the Board of Governors of the Behavioral Sciences Center of Nova University on an avocational basis and is editor of the journal, PSYCHOTHERAPY IN PRIVATE PRACTICE. Dr. Weitz may be contacted at 7566 Martinique Boulevard, Boca Raton, FL 33433.

PSYCHOLOGICAL TEST ANALYSIS
AND REPORT WRITING
VIA A WORD PROCESSOR

Ken R. Vincent

"A clinician's best efforts on his or her best day when codified in objective form will always be superior to his or her efforts at dynamic interpretation on any other day" (Wiggins, 1973, p. 216). This statement is the cornerstone of much psychological test interpretation in automated form, whether via a fully automated computerized system or any other system of test analysis that is based upon objective rules and precoded statements. Predeveloped rules facilitate analysis time, and precoded statements obviously lessen the test interpretation time. While such a system imposes some constraints upon the user, the relief from the tedium inherent in psychological report writing more than compensates for any limitations.

The approach I will discuss here is a fully codified system of automated interpretive statements for a complete psychological test battery and is an extension of my **SEMI-AUTOMATED FULL BATTERY** (Vincent, 1980a, 1980b, 1981) which is used in tandem with my **MMPI SEMI-AUTOMATED INTERPRETIVE STATEMENTS** (Vincent, 1980c). The **AUTOMATED INTERPRETIVE STATEMENTS FOR THE IMPRESSION, VINCENT BIOGRAPHICAL INVENTORY, AND SUMMARY AND COMMENTS SECTIONS OF THE PSYCHOLOGICAL ASSESSMENT BATTERY** (Vincent, 1982), part of which is included in this chapter, are a series of phrases which, when used with the earlier works, make the interpretation and writing of a complete psychological battery a fully codified system.

In compiling a report using automated interpretive statements, a psychologist first scores the test data up to the interpretation stage. Then, referring to the interpretive statements for the tests and other sections used, he or she abstracts the appropriate statements using predetermined rules where applicable and works through the entire report, writing down the codes for the statements used. The clinician may vary from the standard format to add low frequency statements to the test battery as appropriate on those items or tests which have not been codified. In my experience with using the standard format, only a half dozen sentences need to be written for a typical three page psychological report.

The system shown here has cut my time spent in analysis and report writing per battery from about an hour down to an average of 25 minutes, with a comparable reduction in the amount of time required for the report to be typed. In preparing the report, I write down the appropriate call letters on the Work Sheet, along with any additional interpretive sentences or statements that need to be made. The secretary then refers to the Work Sheet and merely calls up the numbers for the appropriate sentences. One call number centers the report and blocks out the name and identifying information on the patient, along with the tests used in the author's standard full battery. Two to four call numbers result in up to a page and a half of Minnesota Multiphasic Personality Inventory (MMPI) analysis on this system. The system can be used even without an automated typing system by a psychologist who either furnishes the prepared interpretive statements in booklet form to a secretary or dictates the statements verbatim.

I have included below an example of a completed Work Sheet, followed by the report that this brief amount of information generated, using the automated system. Psychologists wishing to use such a system, but who use different tests or even a different report format, could use the example and guidelines enumerated at the end of the report in building their own system.

TABLE 1: WORKSHEET

FORMAT # _____1_____

NAME: _Jane Doe_   REFERRAL: _Dr. Smith_
RACE: _____W_____   AGE: _____39_____
MARITAL STATUS: _____M_____   EDUCATION: _H.S. + 3 yr Coll._
DATE: _____3-2-82_____   DATE OF EXAMINATION: _____3-27-82_____
PLACE OF EXAMINATION: _Memorial_

IMPRESSION:

_____1, 17, 21, 28, 34, 55, 79, 80._____

VINCENT BIOGRAPHICAL INVENTORY: _3, 6 yr. old son, she has an 18 yr old son and 24 yr old adopted son; 31, 39, 73: the first of twins, having a twin brother, 99, 119, 130, 133: 72 (cancer) 134, 136: her father, uncle and grandfather, 137: her father 157: "neck pain", 163: following death of her daughter 9 yrs. ago. She has had 4 miscarriages, 167: "neck pain, shoulder pain + numbness in my right hand."_

TEST RESULTS:

Intellectual Assessment:

_1_ : IQ: Verbal: _109_   Performance: _103_   Full Scale: _106_

_____ : WRAT:
      Reading: Grade_____, _____%
      Arithmetic: Grade_____, _____%

_____11, 120, 135_____

Personality Assessment:

HOLTZMAN INKBLOT TECHNIQUE: _A-1, 103, 108, 129_

LOEVINGER SENTENCE COMPLETION BLANK: _IV. The pt. is a lit histrionic._
_B-13, B-21, C-4, D-9, E-11, E-20, F-9, G-1, G8, H-3._
The pt. sees her main problem as neck pain.

SRRS or LESA: _3, 6-7, 6-30, 6-35, 6-43._

MMPI: _Sect. I: 9, Sect. II: 13, 13(a), 13(y)_

Other:

DSM III:

Axis I: _Psychogenic Pain vs. Psychological factors_
affecting physical problem

Axis II: _Histrionic personality_

Axis III: No data.

Axis IV: Psycho-Social Stressors for Past Year: _health, educational,_
and other interpersonal severity: Moderate.

Axis V: Highest Level of adaptive Functioning for Past Year: _fair_

SUMMARY AND COMMENTS:
8, 45, 50, 51, 91, 101, her inability to complete
formal schooling was a major blow to her, 109,
_121, 122_

TABLE 2: PSYCHOLOGICAL REPORT

NAME:	Jane Doe	Referral: Dr. Smith
RACE:	Caucasian	
AGE:	39	
MARITAL STATUS:	Married	
EDUCATION:	High School + 3 Years College	

Date:	3/2/82
Date of Examination:	3/2/82
Place of Examination:	Memorial Hospital

INSTRUMENTS USED:

Wechsler Adult Intelligence Scale (WAIS)
Bender Motor Gestalt Test
Holtzman Inkblot Technique
Loevinger Sentence Completion Blank
Social Readjustment Rating Scale
Minnesota Multiphasic Personality Inventory (MMPI)
Vincent Biographical Inventory
Psychological Interview

IMPRESSION:

Ms. Doe is a stout woman of medium build, who was attired in bedclothes. She has dyed blonde hair and wore glasses. She was pleasant and cooperative during the evaluation, and was quite verbose.

VINCENT BIOGRAPHICAL INVENTORY:

She currently lives with her husband and six year old son. She has an 18 year old son and a 24 year old adopted son. She relates her marriage is happy. She reports being married once previously.

Developmentally, she reports being the first of twins, having a twin brother. She reports having frequent crying spells and being easily upset as a child. She relates no significant educational problems. Regarding her family of origin, her father died at age 72 of cancer, and her mother is still living. She reports a history of alcoholism in her family (her father, uncle, and grandfather). She also relates her father had a drug problem. She relates a chronic health problem with neck pain. She reports previous psychiatric hospitalization for depression following the death of her daughter nine years ago. She has had four miscarriages.

She relates the reason for her hospitalization as "neck pain, shoulder pain, and numbness in my right hand."

TEST RESULTS:

Intellectual Assessment

On the WECHSLER ADULT INTELLIGENCE SCALE the patient scored as follows:

Verbal IQ: 109   Performance IQ: 103   Full Scale IQ: 106

On the WAIS the patient's overall performance was indicative of an individual whose intellectual ability was in the range of average intellect. The patient's subscale configuration on the WAIS was generally not indicative of behavioral correlates associated with organicity. The patient's performance on the Bender Motor Gestalt Test was negative.

Personality Assessment

On the HOLTZMAN INKBLOT TECHNIQUE the following was indicated: The patient is fearful of hypocrisy in others and feels they may be presenting a facade and are not what they seem to be. The patient feels sexually inadequate and fears abandonment. Anxiety and tension are present; emotional lability and excitability are likely.

Innovations In Clinical Practice: A Source Book

On the LOEVINGER SENTENCE COMPLETION BLANK the patient's overall performance depicts an individual whose ego development is at the conformity level, which is the level of the majority of the general population. Emphasis is on conformity and external rules, law, order, and authority. The patient's outlook is traditional and in line with the values and mores of the polite middle class. The patient stresses helping, belonging, social niceness, and social acceptability.

The patient is a bit histrionic. She is quite preoccupied with health concerns and with weight problems. She sees herself as very feminine and is quite traditional regarding male-female sex roles. She appears close to her mother; she was close to her father and mourns his loss. She appears close to her spouse. She is quite concerned about their children and worries about being a good parent. She is very family-oriented and places a heavy emphasis on family responsibilities. She wants desperately to prove herself and succeed at something, but is apt to feel inadequate in doing so. She sees her main problem as her neck pain.

On the SOCIAL READJUSTMENT RATING SCALE the patient's overall performance is indicative of an individual who has incurred a moderate amount of stress in the past year, the most significant of which is: major change in eating habits, ceasing work outside the home, major personal illness, and ceasing formal schooling.

On the MMPI the patient produced a valid profile and the patient's validity scale configuration depicts an individual who responded to the test items in a defensive fashion and who is apt to be lacking in self insight, intolerant of deviant belief systems, and to be shy, inhibited, and socially anxious. This profile type is most often encountered in neurotic individuals but, when attained in a seriously disturbed patient, it is apt to reflect a general lack of awareness on the patient's part as to the seriousness of his or her condition.

Patients with this profile type are usually seen as neurotic and manifesting physical complaints. A wide variety of physical symptomatology is apt to be presented, including: back pain, headaches, gastro-intestinal difficulties, as well as occasional numbness or tremors. These patients are occasionally seen as depressed and anxious, but most likely convert their difficulties into functional physical complaints. These patients are usually egocentric, immature, and suggestible and have longstanding and inordinate needs for sympathy, affection, attention, and reassurance. Few of these patients are incapacitated by their illnesses, at least in regard to doing pleasurable activities. These patients have a strong need to see and interpret problems in living as sociably acceptable. They typically make excessive use of the defense mechanisms of repression, denial, and somatization. Secondary gain for their illnesses is apt to be operating in the form of either manipulation for the attention of close family members or avoiding responsibilities.

These patients manifest physical problems of all sorts. This is the mean profile type for patients evidencing low back pain, early onset asthma, pseudo-neurologic conditions (including pseudo multiple sclerosis), and female urethral syndrome. In addition to the above-mentioned categories and gastro-intestinal and cardiac complaints, virtually no organ system is immune. These patients are almost always seen as neurotic and evidencing psychogenic pain, psychosomatic difficulties, conversion hysteria, or anxiety.

As there is always the possibility that the patient may be evidencing actual physical pathology in conjunction with functional symptomatology, the following is a breakdown of the probabilities of functional physical complaints being evidenced in any individual patient and is based on studies done at the Mayo Clinic on patients of this profile type. For individuals of this profile type who are the same age and sex as the patient, two-thirds were seen as having primarily functional problems, one-tenth presented a mixed picture, and one-fourth were seen as having primarily physical problems.

DIAGNOSTIC IMPRESSION:

DSM-III:

Axis I: Psychogenic Pain versus Psychological Factors affecting physical condition.

Axis II: Histrionic personality.

Axis III: No data.

Axis IV: Psychosocial stressor for past year: health, educational, and other interpersonal. Severity: moderate.

Axis V: Highest level of adaptive functioning for past year: fair.

SUMMARY AND COMMENTS:

The patient appears to be suffering from a mixture of anxiety and somatization. She is an emotionally unstable, emotionally labile, overdramatic individual who is easy prey for stress. She is a passive person who is desirous of support. She is an individual of average intelligence. Her overall level of ego-conscience development is good. Her inability to complete her formal schooling was a major blow to her.

Psychotherapeutically, she will probably profit best from a treatment approach that emphasizes developing a more assertive and modulated stance toward life. Additionally, she needs to be coaxed back into becoming active in the business of living, and sick role behavior needs to be discouraged.

Ken R. Vincent

Ken R. Vincent, Ed.D., Psychologist

HOW TO DEVELOP AN AUTOMATED REPORT

Interested readers who possess a word processor can develop their own report preparation system. (Of course, it is also possible without a word processor if you develop a list of coded statements to guide your secretary). An important aspect of this approach is that it permits each clinician to develop a system which reflects a personal report style. If you want to develop a system, a good place to begin would be with a careful analysis of your past reports. To utilize an automated system, you will need to follow a reasonably consistent format.

Your next goal will be to develop statements for each section of your reports. The list of statements will need to include a whole range of possible statements, descriptions, test results, conclusions, recommendations, and so on for the client population with which you work. Once your statements have been developed, they will need to be saved so that they can be integrated into your reports. This process will vary, depending on your word processing software. In most programs, each statement will be assigned a corresponding code and file name. This will allow the coded statement to be rapidly inserted at the appropriate point in a report.

DEVELOPING INTERPRETIVE STATEMENTS

The following are brief suggestions for developing interpretive statements:

1. If your reports include detailed results from specific tests, you will need a supply of all the previous research on the instrument to be automated or, at least, the major reviews of the tests plus the landmark articles. In the case of client descriptions, you will want to make a systematic analysis of potential descriptions.

2. You should be thoroughly familiar with the test instruments which you wish to automate. The more experience you have with a test instrument, the better you will know its quirks and will have dealt with low frequency profiles and responses. After you have integrated all the data available on an instrument and formulated appropriate interpretive phrases, you will need to draw on experience to fill in the gaps of interpretation with your clinical experience.

3. One of the best sources of personalized lucidity is to reanalyze your old psychological test reports and abstract those statements that are clear and succinct. Such statements can then be extracted and codified to describe specific test score patterns. In this way, your reports will always reflect your best efforts at interpretation, since you have already formulated your best work.

4. When building something new, such as your own social history, or developing a checklist of history, needs, or behaviors for your own setting or a special situation, (e.g., dialysis patients), try to get ideas from as many related types of systems, tests, or checklists as possible through a literature review. By analyzing the best attempts of others to build a system, you can develop an even better one. Also, relevant structured evaluation instruments, rating scales, and checklists can give you ideas on how to build something totally unique and superior.

5. At this point, you may wish to review your efforts and think of any other coded statements that can be added.

6. Next, use your system in rough form for about 50-100 cases, continually revising your statements as you go. At this point, you should have a coded list of high quality statements that will serve you well, though the revision process goes on forever. You may wish to update your narrative as ideas come to you or to simply make notes and periodically (about once a year) update your program.

7. Continue to collect articles on the tests you use and update the hard data (as opposed to the narrative) every few years.

You now have a system that should save you time and produce a better product.

SAMPLE STATEMENTS

The following list contains some sample statements drawn from THE SEMI-AUTOMATED FULL BATTERY (Vincent, 1980a, 1980b, 1981) which pertain to the patient's appearance. From this partial list you can get a sense of how the statements merge together to form a complete sentence. Statements in other sections of the report are of necessity much more complex and lengthy. However, the ones listed here should give you an idea of how to develop statements for automation.*

IMPRESSION

APPEARANCE STATEMENTS

1. The patient is a man
2. The patient is a woman
3. The patient is an adolescent boy
4. The patient is an adolescent girl
5. The patient is a middle-aged man
6. The patient is a middle-aged woman
7. The patient is an elderly man
8. The patient is an elderly woman
9. who was casually attired
10. who is petite
11. who is huge
12. of short stature
13. of medium height
14. who is tall
15. and emaciated.
16. and of thin build.
17. and of medium build.
18. and of muscular build.
19. and of chunky build.
20. and obese.
21. The patient was well dressed and groomed.
22. The patient was casually attired.
23. The patient was attired in bedclothes.
24. The patient was unkempt and slovenly attired.
25. The patient had sandy blonde hair.
26. The patient had light brown hair.
27. The patient had brunette hair.
28. The patient had black hair.
29. The patient had an Afro.
30. The patient had bright red hair.
31. The patient had a mustache.
32. The patient was unshaven.
33. The patient was bald.
34. which was thinning.
35. which was laced with grey.
36. which was a wig.
37. The patient had a tatoo.
38. The patient had braces on his or her teeth.
39. The patient had several teeth missing.
40. The patient walked with a cane.
41. The patient was in a wheel chair.
42. The patient had an obvious motor impairment.

---

*Statements from THE SEMI-AUTOMATED FULL BATTERY, copyright 1981, by Ken R. Vincent are reprinted by permission of the author.

43. The patient was receiving an IV which compromised the testing somewhat.
44. The patient stuttered.
45. The patient had an obvious speech impediment.
46. The patient was hard of hearing.
47. The patient was quite hard of hearing and this made the testing difficult.
48. The patient wore glasses.

TEST BEHAVIOR

49. The patient was pleasant and cooperative during the evaluation.
50. The patient was despondent during the evaluation.
51. The patient was overtly cooperative during the evaluation.
52. The patient was anxious during the evaluation.
53. The patient was defensive during the evaluation.
54. The patient was generally uncooperative during the evaluation.
55. The patient was hostile and suspicious during the evaluation.
56. The patient was restless.
57. The patient was agitated.
58. The patient was quite verbose during the evaluation.
59. The patient was emotionally labile during the evaluation.
60. The patient was overdramatic and emotionally labile during the evaluation.
61. The patient was withdrawn during much of the evaluation.
62. Many of the patient's verbalizations were loose, disjointed, and bizarre.
63. Some of the patient's responses were a bit unusual.

SUMMARY

Computers and word processors will continue to play an increasingly important role in psychological testing and report generation. This chapter has described procedures for developing an automated system to generate psychological reports after tests are administered and scored by the clinician in a traditional fashion.

Computer programs also exist that will score as well as interpret tests using data supplied by the clinician. Additionally, a number of fully automated testing programs are currently available. When these programs are used, the client actually sits at a computer terminal and responds to test items as they are presented on the screen. After the tests are administered, the computer scores the tests and generates a report. However, even when fully automated systems are used, there will be a significant number of clients who, for various reasons both psychological and physical, will be unable or unwilling to take psychological testing via the fully automated system. Also, there are tests (such as neuropsychological instruments and the Wechsler performance scales) which do not lend themselves to full automation.

For many busy clinicians, the overall savings in time and the more consistent quality of test reports achieved by the use of automated and semi-automated systems should more than offset the time and expense required to develop such systems.

Ken R. Vincent, Ed.D., is currently a staff psychologist at The Hauser Clinic & Associates in Houston, Texas. He is senior author of the MMPI-168 CODEBOOK and author of numerous publications in the area of psychological diagnosis and assessment and the computerization of psychological testing. Dr. Vincent can be contacted at 7777 Southwest Freeway, Suite 1036, Houston, TX 77074.

RESOURCES

Vincent, K. R. Semi-automated full battery. JOURNAL OF CLINICAL PSYCHOLOGY, 1980, **36**, 437-446. (a)

Vincent, K. R. SEMI-AUTOMATED FULL BATTERY. Houstin, TX: Psychometric Press, 1980. (b)

Vincent, K. R. MMPI SEMI-AUTOMATED INTERPRETIVE STATEMENTS. Houstin, TX: Psychometric Press, 1980. (c)

Vincent, K. R. Using a word processor to expedite psychological testing. COMPUTERS IN PSYCHOLOGY-PSYCHIATRY, 1981, **3**, 8-9.

Wiggins, J. S. PERSONALITY AND PREDICTION: PRINCIPLES OF PERSONALITY ASSESSMENT. Reading, MA: Addison Wesley, 1973.

OTHER MATERIALS

The handbooks and materials listed below are all available from Psychological Softwear Specialists, 1776 Fowler, Suite #7, Richland, WA 99352.

AUTOMATED INTERPRETIVE STATEMENTS FOR THE IMPRESSION, VINCENT BIOGRAPHICAL INVENTORY, AND SUMMARY AND COMMENTS SECTIONS OF A PSYCHOLOGICAL ASSESSMENT BATTERY by Ken R. Vincent.

THE SEMI-AUTOMATED FULL BATTERY by Ken R. Vincent.

MMPI SEMI-AUTOMATED INTERPRETIVE STATEMENTS by Ken R. Vincent.

VINCENT BIOGRAPHICAL INVENTORY by Ken R. Vincent.

Computer systems and software for administering, scoring, and interpreting psychological tests:

Psychological Assessment Resources, Inc., P.O. Box 98, Odessa, FL 33556. Administration, scoring, and interpretive software including structured interviews, the Beck Depression Inventory, the MMPI, and 16PF. Other software is available for scoring and interpreting the WISC-R, WAIS-R, Bender-Gestalt, and Rorschach.

Psych Systems, 600 Reisterstown Road, Baltimore, MD 21208 and Compu-Psych, Inc., One Liberty Plaza, Liberty, MO 64068. Complete hardware and software systems for test administration, scoring, and interpretation of a large number of tests.

Psychometric Systems, 7500 Beechnut, Suite 308, Houston, TX 77074. Administration, scoring, and interpretation for an objective full psychological battery including: Clark Vocabulary Scale (IQ), Schedule of Recent Experience, Vincent Biographical Inventory, Beck Depression Inventory, and MMPI.

HOW TO IMPROVE THE MARKETING OF THERAPY SERVICES*

Herbert E. Klein

Even a normally busy therapist can hit a slow period, especially during economic doldrums. If the recession has dried up some of your regular sources of referrals, may be time to revitalize your practice. The following is a discussion of approaches that may help. After a brief introduction of ten different techniques, the contribution will focus on three approaches in more detail. While all the techniques might not apply to you, a number of them may prove useful. In some cases, you will be reminded of successful practice-building ideas you used in the past that should be dusted off and tried again. Many of the specific points listed in the first section are based on the experience of John K. Effren, psychologist and president of a consulting group, Professional Practice Developers of Englewood, New Jersey.

TEN WAYS TO REVITALIZE YOUR REFERRAL SOURCES

Here is a brief explanation of ten marketing ideas and some specific advice that will help you use them effectively.

1. Acknowledge that you need patients. Unless you tell them otherwise, your friends and even close colleagues may feel you do not need referrals, so you may have to remind them that you have practice hours to fill. In many cases, there is a very low correlation between the actual clinical competence of a therapist and his or her office activity; sometimes even the best therapists see their referrals decline for a while. Therefore, you should not be shy about letting other people know you are interested in more referrals.

2. Take on a trade name. Even if you have only two rooms, you can recruit one or more colleagues and set up a professional center. Patients are often attracted to group practices because they feel the practitioners are more competent. It may cost only $20 to register yourself as "The Center for Marriage and Family Counseling," or the "Greenville Psychotherapy Institute." Stay away from the word "clinic," however, since clinics fall under state regulations in many localities.

3. Announce your existing practice, or the formation of a new center or group. You have to build your image or at least have your name visible. A tasteful announcement in local newspapers is an inexpensive way to do it.

---

*Copyright 1983, Ridgewood Financial Institute, Inc. Adapted by permission.

Recent Federal laws mean that every state and every professional society should be permitting this type of announcement. Do not forget the telephone yellow pages, either. Phone book ads are one of the very top sources of referrals for many psychotherapists, whether it is just a name and number or a small display ad. What often makes phone book ads so effective is anonymity. A patient may not ask for a referral to a sex therapist, for example, but would look in the phone book. In a crisis, even sophisticated and intelligent people may not take the time to call their physician, but will check the phone book if they need someone right away. Also, many phone directories provide cross referencing, which allows you to put an eye-catching display ad under psychologist, for example, and then have your name and a cross reference under marriage counseling or some other category. Many large counties or metropolitan areas also have split phone books, which means you can target your ad to a specific 25 or 30 mile radius. (Details on yellow page advertising are discussed below.)

4. Rip up your resume, at least as a tool for promoting your practice. Many consultants find that it usually pays to develop an attractive, tasteful brochure, instead. It does not have to be elaborate, but it should be typeset on good paper. If possible, pay a graphics specialist to design a distinctive logo for you. Also, consider printing two brochures, one for the general public and one for other professionals. List all the major services you provide, but do not include every specialized clinical technique that comes to mind. Many people may feel that it is unlikely you can be an expert in everything.

5. Offer free lectures and workshops. Check the phone book for the names of local social service organizations, fraternal groups, athletic associations, cultural groups, churches, synagogues - there are so many, you will never have time to contact them all. For example, you can call some of the groups and say you or your center are sponsoring a series of talks in the interest of educating the public in various mental health areas, and you have selected this group as one to which you would like to offer your services, free of charge.

Do not try to sell yourself over the phone. Give a little information, just enough to gain an appointment. For example, say, "We're busy people and we're offering this in our free time to a few selected groups in your area. We'll be speaking with people next Wednesday and we have a half-hour open at 11 o'clock. Can you meet with us then?" This approach is much more positive than saying, "I'm new in town and I'm trying to build my practice."

At the meeting, your goal is to find the area of interest of the person to whom you are speaking. Suggest a lecture or workshop topic of wide general interest (e.g., sibling rivalry, attachment or loss, how to stop smoking). These are easy topics to sell, since people today are so interested in mental health. Your goal is a short, lively, even amusing presentation.

The key is not to bore the public with academic research material. What generates referrals is not lectures, but audience participation. That arouses interest in you. Make your presentation about 35 to 40 minutes, and then allow another 35 to 40 minutes for audience participation. If it is natural for you, be funny. Violate their stereotypes. Walk around in the group. Take questions. Invite people to call you at your office for more information. Of course, make your brochures available so they will have your phone number. And, after your presentation, be sure to stay at the podium, at the back of the room, or at the coffeepot. Much of the best contact begins after the talk is over.

6. Contact large corporations. Do not be scared off by the name IBM or Exxon. There are real live people behind those fancy desks and they may not have staff at a local office to provide the services they need. Call the large firms in your area and offer to provide short, lively programs on, for instance, alcohol and substance abuse or stress. Those are powerful buzz words because industry is very concerned about cutting down on their medical costs. Very often a large firm will pay a psychotherapist anywhere from $1,000 to $4,000 for a comprehensive workshop about stress directed to upper and middle-level staff. Remember, when you are offering these types of services on an introductory basis, it is best to be as clear as possible about your suggestions. For example, you might say, "We're offering certain groups 1 or 2 hours of our time on a no-fee basis as an introduction to our work. Our purpose is to gain a continuing relationship with your company, with the hope that you'll contract our services in the future."

Everyone is perfectly willing to take something for free, although they may think in the back of their minds that they will never pay for other programs. But if you are effective, you often have a chance to go on to collect fees later. Many large corporations and government agencies call on outside professionals for continuing education programs, psychological testing of new or potential employees, and direct psychotherapeutic services. Even the armed forces often subcontract for local services and seminars. If you do not gain contracts of this type, remember that you may have attracted potential clients for therapy.

7. Use the major media; newspapers, radio, television. Obviously, this is not for everybody, but many more therapists could use it successfully than do. For example, you can call the health editor or writer of a major local newspaper; for small papers, call the editor or managing editor. Call the program director of radio stations (FM is usually better than AM). Cable TV outlets are rapidly becoming another good source of exposure. Remember, the media need you just as much, if not more, than you need them. They are always looking for information to fill newspaper space and air time, and you can benefit from it. Again, in your initial phone conversation, provide a little general information and ask for an appointment. Then, at the meeting, outline a simple program.

For radio or TV broadcasts, you can use one of three formats: phone-in, where you answer questions from listeners; one-on-one direct interview; or audience participation. The last is usually the best, and it takes relatively little preparation. It is often acceptable to give the cable station free rein to plan the program for you. You should, however, demand the right to review any promotional copy to insure that you are represented in an ethical and professional way.

8. Piggyback with other organizations. Associating yourself with known names like the American Cancer Society, the American Lung Association, the National Multiple Sclerosis Society, and other groups can aid you, and helps them reach out to the public. As part of your media approach, many of these organizations will join with you to provide free brochures or additional publicity when you offer programs of mutual interest to them.

9. Send business gifts. A calendar, an attractive paperweight, or any durable object of some value is not likely to be thrown away. People like "transitional objects." They like to touch things on their desk. Although an object may not bring you immediate referrals, just seeing that object with your name on it is very useful when an occasion for referral does arise.

10. Provide a unique service. Clinical therapists often appear similar to potential clients, so you need something to set you apart. Anything unique will make you more attractive, whether it is an enormous tropical fish tank or even a sandbox for children in your waiting room, a newsletter prepared just for your clients, or a willingness to provide "mobile therapy" in homes, hospitals, or nursing homes for patients with chronic illnesses.

Starting with these ten ideas, and some of your own as well, you can revitalize your practice. That is the reason why some practices prosper while others have only limited growth. If you think you do not have the time or the skills to use these ideas yourself, think again. A relatively simple approach that takes just a few hours of your time can produce startling results over a period of time.

AN EFFECTIVE WAY TO MAKE PERSONAL CONTACTS

The best way to get referrals is to give referrals. This may sound unrealistic when you have office hours to spare, but do not be deterred. Below are some suggestions on how to use this technique.

Begin by contacting potential referral sources in your area: family physicians, internists, gynecologists, neurologists, reconstructive dermatologists, podiatrists, even your local police chief or juvenile detective. Explain that you are putting together a list of professionals to whom you can send referrals, and ask to set up a short meeting. Invite yourself to their office. Most professionals will agree to a half-hour appointment.

Target your approach to each person's particular interests. Perhaps it is a family physician who specializes in geriatric medicine. Then you might discuss family counseling with sons and daughters of the aged. With a reconstructive dermatologist, you might discuss therapy for victims of serious accidents. Find that individual's interest and reverse the interview situation. Do not offer your services; ask about theirs.

One consultant calls this approach "the negative close." Its power is that it is not direct soliciting. It is a way of providing information about your own practice without having to sell yourself. "Referral is an ephemeral thing," he explains, "and many of your colleagues have numerous occasions to refer, and would be glad to, but they just don't think of it. By contacting them directly, you simply lower the threshold and make referrals more likely to occur." When you receive referrals, quickly send a short, handwritten note on your office stationery.

Once you have established ties with colleagues, your referrals will increase - but not immediately. It may be months before you see the fruits of your labors.

SHOULD YOU INVEST IN THE YELLOW PAGES?

Professional advertisements range anywhere from direct-mail announcements to 60 second radio spots or full-page displays in local newspapers. According to a recent survey of several **PSYCHOTHERAPY FINANCES** consultants, most therapists prefer to stick to rather modest ads in the telephone company's yellow pages. For many, however, a more substantial investment in phone book advertising can lead to an increase in referrals. Below is their advice on how to play your ads.

If you have a business phone, you automatically receive a one-line name, address, and phone number listing in the local and county yellow pages. After that, the choice is yours, within some limits. Most notably, some phone companies prohibit anything more than a simple name-address-phone listing under their "Psychologist" and "Psychiatrist" headings. However, the field can be wide open for listings under Clinics, Counseling Service, Educational Consultants, Marriage and Family Counselors, Personal Problem Consultants, Social Workers, and others.

Boldfaced type is the least expensive addition. It can be used for your name only, or for your name and phone number. In most localities, boldface for your name will run $3 per month. With boldface for name, address, and phone number, it is about $10 to $12 per month. Yellow pages ads are charged by the month, for the life of the book (usually 12 months).

Tasteful and professional display ads can be effective. A small one to two inch in-column ad with a thin line around it sells for about $60 to $70 per month in most county books. With a quarter-column box ad, your bill rises as high as $100 per month. A larger half-column ad, running two columns across brings the tally to about $150. Add on extra for full column or quarter-page size, for special graphics, or even for an eye-catching color listing (some yellow pages directories have added red printing).

What do you get for $1,000-plus per year? According to one consultant, every $1,000 you invest can generate a return of $6,000 to $7,000 in new business, depending on your locale. "Can you tell me another source of advertising that gives you this kind of return?" he asks rhetorically. Yellow pages ads are clearly an excellent value. The cost is actually pennies per home.

You should be aware that the advertising companies which produce the yellow pages offer many free services. They will prepare two or three sample lay-out sketches and logos for you to choose from, or they will show you samples from books in other areas of the country to give you ideas. In addition, you also get to keep the art work for use in other ways. And, in addition, you will receive 2,000 free copies of the ad, which can be used as a flyer in any mailings you do.

Dr. Ron Lechnyr, an Oregon clinical social worker, is one therapist who is enthusiastic about the yellow pages: "I think a lot of therapists enter practice hoping to have the minimal amount of expense possible, so they are real cheap about their advertising in the telphone book, and then they are very disappointed about what they get." You get what you pay for, Lechnyr finds. "You can't just have your name and a phone number. You have to let people know, clearly, who you are and what you do. For example, I have a doctorate in social work, but the public doesn't know what that means. So I put down Doctor of Psychiatric Social Work."

Lechnyr takes two main listings (both box ads) under the Marriage and Family Counselors heading. One is his own name listing and the other is his group psychotherapy practice. He has additional listings under Counseling, Biofeedback, Hypnosis, and Social Work. One problem was that a heading existed for Psychiatric Social Worker, but not for Clinical Social Worker. Although the yellow pages sales staff will not always create new headings, they will often add on to related listings, so Lechnyr was able to obtain the additional Social Worker listing, as well as one under Biofeedback Therapist (there had already been a heading for Biofeedback Equipment).

Psychotherapist Mark Lewin of Buffalo, New York, also advertises, but for a different reason. He finds that people often get a referral and then forget the therapist's name, so they will use the yellow pages to jog their memories. "As far as this recall aspect, it's dangerous not to have a listing," Lewin says. "And remember, your ad isn't only for new clients. It's also for the gate keepers - the lawyers, physicians, and others who can give you referrals. They'll often check the book for your address and phone number."

What if you want to discourage self-referrals? Washington, D. C. therapist Richard Mikesell does, but he still pays for a listing. "I run an ad, not to stimulate business, but as a referencing tool," Mikesell explains. "It's really for people who already know about me, just to make it easy for them to find me." But if someone calls "cold," Mikesell refers them to the District of Columbia Psychological Association. "People who call blind out of the yellow pages - perhaps they like the name Mikesell better than Jones - generally are not sure what they want. I would prefer to have a referral service deal with them."

Even though Mikesell has a yellow page listing he shuns display ads. "When I needed window glass for my car, I looked under glass dealers in the yellow pages. But I'd be pretty leery about looking for something personal. Would you look in the yellow pages for a brain surgeon?" Mikesell has two basic complaints against large display listings. First, they may have a reverse effect: "If a patient is considering going to a therapist and then sees a big splashy ad in the yellow pages, he's going to wonder how come the therapist is resorting to something like that." In addition, Mikesell does not like the patients he has gotten through the yellow pages: "I find that many of them turn out to be no-shows, or just come in once."

Like Mikesell, other psychotherapists balk at the idea of selling themselves very hard through advertising, often fearing what their colleagues might think. John Effren, and others who strongly favor promoting practices, say that that is not realistic. "Since the FTC rules to permit professional advertising," argues Lechnyr, "people aren't as uptight about it." Advertising has become very acceptable, and in many cases it is the yellow pages that work best for therapists. Lechnyr, for example, has been on TV 37 times and mentioned in newspapers even more frequently, with very little benefit for his practice. "Everyone thinks doing workshops and getting your name in the papers and on TV brings people in, but it doesn't. It's the yellow pages that really pull."

MAXIMIZING RESULTS FROM PUBLIC SPEAKING

A basic technique for building your reputation in your home community, and ultimately increasing sources of referrals, is to invest as much time as possible in making presentations to various local organizations. For the therapist new to private practice, this often turns out to be the key to gaining recognition and ultimately building a successful practice. But even many established therapists find that keeping their names before the public in a variety of ways is both a worthwhile public service and an effective way to keep appointment books filled when other referral sources slow down.

Therapists who use this approach, however, rarely find it results in immediate change. If you give a talk to a local chapter of Parents Without Partners, for example, or run a seminar on teenage problems for a church group, you probably would not find your telephone ringing off the hook the next day. But your practice will benefit in the long run. Weeks or even months later, new patients will tell you they or a friend were favorably impressed with your presentation.

In addition, increasing your exposure in the community by making public appearances will bring you into contact with the sponsoring groups and their leaders. And people who serve as presidents and chairs of local organizations, as well as the clergy who are often involved, can become the "gate keepers" who steer referrals your way when someone asks for advice.

Naturally, the types of groups you want to reach and the nature of your involvement (a speech, a workshop, a professional resource person at a meeting) will depend on your own professional expertise and abilities as a communicator. The following suggestions will help you review some of the basics involved in working with local groups and outline a number of practical tips developed by several therapists who have found this approach worthwhile.

WHAT TYPES OF GROUPS SHOULD YOU APPROACH?

Our best advice here is probably to look at the obvious places first, trying to keep your own background and specialized training in mind. If you have a personal or professional edge, use it. For example, a marriage counselor in northern New Jersey found that despite a great deal of competition, he quickly became a favorite speaker at Roman Catholic church groups in the area. The fact that he and his family were active church members won him an enthusiastic response from these groups. Similarly, a clinician in Oregon found a receptive audience for talks about the use of biofeedback equipment in pain control among various health care groups, including medical technician students at local community colleges. His reasoning: Awareness of the uses of biofeedback by all health personnel will eventually lead to referrals to himself and other practitioners.

Chances are your approach will be more general: adult education groups; self-help organizations; YMCA and YMHA programs; churches; professional organizations; veterans groups; hospital staff training programs; Lions clubs; Rotary, and so on. A little research in your community will turn up more real possibilities than you would probably guess.

HOW DO YOU GET STARTED?

Among ways suggested to us, the most efficient and practical in many situations is a phone call to the president or program chairman of the group in which you are interested. Here is a simple approach to consider: (a) introduce yourself quickly; (b) explain that as part of your community relations program you would like to make a presentation to appropriate organizations; and (c) you want to set up an appointment to talk about it. As in a job search, explain that the purpose of the call is to set up an interview, not to try to pin anything down.

You will find that the bigger the organization, the more important it is to get to the top person, or as close to the top as possible. Otherwise, any ideas you present are likely to bounce around and get lost in the shuffle. You are also likely to find that many community groups are poorly organized and frustrating to get started with. As Ari De Levie, Ph.D., a New York therapist, has found, "Initial contacts are often a problem, and people tend to break appointments or not follow up on what you discuss." The point is, you must be persistent and follow up meetings with phone calls and letters to keep the process moving.

IS IT A GOOD IDEA TO CHARGE A FEE?

Usually not. Consultants I have spoken to agree that you should consider this type of activity a marketing and community education program. Keep it separate from any seminars or workshops that you may run on a fee basis. Of course, if a group routinely pays an honorarium to its monthly luncheon speaker, you would accept it. You might also accept a situation where the group itself charges a small admissions fee to build up its own treasury, even if you do not get paid.

SHOULD YOU GET INVOLVED IN PROMOTING YOUR PRESENTATION?

Wherever possible, say the consultants. "Too often," says De Levie, "a group will set up a meeting and then drag its feet on promoting it. I've also seen situations where they've left out the name of the speaker on the program." In some cases, you may even want to do an announcement yourself to members of the group to make sure there is a good audience. While that is rare, you should certainly try to make sure that the organization's own mailings or other promotional efforts do an effective job in "selling" your appearance. Do not be shy about suggesting an interesting title for your talk or writing a short paragraph or two of explanation that will help attract an audience. After all, if you are doing the work to prepare a talk you want a good audience to hear it. If the organization does its own announcements of your presentation, you should ask to review the material to make sure it is professional and does not contain misleading claims.

FINAL POINT

One of the biggest mistakes that therapists make when they decide to talk to community groups is failing to follow up on their initial effort. If your first contact with a group in which you are interested fails, try again a few months later; sometimes the annual change in officers will bring in someone who is more responsive to you. You may also find that talking to a group once seems to have little or no impact, and you have to return several times before you see any referrals develop. Whether or not you actually make a presentation to an organization, make an effort to keep up with the "gate keepers." Drop them a note if you start a new professional service or arrange to see them occasionally for lunch. Your efforts may increase your chances for a long and successful private practice.

Herbert E. Klein is currently the editor and publisher of PSYCHOTHERAPY FINANCES. He is also president of Ridgewood Financial Institute, Inc., a company which publishes newsletters and books for psychotherapists, attorneys, and other professionals. He formerly served as the financial editor of MEDICAL ECONOMICS. Mr. Klein may be contacted at 500 Barnett Place, Ho-Ho-Kus, NJ 07423.

RESOURCE

PSYCHOTHERAPY FINANCES, published monthly by Ridgewood Financial Institute, Box 509, Ridgewood, NJ 07451. $39 per year.

INDEPENDENT PRACTICE: CHECKLIST AND RESOURCES GUIDE

Peter A. Keller and Lawrence G. Ritt

Planning and managing an independent clinical practice is a challenging task. Many new practitioners naively assume that they can begin independent practice simply by finding suitable office space and letting the community know their services are available. In reality, nothing could be further from the truth; successful practice management requires clinical expertise, sound business management skills, and the personal temperament to find satisfaction working independently. For every successful practitioner in a given community, there are likely to be several others who maintain marginal practices because of failures or oversights in one or more of these areas.

While we are aware of no research which specifically focuses on private practice success, it can be presumed that there is a direct correlation between careful planning and success. The successful practitioner is likely to be the one who maintains high quality clinical services, effective relationships with referral sources, and sound management practices.

In preparing this article, we reviewed a number of books that deal with private practice issues (see annotated bibliography). We then developed the "Independent Practice Checklist" to help clinicians considering independent practice evaluate their readiness for such an enterprise and to allow current private practitioners to evaluate their existing practices.

No norms or formal scoring procedures are applicable to this checklist. It is intended only as a self-evaluation tool for the clinician. It provides opportunities for you to rate the adequacy of your preparedness on numerous issues.

Completion of the checklist may lead naturally to questions about management of the independent practice. The annotated bibliography which follows provides information regarding several valuable sources of material on independent professional practice. Readers can also obtain useful information on practice management through appropriate workshops offered by experienced practitioners and discussions with colleagues who already manage successful practices.

INDEPENDENT PRACTICE CHECKLIST

Use the following list to review your practice plans and management by placing a check mark in the appropriate columns.

	Yes	No/Not a Problem	No/Needs Attention

The Decision to Enter Independent Practice

1. Am I adequately trained for independent practice? ___ ___ ___

2. Do I have adequate savings for the personal and family financial transition? (6 to 18 months with little or no income) ___ ___ ___

3. Do I have adequate financial resources to open an office? ___ ___ ___

   Office Rent: ___ ___ ___
   Office Modification, Decoration: ___ ___ ___
   Furniture: ___ ___ ___
   Secretarial Services: ___ ___ ___
   Stationary, Forms, Testing Supplies: ___ ___ ___
   Telephone Services: ___ ___ ___
   State, County, City Licenses: ___ ___ ___
   Office Fire, Theft, Accident Insurance: ___ ___ ___
   Professional Liability Insurance: ___ ___ ___
   Office Overhead & Disability Insurance: ___ ___ ___

4. Can my family support or tolerate a time-consuming, expensive transition? ___ ___ ___

5. Can the community support my practice? ___ ___ ___

6. Have I cultivated or can I cultivate enough referral sources? ___ ___ ___

7. Should I begin practice in association with colleagues? ___ ___ ___

8. Could I purchase an established practice? ___ ___ ___

9. Do I have the organizational skills to manage a small business (i.e., practice)? ___ ___ ___

10. Would I enjoy working independently? ___ ___ ___

11. Have colleagues and potential referral sources given me feedback that supports my going into independent practice? ___ ___ ___

Planning the Practice

1. Are my areas of competence clearly defined for the public and referral sources? ___ ___ ___

	Yes	No/Not a Problem	No/Needs Attention

2. Is there any reason to incorporate? ___ ___ ___

3. Have I considered how to let people know of my practice?

Yellow-Page Listings (What Titles?): ___ ___ ___
Formal Announcements for Mailing: ___ ___ ___
Newspaper Announcements: ___ ___ ___
Personal Letters to Key Sources: ___ ___ ___
Consistency with Professional Standards: ___ ___ ___
Press Releases (Articles): ___ ___ ___
Availability for Speaking: ___ ___ ___
Other: ___ ___ ___

4. Do I have office space that is conducive to a successful practice?

Accessible Location in Community: ___ ___ ___
Location in Appropriate Professional Building: ___ ___ ___
Security and/or Alarm Systems: ___ ___ ___
Within Zoning Regulations: ___ ___ ___
Adequate Space and Design: ___ ___ ___
Soundproofing: ___ ___ ___
Desirable Lease Negotiated: ___ ___ ___
Storage Space: ___ ___ ___
Janitorial: ___ ___ ___
Utilities: ___ ___ ___
Grounds Maintenance: ___ ___ ___
Lighting: ___ ___ ___
Others: ___ ___ ___

5. Do I have appropriate licenses?

State (Including Professional Licenses): ___ ___ ___
City and County: ___ ___ ___

6. Is my insurance adequate?

Professional Liability: ___ ___ ___
Office Fire, Theft, Accident: ___ ___ ___
Office Overhead: ___ ___ ___
Disability Income: ___ ___ ___
Medical: ___ ___ ___
Life: ___ ___ ___

7. Have I considered what telephone services I'll need?

Adequate Number of Phones: ___ ___ ___
Adequate Number of Lines: ___ ___ ___
Answering Service or Machine: ___ ___ ___

	Yes	No/Not a Problem	No/Needs Attention
Intercom System:	___	___	___
Own or Lease the System:	___	___	___

8. Have I considered what office equipment I'll need?

Typewriter:	___	___	___
Copier:	___	___	___
Microcomputer System:	___	___	___
Dictation System:	___	___	___
Audio Recording Equipment:	___	___	___
Video Recording Equipment:	___	___	___
Other:	___	___	___

9. What office furnishings will I need?

Waiting Room Tables, Chairs:	___	___	___
Secreterial Desk, Chairs, Tables:	___	___	___
Filing Cabinets (Locking):	___	___	___
Small Refrigerator:	___	___	___
Coffee Maker:	___	___	___
Desk and Table Lamps:	___	___	___
Table and Chairs for Testing Room:	___	___	___
Professional Desk and Chair:	___	___	___
Book Cases:	___	___	___
Storage Cases:	___	___	___
Client Seating:	___	___	___
Reclining Chair:	___	___	___
Art Work:	___	___	___

10. What professional supplies will I need and do I know where to purchase them?

Waiting Room Magazines:	___	___	___
Toys for Play Therapy:	___	___	___
Other:	___	___	___
Testing Supplies:	___	___	___

Managing the Practice

1. Are my announced practices and policies consistent with the established standards for service providers in my profession?   ___   ___   ___

2. What management systems and forms will I use?

Accounting System:	___	___	___
Billing System:	___	___	___
Payable System:	___	___	___
Insurance Claim System:	___	___	___
Pegboard or "One Write" System:	___	___	___

	Yes	No/Not a Problem	No/Needs Attention

3. Will I need the help of:

    A Management Consultant: ___ ___ ___
    Accountant/Bookkeeper: ___ ___ ___

4. What stationary and forms will my practice require?

    Correspondence Stationary and Envelopes: ___ ___ ___
    Note or Memo Forms: ___ ___ ___
    Intake Data Forms: ___ ___ ___
    Screening and History Questionnaires ___ ___ ___
    Mental Status Data Form: ___ ___ ___
    Progress Summary Forms: ___ ___ ___
    Release Forms: ___ ___ ___
    Office Information/Policy Statements: ___ ___ ___
    Insurance Collection Forms: ___ ___ ___
    Client Satisfaction Questionnaire: ___ ___ ___
    Guarantor's Statement: ___ ___ ___
    Specific Assessment Forms: ___ ___ ___
    Other Forms: ___ ___ ___

5. Is my office staff trained for:

    Scheduling Appointments: ___ ___ ___
    Bookkeeping: ___ ___ ___
    Paying Bills: ___ ___ ___
    Filing Insurance Claims: ___ ___ ___
    Routine Questions: ___ ___ ___
    Difficult Clients: ___ ___ ___
    Dangerous Clients: ___ ___ ___
    Suicidal Clients: ___ ___ ___
    Other Emergencies: ___ ___ ___
    Other: ___ ___ ___

6. Do I have consistent office management policies and systems to handle:

    Billing: ___ ___ ___
    Insurance Reimbursement: ___ ___ ___
    Collections: ___ ___ ___
    Bookkeeping: ___ ___ ___
    Security Against Thefts
      (e.g., Bonded Employees): ___ ___ ___

7. Do I have consistent clinical policies to handle:

    Releasing Information: ___ ___ ___
    Allowing Clients to see Records: ___ ___ ___
    Handling Confidential Information: ___ ___ ___
    Management/Disposal of Old Records: ___ ___ ___

Innovations In Clinical Practice: A Source Book

	Yes	No/Not a Problem	No/Needs Attention

Informing Clients about Confidentiality: ___ ___ ___
Requesting Confidential Information: ___ ___ ___
Making Medical Referrals: ___ ___ ___

8. Do I have a system for developing
    clinical records that include:

    Adequate Screening and Development
      of a Data Base: ___ ___ ___
    Mental Status Evaluation: ___ ___ ___
    Information from Previous Treatment: ___ ___ ___
    Level of Functioning Evaluation: ___ ___ ___
    Clear Problem Definitions: ___ ___ ___
    Diagnosis: ___ ___ ___
    Long Term Goals: ___ ___ ___
    Intermediate Objectives: ___ ___ ___
    Statement of Planned Services: ___ ___ ___
    Updated Record of Service Contacts: ___ ___ ___
    Evidence of Regular Review of Problems,
      Progress, Goals: ___ ___ ___
    Appropriate Release Forms: ___ ___ ___
    Ongoing Progress Notes: ___ ___ ___
    A Method for Measuring Goal Attainment: ___ ___ ___
    Discharge Summary (If Client Is
      Terminated): ___ ___ ___
    Plan for Follow-up of Discharged Clients: ___ ___ ___

9. Can I insure that my clinical records
    will be:

    Legible: ___ ___ ___
    Orderly (i.e., Follow a Planned Format): ___ ___ ___

10. Do I have a plan to keep my collection
    rates within an acceptable range?

    Payment at the Time of Visits: ___ ___ ___
    Automatic Review of Delinquent Accounts: ___ ___ ___
    Clear Collection Policies: ___ ___ ___

11. Do I have a plan to keep my financial
    records up to date? ___ ___ ___

12. Do I routinely seek feedback from clients
    regarding my professional practices? ___ ___ ___

13. Do I have a plan to maintain time for:

    Attending Workshops and Seminars: ___ ___ ___
    Reading Professional Publications: ___ ___ ___
    Engaging in Other CE Activities: ___ ___ ___

	Yes	No/Not a Problem	No/Needs Attention

<u>Professional Development:</u>

1. Will I consult with colleagues and obtain outside supervision as appropriate? ___ ___ ___

Peter A. Keller, Ph.D., is currently an Associate Professor of Psychology and the Graduate Psychology Coordinator at Mansfield University. He is also the Senior Editor of the Professional Resource Exchange, Inc. He holds a doctorate in clinical psychology. Dr. Keller may be contacted at P. O. Box 453, Mansfield, PA 16933.

Lawrence G. Ritt, Ph.D., is currently in private practice and is also an adjunct Associate Professor in the Department of Clinical Psychology at the University of Florida. In addition, Dr. Ritt is the Publisher of the Professional Resource Exchange, Inc. He holds a doctoral degree in clinical psychology. Dr. Ritt may be contacted c/o the Professional Resource Exchange, Inc., 635 South Orange Avenue, Suite 4-5, Sarasota, FL 33277-1560.

PRACTICE MANAGEMENT RESOURCES

American Psychological Association. STANDARDS FOR PROVIDERS OF PSYCHOLOGICAL SERVICES. Washington, DC: Author, 1977. Available from American Psychological Association, 1200 Seventeenth Street, NW, Washington, DC 20036.

These standards adopted by the American Psychological Association establish minimally acceptable levels of psychological services applicaple to all providers of such services. Clear standards of accountability are included. Anyone in independent or institutional practice should be thoroughly familiar with these standards.

Browning, C. H. PRIVATE PRACTICE HANDBOOK (2nd ed.). Los Alamitos, CA: Duncliff's International, 1982. Available from Duncliff's International, 3662 Katella Avenue, Suite 218, Los Alamitos, CA 90720. $24.95 Hard-cover - $19.95 Soft-bound.

This is the second edition of a 233 page volume prepared by a practicing psychologist. The book has a detailed table of contents but no index. In addition to the requisite chapter on deciding to enter independent practice, the book focuses on developing referrals and recognition in the community. There are many valuable suggestions in this regard. It contains a number of practical checklists and examples of material used in the author's practice. It is, perhaps, lightest on clinical management issues. The final chapter, titled "A Personal Discovery," contains personal revelations of a religious nature not discussed throughout the previous chapters.

Keller, P. A. & Ritt, L. G. INNOVATIONS IN CLINICAL PRACTICE: A SOURCE BOOK (Vol. 1). Sarasota, FL: Professional Resource Exchange, 1982. Available from the Professional Resource Exchange, Box 15560, Sarasota, FL 33579.

This is part of a series for clinicians available in either looseleaf or hard-bound editions. The volume is divided into five sections, one of which deals with practice management issues. Another contains forms and instruments for use in the clinical office. Most of the material can be copied without further permission.

Kissel, S. PRIVATE PRACTICE FOR THE MENTAL HEALTH CLINICIAN. Rockville, MD: Aspen Systems Corporation, 1983. $26.95.

Lewin, M. H. ESTABLISHING AND MAINTAINING A SUCCESSFUL PRIVATE PRACTICE. Rochester, NY: Professional Development Institute, 1978. Available from the Professional Development Institute, 756 East Main Street, Rochester, NY 14605. $25.00 Hardbound.

This large-format, 177 page manual is written by a practicing clinical psychologist who has managed a professional corporation practice. Seventeen chapters address issues ranging from the compatability of one's personality with private practice to record keeping and establishing and collecting fees. Parts of the volume are in a workbook format, including such things a business plan and financial work sheets. Examples of referral and evaluation forms are included.

Pressman, R. M. PRIVATE PRACTICE: A HANDBOOK FOR THE INDEPENDENT MENTAL HEALTH PRACTITIONER. New York: Gardner Press, 1979. Available from Gardner Press, 19 Union Square West, New York, NY 10003.

This volume was written by a practicing psychologist in collaboration with two psychiatrists. The book is divided into ten chapters with an annotated bibliography (146 pages) and 12 appendices (76 pages). The appendices include information on licensing regulations, ethical standards, and sample reports and forms. The book is introductory in its approach, beginning with the decision to enter independent practice and moving on to basic steps in practice development, relating to referral sources, management issues, clinical records, and legal issues.

PSYCHOTHERAPY FINANCES. A monthly newsletter available from Ridgewood Financial Institute, Box 509, Ridgewood, NJ 07451. Subscription $39.00 per year.

This newsletter contains practical infomation on such things as insurance reimbursement, retirement planning finances, new area of practice, and so on. The focus is on financial issues. Each year a survey of current fees is reported. There is also a regular section which deals with reader questions.

Shimberg, E. THE HANDBOOK OF PRIVATE PRACTICE IN PSYCHOLOGY. New York: Brunner/Mazel Publishers, 1979. Available from Brunner/Mazel Publishers, 19 Union Square, New York, NY 10003. $15.00.

Written by a practicing clinical psychologist, this 104 page book covers the basics of private practice management. It includes the expected chapter on the decision to enter private practice, discusses various types of practices (e.g., partnerships, groups, and corporations), establishing and running the office, fees, and so forth. The treatment of each topic is concise.

Weitz, R. (Editor). PSYCHOTHERAPY IN PRIVATE PRACTICE. A quarterly journal available from The Haworth Press, 28 East 22 Street, New York, NY 10010. Personal Subscriptions $24.00 per year.

This is a new journal introduced by the publisher in Spring of 1983. It is described as striking a meaningful balance between therapy approaches, business matters, and administrative concerns.

HOW TO ESTABLISH AND COLLECT CONSULTING FEES*

Robert E. Kelley

An optometrist once told me how he determines his fee. He calls it the "Blink Method," noting that it follows the rule of a free market system. At the end of each glass fitting examination, he looks his patient in the eye and tells him, "It will cost thirty dollars...." While saying this, he watches if the patient blinks. If no blink occurs, he quickly adds "...for the frames. There is an additional thirty dollar charge...." Again, he looks for the blink. If none is forthcoming, he continues "...for each lens. The lens grinding costs fifteen dollars...." He continues to add on charges until the patient blinks. At that point, he figures that he has charged what the market will bear.

Your fees are your revenue and your proof that you can make it as a consultant. Unfortunately, the public (and potential consultants) do not understand fees very well. The media reports that consultants charge anywhere from $100 per hour to $2,000 per day. The public mistakenly assumes that those rates are pure profit. With some quick calculations using 2,000 work hours per year times $100 per hour, they arrive at an annual income of $200,000 per year. The public then splits into two groups, each group drawing its own conclusions. The first group concludes that they would like to be consultants. The second group decides that consultants overcharge for their services. Neither group fully comprehends the relationships of fees to revenues and to the expenses incurred to generate that revenue.

This contribution discusses how fees fit into your consulting practice. (The information presented is the result of numerous discussions with successful consultants.) Specifically, all the business elements included in your fee will be explained. Then, using a common formula, you will be able to determine your exact fee. In addition, various fee arrangements will be discussed, and guidelines for collecting your fees (an essential task for a successful practice) will be provided.

THE FEE

At the base of most fee structures is the consultant's billing rate. Your billing rate is the dollar amount that a client pays for a specified time

---

*This contribution is adapted from CONSULTING: THE COMPLETE GUIDE TO A PROFITABLE CAREER, by Robert E. Kelley (New York: Charles Scribner's Sons, 1981). Copyright© 1982 by Robert E. Kelley. All rights reserved.

period. The time period is usually an hour or a working day. For example, you might state your billing rate as $40 per hour or $320 per day. When expressed as a daily rate, it is called a "per diem." For most consulting firms, the billing rate is the cornerstone of their fee structure and their revenues. As such, it is important to understand all that is included in the billing rate.

Your billing rate must take into consideration the following eight items: (1) salary; (2) employee benefits; (3) overhead expenses; (4) profit; (5) competition; (6) economic conditions; (7) bad debts; and (8) fairness to you and your clients. By evaluating each of these items, you can determine your fee. Each item will now be explored more fully.

SALARY

Your salary is your worth as a labor commodity on the open market performing the same services you provide as a consultant. In other words, how much would a company pay you to use your skills full time? If you are now working full time, your current salary may or may not represent your true worth. Research shows that many people are underemployed and underpaid. Moreover, most salaries increase as a result of a job change from one position to another. In any case, make a note of your current salary prospects if you worked full time for someone else.

If you have a difficult time determining a salary figure, then consider the following four items:

1. What is the value of your service to the client? Will your clients lose money by not utilizing your services, or will they make considerably more money with your help? In either case, how much money? Will they gain either short-term or long-term benefits or both?

2. What client responsibilities will you assume as a consultant? Will your actions and recommendations considerably shape the fate of the client's company?

3. What skills are required for your services? Is there a large or short supply of those skills? The economics of high demand and short supply result in higher salary.

4. What are your previous education and experience costs? Did you spend years in graduate training or apprentice at minimum wage many years? High past costs are generally recouped in your current salary.

Your salary plays an important role in determining your billing rate. If need be, interview either consulting firms or companies to obtain your salary range. Once you have this dollar figure, you can use it in the formulas presented later in this chapter.

EMPLOYEE BENEFITS

Benefits are the "extras" you receive from an employer, above and beyond your salary. Benefits are normally tax free. For most employees, benefits amount to 25-60% of their salary. In other words, they receive an extra 25-65%

income, tax free. Benefits include such items as (a) insurance (health, life, liability, legal), (b) training, on and off the job, (c) vacation, (d) sick leave, (e) pension, (f) unemployment insurance, and (g) payroll taxes.

Many consultants include benefits as part of overhead, which is covered in the next section. Some prefer to separate them. This forces you as a business owner to think about the "extras" you will provide for yourself and any future employees. Moreover, you can see the relationship between the dollar cost of benefits and your billing rate. You might find that certain benefits are too costly because they elevate your billing rate to an uncompetitive level.

OVERHEAD EXPENSES

Overhead represents the expenses incurred in operating a business. When analyzing your expenses, you must separate them into two categories. One category involves expenses that are directly related to business operations. This category is overhead. For example, rent, fire insurance, and typing costs for correspondence are overhead. The second category includes expenses incurred while serving your client. For example, long distance calls made on a client's behalf are client expenses, not overhead. Normally, you bill these expenses to the client. Do not include them as part of your monthly operating costs (overhead).

Monitor the following expenses to insure that you are not inadvertently absorbing client expenses.

Typing. Typing performed for client projects is billed to the client. Some consulting firms bill as much as 50% of all typing.

Telephone. Client-related calls are billed to the client. Nonclient-specific calls are overhead. Remember to invoice the client for time you spend on client-related calls.

Automotive. Miles accumulated while working on a client project are billed at the most recent Internal Revenue Service rate.

Travel. Travel includes transportation, hotels, meals, tips, and any other appropriate expenses. Client-related travel is billed directly to the client. All other travel is overhead.

Postage and Delivery. Whenever material other than monthly statements is sent to clients, you bill the client. Postage and delivery not chargeable to clients is overhead.

Duplicating. Labor and machine costs of duplicating for clients is billed accordingly.

Securing Projects. Many costs are incurred when you negotiate and secure new consulting engagements. Labor, typing, travel, and duplicating costs add up when you write proposals and make presentations. Some firms inform potential clients at the outset that they bill these expenses. Other firms recover these expenses after securing the engagement. Fewer and fewer firms are willing to absorb these costs as overhead.

PROFIT

Profit is your reward for business risks and ownership. It is above and beyond your salary for labor. Profit generally ranges from 10-50% of your salary, plus benefits, plus overhead. Business owners often make a critical mistake concerning profits. They confuse their salary with their profit. When they receive $30,000 net income from their business each year, they declare a $30,000 profit. In truth, that $30,000 represents both salary and profit. They must subtract what they could have made working for someone else. What remains is their profit and reward for the work, responsibilities, headaches, and risks of being a business owner. You must determine what profit level you require for doing the same.

COMPETITION

When establishing your billing rate, you must be cognizant of the customs of your community and other consultants. Three factors determine your competitive position. First, what are your successful competitors charging? Second, what will your clients pay? Third, what minimum and maximum levels are you willing to accept? The answers to these three questions will give you lower and upper limits for your billing rate. You can then compare these limits to the rates needed to meet your salary, benefits, overhead, and profit. If your rate does not fall within the limits, then you will find it impossible to operate your business without some adjustments.

To obtain the information necessary to answer the above questions, ask bankers, lawyers, accountants, and other consultants. They generally know the customs of your business community and can be very helpful. Also contact your professional colleagues for information. The rates for your community or type of consulting may vary considerably.

You must consider your potential clients' perceptions of your fee. On the one hand, client resistance to consulting fee levels is more widespread now than previously. Managers and owners of client organizations are comparing their own visible compensation levels with consulting fee rates. In addition, they seek to reduce high costs in this time of economic difficulty. Unless they clearly foresee benefits that will exceed your fees, they will do without your services. On the other hand, clients familiar with consultants know the acceptable fee range. If your fee is too low, they will assume either that you are a "greenhorn" or that your quality is as low as your price. In either case, they will not engage you unless your reputation is well known and respected.

As you can see, your client's perception of a fair price is important. Again, ask your local network of bankers, accountants, lawyers, and professional colleagues. You might conduct a survey of potential clients. Ask what they have paid consultants in the past and what they consider a fair price. Another opportunity to find this information occurs during project negotiations. Whenever you discuss a potential consulting project, you should ask three questions: Have they ever used consultants before? Were they satisfied? What was the nature of the fee arrangement? You will then have rate information for this particular client along with any biases the client has toward consultants.

ECONOMIC CONDITIONS

Your billing rate must take into account not only your clients and competitors, but also the economic conditions that affect you. How are inflation and the recession affecting you? At what rate are your costs rising or falling? How does this compare with the way your clients and competitors are affected? Economic conditions might justify adjustments in your billing rate.

Consider also your current financial position. This includes your solvency philosophy, your growth philosophy, and your profit philosophy. For example, if you are just making ends meet, then an increase in your billing rate may be necessary. On the other hand, if you are content with making a modest profit, you may even lower your rates.

BAD DEBTS

Bad debts affect every business. A bad debt occurs when you are not paid for services you provided. You can determine your total bad debt rate by subtracting the total fees you collect from the total fees you bill. Bad debts are also expressed through a percentage known as your collection rate. To determine your collection rate, you divide your total fees collected by your total fees billed:

$$\text{Collection rate} = \frac{\text{Total fees collected}}{\text{Total fees billed}}$$

Bad debt rate = 100 minus your collection rate

Professional firms experience bad debt rates from 5-40%. Very few firms collect all their bills. Most try to maintain a 90-95% collection rate, or, in other words, a 5-10% bad debt rate. Some large firms become alarmed when their collection rate falls under 85%. Few businesses can absorb a 15% revenue loss after paying the operating costs to generate that revenue.

FAIRNESS TO YOU AND YOUR CLIENTS

After considering all the above items (your salary, benefits, overhead, profit, competitive position, economic conditions, and bad debts), you must then make an ethical judgment. What do you think is fair to your clients and to your firm? At what point will your billing rate be excessive, creating an unwarranted burden on your clients? Can you truly justify the value you give with the monetary value you receive? On the other hand, are you selling your services too cheaply? Are you cheating yourself? Many professionals undersell themselves to avoid being rejected by potential clients. They interpret the rejection not in relation to their billing rate but as a reflection of their professional skills. Consequently, they underbid in an effort to maintain their professional pride. This is a self-defeating transaction.

Your billing rate is part of an exchange. Research shows that equitable exchanges are the only ones that produce satisfaction for both parties. If you as a consultant feel cheated, then you will attempt to achieve equity by reducing the quality of your work. If your clients feel cheated, then they will either attempt to extract extra services for the same price or refuse to pay. Thus, you serve everyone's best interest by deciding on a fair price and sticking to it. As a result, you can perform your services without the psychological handicap of a guilty conscience.

The billing rate is the cornerstone upon which most consultants build their fee structures. Your billing rate requires you to make important calculations and to exercise good judgment. Some calculations will be precise, such as the dollar amount of your salary, benefits, overhead, and profits. Other calculations will be estimates, such as your competitive position, the economic conditions, and your bad debt rate. You must translate the sum of these calculations into an exact dollar figure: your billing rate. You then make a moral decision as to whether that rate is fair to both yourself and your clients.

HOW TO CALCULATE YOUR BILLING RATE

In the previous section, I explained the elements included in your billing rate and methods to determine a dollar figure for each element were suggested. In this section, you will learn how to plug those dollar figures into the most common formula used by consultants to calculate their billing rates. Other formulas may be found in Kelley (1981).

Before the formula is presented, two more important terms need to be defined: billable hours and utilization rate. Billable hours are the number of working hours you bill to clients. A weekly rate of 40 hours multiplied by 52 weeks per year equal 2,080 working hours per year. As a full-time consultant, you will work at least that many hours each year, but not all will be on client projects. You will spend some time answering correspondence, administering your practice, keeping up in your field, recovering from sickness, and taking vacations. Seasoned consultants devote 15-20% of their time marketing their services to secure new projects. Most of these hours are nonbillable hours. For full-time consultants, the average number of billable hours ranges between 1,300 and 1,700 hours.

Your utilization rate tells you what percent of your total working hours you bill to clients.

$$\text{Utilization rate} = \frac{\text{Billable hours}}{\text{No. of total working hours available}}$$

To determine the utilization rate, you simply insert the appropriate numbers. For example, based on a 40-hour work week, and allowing for 2 weeks vacation (or 80 working hours), full-time consultants have 2,000 total work hours available each year. If they bill 1,300 hours each year to clients, then 1,300 divided by 2,000 equals a 65% utilization rate. With 1,700 billable hours, the consultant has an 85% utilization rate. If you plan to consult part time at 10 hours per week, and you bill for 5 hours each week, then your utilization rate is 50%. Your utilization rate quickly tells you how much of your time clients are directly paying for and how much you must absorb as overhead.

The majority of consulting firms rely on the "Rule of Three" to calculate their billing rates. This rule utilizes your salary requirement as its base. In addition, it assumes that every consultant generates overhead and benefits that equal his or her salary. Moreover, each consultant should produce a profit that equals his or her salary. Multiply each consultant's salary requirement by 3 to arrive at total yearly revenues. One-third of these revenues pays for salaries, another third pays for overhead and benefits costs, and the last third is profit. The total yearly revenues are divided by your yearly billable hours to calculate your hourly billing rate. Thus,

```
    1/3 = Salary of consultant
  + 1/3 = Overhead plus benefits
  + 1/3 =   Profit
        = Total yearly revenues
```

Then:

$$\text{your hourly billing rate} = \frac{\text{Total yearly revenues}}{\text{Yearly billable hours}}$$

Example:

```
If Salary      = $20,000
then Overhead =  20,000
Profit        =  20,000
Total         = $60,000 = 3 x $20,000 Salary
```

If your yearly billable hours = 1,500 hours, then:

```
Total yearly revenues  = $60,000
Yearly billable hours  = 1,500 hours
```

Then:

```
hourly billing rate    = $40/hour
and daily billing rate = $40/day x 8
                       = $320/day
```

The Rule of Three is a simple and quick method of calculating your billing rate. You only need to know your annual salary requirements and the number of hours you can bill to clients each year. The more hours you can bill, the less you need to charge to maintain your profit level. The fewer hours you bill, the more you must charge per hour. However, if your salary requirements and billable hours are within the average range, then your billing rates will compare with the average.

FEE ARRANGEMENTS

Up to this point, your billing rate has been used in determining your fee because it is the predominant method. However, other fee arrangements exist.

Many consultants use different fee arrangements, depending on the nature of the project. For the majority of their consulting work, they charge an hourly or daily rate. For other projects, such as government projects, they might charge a fixed fee.

Before the different fee arrangements are presented, there are three guidelines to be considered pertinent to their use. First, the ethical codes of many professions prohibit certain types of fee arrangements. Check with your own professional associations to insure that your fee arrangements comply with their codes of ethics.

Second, since fee arrangements are business transactions, they contain an element of risk. In most cases, either you or the client carry the risk. The party that assumes the risk stands to win or lose the most. For instance, if you promise to perform a project for a fixed dollar amount of $5,000, you carry the risk. A budget overrun of $2,000 leaves you absorbing the extra cost. However, performing the project for only $3,000 rewards you with a $2,000 difference. Consequently, you must analyze your fee arrangement with regard to this risk factor.

Third, you may want to use a fee arrangement that is familiar to your client. For example, most lawyers charge by the hour. So, when you consult to lawyers, you should charge by the hour. In essence, you should try to speak your client's language if at all possible. It avoids misunderstandings and helps the clients incorporate your fees into their own budgetary processes.

These guidelines are reflected in the most commonly used fee arrangements discussed below. More specialized fee arrangements can be found in Kelley (1981).

HOURLY OR TIME CHARGES

Hourly or time charges involve multiplying your billing rate by the number of hours you work for the client. As I have mentioned previously, this is the most basic and common fee arrangement. All you need is your standard billing rate and a method to keep track of how you spend your time. With time charges, the clients assume the risk, and consultants know they will be paid for time spent. The risk factor is that the project may require more time than initially perceived and the client could face a substantial bill.

FIXED FEES

Fixed fees occur when a particular service is performed for a fixed dollar amount. When a lawyer quotes an absolute price to write your will, this is a fixed fee. Many government contracts require fixed-fee agreements. As a consultant, you should utilize a fixed fee only when you have effective cost control of the project. You must be able to estimate your time and costs with a high degree of accuracy. As a general rule, do not use fixed fees for projects with which you have little experience. You should have performed a similar project at least once to charge a fixed fee.

In fixed-fee arrangements, the consultant carries the risk of budget overruns and the reward for budget underruns. If you quote a certain fee and it requires more time than expected, you absorb the difference. For this reason, clients prefer fixed fees for novel and complex problems. In these situations the risk of a budget overrun is great. Experienced clients prefer to have the consultant carry the risk through fixed fees. The consultant prefers to have the client assume the risk through hourly time charges.

BRACKET FEES

A bracket fee combines fixed fees and time charges. In essence, the consultant works on an hourly basis, but his or her fee cannot exceed a specified dollar amount. Bracket fees protect the client from budget overruns. Also, since the consultant only charges for time spent on the project, the client is rewarded by any budget underruns. Cost-conscious government agencies have increased their use of bracket fees in the last few years.

CONTINGENT FEES

You collect contingent fees once you obtain a successful result for your client. Lawyers commonly use contingent fees in medical malpractice suits. They are paid only if they win. They will usually take a percentage of the awarded settlement. Some executive search firms charge a percentage of an executive's salary after placement. If they do not place the executive, they receive no fees.

Contingent fees are considered unethical by many professional associations and would generally not be appropriate for mental health consultants. The major reason is that they can pose a conflict of interest for the consultant. The objectives of the consultant and client may differ when payment is dependent on successful results. Consequently, it is assumed that you can charge for time and skills, but not for specific results.

VALUE OF ASSIGNMENT FEES

Some consultants may perform projects that have intrinsic value beyond the number of days or hours consumed. Value of assignment fees are additional payments for such projects. For example, consultants that turn around a troubled business have performed a valuable service not only for the client, but also for the client's employees, creditors, customers, and community. Generally, they charge a substantially higher fee than if they relied solely on time charges. These fees can be either fixed amounts or percentages. Again, such fees would not generally be appropriate for mental health consultants.

RETAINER FEES

Retainer fees have several meanings among consultants. This may describe an advance payment to "retain" your services for a particular project. In this respect, it is a sign of faith on the client's part to use your services and to insure payment.

In a slightly different sense, retainers are used to guarantee your availability during a time period, even though the client may not use your services. For example, if you have a small practice, you may be working on a large, time-consuming project for Client A. If Client B calls, you may not be available to meet that client's needs. If Client B wants to avoid this situation, then he or she may pay retainer fees on a regular basis. Calculate the retainer by the amount of money you require to forego other opportunities, normally a sizable amount (i.e., 10 to 25% of your income).

Consultants also use retainers as an arrangement to provide specified services for a fixed fee for a period of time. In this arrangement, you spell out the services and the time period. Services outside the retainer agreement are billed separately. For example, if you consult in the area of executive counseling, you may counsel a certain number of hours each week. Thus, it is important for both you and the client to define your use of retainer fees.

LIMITING FEE COLLECTION PROBLEMS

Knowing how to determine your fee is a major step in generating revenues to support your consulting practice. Securing and performing consulting work is the next major step. As scientists say, however, these are necessary but not wholly sufficient steps for successful practice. The third step is the collection of the revenues generated. Without successful fee collection, you cannot meet your own bills. Oddly, new consultants often ignore fee collections until it is too late; they make three mistakes that can put them out of business:

1. When they first open their practice, they "carry" too many clients. They perform the work and allow clients to defer payment. As a result, they have little incoming cash to meet their business or family obligations.

2. They do not watch their collection rate. As mentioned earlier, the collection rate is crucial to profitability. If they do not monitor their collection rate, they have no way of knowing when it falls to dangerous levels.

3. They do not follow up on unpaid bills. Many people are reluctant to ask for money, yet avoiding the topic creates a desire in both parties to avoid each other. The best way to handle such situations is by gentle reminders. When those fail, you must sit down with the client to work out mutually acceptable arrangements.

Since the success of your practice depends on successful fee collections, devote considerable attention to it. Toward this end, most professionals follow three general rules: (a) avoid the problem; (b) limit your exposure to bad debts; and (c) review your billing and collection practices.

AVOID THE PROBLEM

You can avoid many fee collection problems through good front-end communications. As early as possible, obtain a mutual understanding with your client concerning the fee. As a general practice, discuss your fees during the first meeting. Also, indicate how and when billing occurs. Then, follow up your conversation with a letter reviewing your mutual understanding. In this way, you avoid confusion and disputes at a later date.

Remember that many clients have little or no experience with consultants. They do not know how much a particular service will cost, yet they need to know so that they can make budgeting decisions. Not knowing induces anxieties about exorbitant fees. If they have any preconceived fears about high cost, lack of discussion about the fee will heighten the fear. They reason that if the fee were moderate, you would talk about it. Consequently, your silence reinforces their anxieties.

LIMIT YOUR EXPOSURE TO BAD DEBTS

Establish a common understanding before you begin the consulting project. Too many consultants believe that their collection efforts stop there. To improve your collection rate, you must limit your exposure during each step of this process.

You can ease your collection efforts by following guidelines used by many consulting firms. First, involve your client in handling the assignment. Successful consultants include the client at each step of the engagement rather than ignore the client while performing the project. They delegate tasks wherever possible and hold regular progress meetings. They send documents, progress reports, and letters to maintain constant communication. In other words, these consultants try to keep their efforts in the forefront of their clients' minds. If your clients know that you are working hard on their behalf, they will be less likely to withhold payment.

Second, obtain progress payments by billing frequently. There is no reason for you to wait for payment until the project is completed, unless clearly specified by your fee arrangement. Instead, most consultants send monthly bills for work performed to that date. Sending regular and frequent bills produces many benefits. For starters, several small bills are more likely to be paid than one large one, especially for smaller clients. A business can budget $1,000 per month in consulting fees more easily than it can absorb a $12,000 bill at year's end. Another useful effect is that if payment stops, you can stop your work. Thus, you limit your potential losses by withholding your services. In effect, regular payment of your bill provides positive feedback as to how the client values your services. If the client stops payment, you know an important change has occurred. You should deal with this change before you resume the project. A final benefit is that regular statements force you to keep your billing and accounting system in order. When your billing system is sloppy, your collection rate invariably decreases.

A third guideline to improve collections is to bill on time. Timing is critical, particularly if your work produced favorable results. Make sure that your final bill is presented at the conclusion of the project. A former graduate student of mine informally surveyed the billing practices of doctors, dentists, and lawyers. She found that professionals who request payment before the client leaves the office have 90-100% collection rates. Those who send monthly statements average 65% collection rates.

A fourth guideline is to account in detail for all work, time, and expenses related to the client. Note the time, date, and tasks performed, as well as who performed the tasks. In other words, you want to have complete records in case of any disputes. Keeping these records also enables you to budget for similar projects in the future.

A fifth guideline is to send general bills to your client. Usually, you need not provide all the details described in the previous paragraph. Those details are for your records. Instead, most consulting firms send a general bill indicating the phase of the project, the general activities performed, the number of hours, expenses, and the total fee. If the clients request more detailed information, these firms willingly provide it.

The sixth guideline applies to high-risk clients. High-risk clients are those who have a reputation for late or nonpayment or who constantly argue about their bills. For those clients, get disbursements in advance. Many consultants will demand sizable front-end retainers, which they deposit in a trust account. They then subtract their bills from this account. If possible, withhold an essential element that the client needs, such as the final report, until the bill is paid. If you are in doubt about a client's reputation, check with other professionals.

A final guideline is to follow up on your billing. Monitor the payment trends of each client. When this trend begins to change in a negative direction, make note of it. Often it signals financial problems for your client or a client's displeasure with your work. When payments are overdue, send reminders. When the reminders are unheeded, a telephone call is necessary. Inform the client of the situation. In some organizations, your client may not see the bill or realize that payment is overdue. Discuss the late payment with the client to determine the reasons for it. If the client is in a financial bind, set up a meeting to arrange a mutually acceptable payment plan. If no arrangement is possible, stop the project. Send a certified letter to the client informing him or her of your action.

The above guidelines should make it clear that successful collections require constant effort. The best method to insure payment is by making it clear that your services are valuable to the client and that you are working hard to provide that value. Of course, it is difficult to create that perception if neither aspect is true. The next best way to receive payment is to ask for it. If you do not ask, few people will offer it. All of these guidelines, however, must be used intelligently. Rather than rigidly apply them, adapt them to your particular clients and consulting practice.

REVIEW YOUR BILLING AND COLLECTION PRACTICES

Successful billing and collection requires a system. The sooner this system is in place, the better your collection rate will be. Unfortunately, too many professionals fail to examine their own systems. Once it is established, they are slow to change it. They do not check to see if it is working or if their practice now requires a new system.

To prevent this happening to you, review your billing and collection systems on a regular basis. First, examine your billing rate every 6 or 12 months. Modifications are generally required, depending on your costs, competitive position, economic conditions, and your worth as a consultant. Second, review your fee arrangements. What type of fees did you charge? How well did they work for you? What lessons did you learn for future fee arrangements? Third, persons not involved in the projects should evaluate your bills and billing procedures. Did you depart from your standard rates or usual fee arrangement? If so, why? Did you give discounts or extend credit to your customers? How often did this occur and what are your justifications? How did they affect your profits? If you force yourself to answer these questions to someone not involved in the consulting project, then you will receive more objective feedback concerning this aspect of your practice. Since the individual does not have emotional involvement in the project, he or she can provide the outside input necessary to modify the system. Last, examine your collection procedures. Are you billing regularly and on time? Are you following up on nonpayments? What is your collection rate? These questions will give you important insights to improve your collections.

If you follow the three collection rules (avoid the problem, limit your exposure, and review your billing and collection practices) then you will make important strides in improving your collection rates. As in most aspects of life, prevention is easier and less expensive than remedial efforts. The easier you make it for the client to pay, the easier it is to collect. To do this, you must have a system that requires but minimizes continuous effort on your part.

It is important to note that each fee arrangement requires an analysis of the project, the client, and the risk factor. The guidelines and rules are generalities. You must apply them flexibly to your practice.

Regardless of your situation, to secure a profit you must pay attention to three of the concepts presented in this contribution. First, watch your billing rate to make sure it reflects the financial realities facing your practice. You can increase profitability through your billing rate in two ways: charge more or reduce expenses. Both give your billing rate a higher profit margin. Second, watch your utilization rate to insure that you are billing the number of hours required for profitability. If not, you must sell and perform more consulting work. Third, monitor your collection rate to insure that the revenues produced by your billing rate and utilization rate are being collected. If these rates are kept to maximum levels, then profitability should follow.

Robert E. Kelley, Ph.D., is currently a senior management consultant at the Stanford Research Institute. Prior to his present position, he was a visiting scholar at the Harvard Business School and management professor at Portland State University. His training is in industrial-organizational psychology, and he is the author of numerous articles in the areas of strategic planning and implementation, organizational design and growth, and human resources. Dr. Kelley may be contacted at SRI International, IMEG, 333 Ravenswood Avenue, Menlo Park, CA 94025.

RESOURCES

Altman, M. A. & Weil, R. I. MANAGING YOUR ACCOUNTING AND CONSULTING PRACTICE. New York: Matthew Bender & Co., 1978.

Kelley, R. E. CONSULTING: THE COMPLETE GUIDE TO A PROFITABLE CAREER. New York: Charles Scribner's Sons, 1981.

Kubr, M. MANAGEMENT CONSULTING: A GUIDE TO THE PROFESSION. Geneva, Switzerland: International Labour Organization, 1976.

INTRODUCTION TO SECTION III: ASSESSMENT INSTRUMENTS AND OFFICE FORMS

This section of **INNOVATIONS** contains instruments, checklists and forms for practitioners to use to collect and organize information.

Although some of the materials presented here were formally developed and standardized, many were designed by the contributors for use in their own practices. We included these because we feel they can be effectively used by other practitioners, either in their original or modified form. The value of these instruments is dependent on appropriate applications by the clinicians who use them. For the most part, they are not designed to generate the types of inferences often associated with more formalized tests.

In spite of the informal quality of some of these materials, we have attempted to insure that all published instruments include sufficient information to allow readers to evaluate their appropriateness for specific practice needs. Certain basic information, instructions, and interpretation have been included with each contribution and, when necessary, the Resource Section contains sources for more detailed information.

Walker presents an interview guide for use during the initial assessment of child therapy cases. Hendler's contribution is a test for use in the clinical evaluation of clients with chronic back pain. For clinicians involved in forensic evaluations, Lipsitt and Lelos offer an instrument for developing clinical opinions and communicating to the court regarding a client's competence to stand trial. Keller and Murray have developed three questionnaires for clinician use in obtaining feedback regarding their services from clients and other professionals. Rhonda Keller presents a form for collecting intake information from couples in marital therapy. Newman discusses scales that can be used to complement other diagnostic data in determining a client's ability to function in the community. Overall offers both a brief scale for rating the major dimensions of a patient's manifest psychopathology and a brief checklist data form for obtaining psychiatric history and background information.

If you are considering submitting a contribution for possible inclusion in this section of a future volume of **INNOVATIONS**, please write for information on the issues which need to be addressed in preparing assessment instruments.

CURRENT SYMPTOM CHECKLIST FOR CHILDREN

C. Eugene Walker

The Current Symptom Checklist for Children was developed by the author for use in the outpatient Pediatric Psychology Clinic at the University of Oklahoma Medical School and Oklahoma Children's Memorial Hospital. The purpose of this checklist is to serve as an interview guide during the initial diagnostic assessment of child therapy cases. It was our experience that parents often overlooked significant child psychopathology in the initial interview, tending to report the symptoms which were most annoying to them, but neglecting equally important symptoms that did not seem as presssing at the time. They also tended to be unaware of the range of services that could be provided or facilitated by the psychologist and did not mention some symptoms (e.g., encopresis, eating problems, communication problems, organic illness), assuming they were not relevant and that, in any case, those symptoms should be treated by a medical specialist. Of course, as clinical pediatric psychologists, we wanted to be aware of all the symptoms that were present since, in many cases, we could treat them or coordinate a team to treat the full range of problems presented by the child. To get all of this information from the interview, we found we spent a great deal of time simply reviewing with the parents a wide range of possible symptoms and problems that the child might have in order to elicit some response. It occurred to us that the parents could easily fill out a brief questionnaire in the waiting room which would save us time during the interview and guide our questions.

Items for the checklist were derived from numerous sources. First, we reviewed the literature on frequencies of reported symptoms for children seen in clinics similar to ours (Mesibov, Schroeder, & Wesson, 1977; Monnelly, Ianzito, & Stewart, 1973; Walker, 1979). Second, we did a three year chart review of our own cases and the symptomatology presented by the patients we had treated. Third, we examined several published and unpublished checklists which have been employed in our medical center and others throughout the country. Fourth, we drew upon the clinical experience of the faculty in Pediatric Psychology at the University of Oklahoma Medical School. From these sources, a large pool of potential items was generated. These were then classified and sorted into categories. Items were eliminated if they overlapped with others or if they were sufficiently rare that we felt it was unnecessary to include them. We added room at the end of the questionnaire for "other" symptoms so parents could mention any that were not included, or could note any symptoms which may not have fit into the categories we provided.

A concerted effort was made to keep the number of items to a minimum since we did not want to overburden our patients with a long detailed questionnaire that would only delay their appointment and irritate them prior to being seen face to face. In addition, we attempted to state the symptoms in very simple language and short declarative sentences. This was done because many of the patients we see have limited educational backgrounds and find more sophisticated questionnaires beyond their comprehension. There is a strong response bias built into the checklist; all items are stated in such a way that the presence of the symptom would require a "yes" response. We were well aware of the bias involved in using this format but, since the purpose of the questionnaire was to uncover symptoms, we preferred the bias to be in the direction of over-reporting rather than under-reporting. The significance of the symptom is evaluated in the interview.

The purpose of this checklist is strictly to serve as a guide to interviewing. No claims are made for reliability, validity, or other psychometric properties of the instrument. We are currently gathering normative data on the frequency with which the various symptoms are endorsed and the correlations among symptoms (e.g., If a child wets the bed, is he or she also likely to be a thumb sucker or encopretic?), but these data were not available in time for the present publication.

We have found that this instrument saves us considerable time and also gives us some clues about areas to probe during the interview. Often a parent will be having difficulty in an area but be somewhat defensive and reluctant to go into it when asked initially by the interviewer. In the safety of the waiting room, however, dealing only with a paper and pencil instrument, they will more likely note the area as a problem. Thus, we are often alerted to areas that should be pursued even if the patient does not volunteer a great deal of information in the first stages of the interview.

Some therapists in our clinic find it useful to administer this questionnaire again in the middle and at the end of therapy in order to see what changes have taken place. This checklist, which takes approximately ten minutes to complete, can give the clinician a significant amount of information which facilitates the initial assessment of the patient and can be valuable in follow-up assessments, as well.

C. Eugene Walker, Ph.D., is currently a Professor of Psychology and Director of Training in Pediatric Psychology at the University of Oklahoma Medical School. He is also Associate Chief of Mental Health Services and Director of Out-Patient Pediatric Psychology Clinic at the Oklahoma Children's Memorial Hospital. Dr. Walker has authored many articles on clinical psychology and psychotherapy in the professional literature. Dr. Walker may be contacted at O.U. Health Sciences Center, Department of Psychiatry, P. O. Box 26307, South Pavilion - 5SP 138, Oklahoma City, OK 73126.

CURRENT SYMPTOM CHECKLIST

Name_____   Birth Date_____

Date_____   Sex_____

Name of Person Completing Checklist   Relationship_____

_____

Below you will find a large number of statements about your child and the problems he or she is having. Circle "YES" for those that are true of your child **at the present**. Circle "NO" for those that are not true **at present**.

PERSONAL — SOCIAL

1.	My child continually seeks attention.	YES	NO
2.	Often I can see the tension building up in my child.	YES	NO
3.	My child explodes under stress.	YES	NO
4.	My child has nervous habits, like pulling at his (her) clothing, clearing his (her) throat often, sniffing his (her) nose, etc.	YES	NO
5.	My child cries easily.	YES	NO
6.	My child is a thumb or finger sucker.	YES	NO
7.	My child is a worrier.	YES	NO
8.	My child often rocks back and forth.	YES	NO
9.	My child shakes or trembles sometimes.	YES	NO
10.	My child has many or unusual fears.	YES	NO
11.	My child is often angry.	YES	NO
12.	My child is moody.	YES	NO
13.	My child becomes overexcited easily.	YES	NO
14.	My child is hyperactive and restless.	YES	NO
15.	My child becomes hysterical, upset, or angry when things do not go his (her) way.	YES	NO
16.	My child seems sad.	YES	NO
17.	My child has sleep problems.	YES	NO

18. My child has bad dreams.   YES   NO

19. My child walks or talks in his (her) sleep.
     (Underline which)   YES   NO

20. My child gets confused easily.   YES   NO

21. My child has trouble remembering things.   YES   NO

22. My child has difficulty concentrating for any
     length of time.   YES   NO

23. My child complains he (she) never gets a fair
     share of things.   YES   NO

24. My child says people don't like him (her).   YES   NO

25. My child often tends to be very selfish and
     self-centered.   YES   NO

26. My child is very shy.   YES   NO

27. My child is sensitive and has his (her) feelings
     hurt easily.   YES   NO

28. My child avoids competition.   YES   NO

29. My child is often a poor sport and a poor loser.   YES   NO

30. My child often has trouble making friends.   YES   NO

31. My child often seems to have little self-confidence.   YES   NO

32. My child cannot get along with my husband (wife).   YES   NO

33. We frequently have family problems.   YES   NO

34. There is a lot of arguing and fighting in our house.   YES   NO

35. My child expresses concern about something terrible
     or horrible happening to family members or himself
     (herself).   YES   NO

36. My child does not get along with his (her) brothers
     and sisters.   YES   NO

37. My child often expresses strong dislike for home and
     family.   YES   NO

38. One (or more) of my other children has problems, too.   YES   NO

39. My child often says strange things or asks unusual
     questions.   YES   NO

40. My child often does strange or stupid things.   YES   NO

41. My child often says he (she) wishes he (she) were dead or away from it all. YES NO

42. My child has been physically or sexually abused. YES NO

43. My child often has small accidents or injuries. YES NO

BEHAVIORAL

44. My child is a discipline problem at home. YES NO

45. My child is a discipline problem at school. YES NO

46. My child tells tall tales or lies. YES NO

47. My child often throws temper tantrums. YES NO

48. My child has attempted to seriously harm a person or animal. YES NO

49. My child manipulates situations to his (her) own benefit. YES NO

50. My child does sexual things he (she) shouldn't. YES NO

51. My child seems to welcome punishment. YES NO

52. My child disturbs other children: teasing, provoking fights, interrupting others. YES NO

53. My child steals things sometimes. YES NO

54. I often have to spank my child. YES NO

SCHOOL

55. My child is in a special program at school. YES NO

56. My child may have a learning disability. YES NO

57. My child voices an intense dislike of school. YES NO

58. My child does not seem to be learning as he (she) should. YES NO

59. The teachers complain about my child. YES NO

PHYSICAL

60. My child's bowels do not move regularly. YES NO

61. My child is overweight or underweight. YES NO

62. My child is taking medicine now. YES NO

63. My child has had a major illness, operation, or accident. YES NO

64. My child frequently stares blankly into space and is unaware of his (her) surroundings when doing so. YES NO

65. My child has a visual, hearing, or speech problem. (Underline which) YES NO

66. My child has allergies or asthma. YES NO

67. My child has a chronic illness or handicap. YES NO

68. My child often complains of illnesses such as nausea or stomach pain or headaches. YES NO

69. My child sometimes has accidental bowel movements in his (her) clothing. YES NO

70. My child has eating problems. YES NO

71. My child wets the bed. YES NO

OTHER

List any other problems or concerns you have about your child that were not listed above.

_____

_____

_____

_____

_____

_____

_____

_____

_____

RESOURCES

Mesibov, G., Schroeder, C., & Wesson, L. Parental concerns about their children. JOURNAL OF PEDIATRIC PSYCHOLOGY, 1977, **2**, 13-17.

Monnelly, E., Ianzito, B., & Stewart, M. Psychiatric consultations in a children's hospital. AMERICAN JOURNAL OF PSYCHIATRY, 1973, **130**, 789.

Walker, C. E. Behavioral intervention in a pediatric setting. In J. R. McNamara (Ed.), BEHAVIORAL APPROACHES TO MEDICINE: APPLICATION AND ANALYSIS. New York: Plenum Press, 1979.

HENDLER SCREENING TEST FOR CHRONIC BACK PAIN PATIENTS

Nelson Hendler

The Hendler Screening Test for Chronic Back Pain Patients is a brief screening instrument which has been found to be useful in assisting with the clinical evaluation of patients who present chronic back pain. The information obtained from this instrument can be helpful in discriminating between patients who may or may not benefit from surgery, as a therapy for back pain.

This instrument was based originally on data collected by the author from psychiatric evaluations of 387 outpatients and 258 inpatients under treatment at a chronic pain treatment center. Patients were grouped on the basis of their response to treatment of chronic pain. Items were formulated on the basis of the patient's personal and social history and how the different groups responded to questions about their pain. Four categories described ranged from patients with objective pain to those with prior psychiatric difficulties and no identifiable organic basis for pain.

A report in **PSYCHOSOMATICS** (Hendler, Viernstein, Gucer, & Long, 1979) described the findings from subsequent administrations of this instrument retrospectively to 315 patients who reported back pain. Complete physical evaluations were also available on each of the patients, making it possible to correlate the instrument results with the absence or presence of objective medical results. Of the 162 respondents with confirmed physical findings, 83% would have obtained 18 points or less on the instrument. Of the 58 patients with no definable physical problems, 66% would have obtained more than 32 points on the screening test. Follow-up studies involving prospective administration of the instrument have generally supported the predictive value of the instrument, but more work is required before it is fully refined.

In terms of reliability, the most recent form of the test indicates that 91% of test-retest scores with different examiners fall within two points of each other. It is suggested, however, that nonmedical personnel confirm the answers to Items 2 and 4 with medical staff.

While this instrument seems to have substantial clinical value in helping the diagnostician discriminate between various types of chronic pain patients, it should be emphasized that it is not a refined test but a means for the clinical evaluator to collect relevant information from pain patients. Important decisions should not be made solely on the basis of this instrument, and it should not be considered as a substitute for other more formal tests which may be used to evaluate patients in medical settings. Rather, it should be viewed as an aid to the diagnostic process.

Nelson Hendler, M.D., M.S., is currently Assistant Professor of Psychiatry and Neurosurgery in Psychiatry at the Johns Hopkins Hospital. He is also clinical director of the Mensana Clinic. Dr. Hendler may be contacted at the Mensana Clinic, Greenspring Valley Road, Stevenson, MD 21153.

RESOURCES

Hendler, N., Viernstein, M., Gucer, P., & Long, D. A preoperative screening test for chronic back pain patients. PSYCHOSOMATICS, 1979, **20**, 801-808.

Medicomp, Inc., 845 Margaret Place, Shreveport, LA 71101, offers computerized assessment of stress and chronic back pain patients. Their battery includes the Hendler Screening Test for Chronic Back Pain Patients and other relevant instruments available in two integrated batteries.

HENDLER SCREENING TEST FOR CHRONIC BACK PAIN PATIENTS*

Instructions: Each question is asked by an examiner, and the patient is given points according to the response that he or she makes. The number of points to be awarded for the various responses is shown in the column at the right. At the end of the test, the examiner calculates the total number of points. The results are interpreted as explained in the **Key**.

Points

I How did the pain that you now experience occur?
(a) Sudden onset with accident or definable event 0
(b) Slow, progressive onset without acute exacerbation 1
(c) Slow, progressive onset with acute exacerbation without accident or event 2
(d) Sudden onset without an accident or definable event 3

II Where do you experience the pain?
(a) One site, specific, well-defined, consistent with anatomical distribution 0
(b) More than one site, each well-defined and consistent with anatomical distribution 1
(c) One site, inconsistent with anatomical considerations, or not well-defined 2
(d) Vague description, more than one site, of which one is inconsistent with anatomical considerations, or not well-defined or anatomically explainable 3

III Do you ever have trouble falling asleep at night, or are you ever awakened from sleep?
If the answer is "no," score 3 points and go to question IV.
If the answer is "yes," proceed:

What keeps you from falling asleep, or what awakens you from sleep?
IIIA (a) Trouble falling asleep every night due to pain 0
(b) Trouble falling asleep due to pain more than three times a week 1
(c) Trouble falling asleep due to pain less than three times a week 2
(d) No trouble falling asleep due to pain 3
(e) Trouble falling asleep which is not related to pain 4

IIIB (a) Awakened by pain every night 0
(b) Awakened from sleep by pain more than three times a week 1
(c) Not awakened from sleep by pain more than twice a week 2
(d) Not awakened from sleep by pain 3
(e) Restless sleep, or early morning awakening with or without being able to return to sleep, both unrelated to pain 4

IV Does weather have any effect on your pain?
(a) The pain is always worse in both cold **and** damp weather 0
(b) The pain is always worse with damp weather **or** with cold weather 1
(c) The pain is occasionally worse with cold **or** damp weather 2
(d) The weather has no effect on the pain 3

---

*Test copyright 1979 by Nelson Hendler, M.D., M.S. Reprinted by permission.

Innovations In Clinical Practice: A Source Book

V   How would you describe the type of pain that you have?

  (a)   Burning; or sharp, shooting pain; or pins and needles; or
        coldness; or numbness   0

  (b)   Dull, aching pain, with occasional sharp, shooting pains not
        helped by heat; or, the patient is experiencing hyperesthesia   1

  (c)   Spasm-type pain, tension-type pain, or numbness over the
        area, relieved by massage or heat   2

  (d)   Nagging or bothersome pain   3

  (e)   Excruciating, overwhelming, or unbearable pain, relieved
        by massage or heat   4

VI   How frequently do you have your pain?

  (a)   The pain is constant   0

  (b)   The pain is nearly constant, occurring 50%–80% of the time   1

  (c)   The pain is intermittent, occurring 25%–50% of the time   2

  (d)   The pain is only occasionally present, occurring less
        than 25% of the time   3

VII   Does movement or position have any effect on the pain?

  (a)   The pain is unrelieved by position change or rest, and
        there have been previous operations for the pain   0

  (b)   The pain is worsened by use, standing, or walking; and
        is relieved by lying down or resting the part   1

  (c)   Position change and use have variable effects on the pain   2

  (d)   The pain is not altered by use or position change, and
        there have been no previous operations for the pain   3

VIII   What medications have you used in the past month?

  (a)   No medications at all   0

  (b)   Use of non-narcotic pain relievers; non-benzodiazepine
        tranquilizers; or use of antidepressants   1

  (c)   Less than three-times-a-week use of a narcotic, hypnotic,
        or benzodiazepine   2

  (d)   Greater than four-times-a-week use of a narcotic,
        hypnotic, or benzodiazepine   3

IX   What hobbies do you have, and can you still participate in them?

  (a)   Unable to participate in any hobbies that were formerly enjoyed   0

  (b)   Reduced number of hobbies or activities relating to a hobby   1

  (c)   Still able to participate in hobbies but with some discomfort   2

  (d)   Participate in hobbies as before   3

**X   How frequently did you have sex and orgasms before the pain, and
how frequently do you have sex and orgasms now?**

  (a^1) Sexual contact, prior to pain, three to four times a week, with
        no difficulty with orgasm; now sexual contact is 50% or less
        than previously, and coitus is interrupted by pain   0

  (a^2) (For people over 45) Sexual contact twice a week, with a 50%
        reduction in frequency since the pain   0

  (a^3) (For people over 60) Sexual contact once a week, with a 50%
        reduction in frequency of coitus since the onset of pain   0

(b) Pre-pain adjustment as defined above ($a^1 - a^3$), with no
difficulty with orgasm; now loss of interest in sex and/or
difficulty with orgasm or erection ... 1

(c) No change in sexual activity now as opposed to before the
onset of pain ... 2

(d) Unable to have sexual contact since the onset of pain, and
difficulty with orgasm or erection **prior to** the pain ... 3

(e) No sexual contact prior to the pain, or absence of orgasm
prior to the pain ... 4

XI **Are you still working or doing your household chores?**

(a) Works every day at the same pre-pain job or same level of
household duties ... 0

(b) Works every day but the job is not the same as pre-pain job,
with reduced responsibility or physical activity ... 1

(c) Works sporadically or does a reduced amount of household chores ... 2

(d) Not at work, or all household chores are now performed by others ... 3

XII **What is your income now compared with before your injury or the
onset of pain, and what are your sources of income?**

(a) Any one of the following answers scores ... 0

1. Experiencing financial difficulty with family income
50% or less than previously

2. Was retired and is still retired

3. Patient is still working and is not having financial
difficulties

(b) Experiencing financial difficulty with family income only 50%-75%
of the pre-pain income ... 1

(c) Patient unable to work, and receives some compensation so that
the family income is at least 75% of the pre-pain income ... 2

(d) Patient unable to work and receives no compensation, but the
spouse works and family income is still 75% of the pre-pain
income ... 3

(e) Patient doesn't work, yet the income from disability or other
compensation sources is 80% or more of gross pay before the
pain; the spouse does not work ... 4

XIII **Are you suing anyone, or is anyone suing you, or do you have an
attorney helping you with compensation or disability payments?**

(a) No suit pending, and does not have an attorney ... 0

(b) Litigation is pending, but is not related to the pain ... 1

(c) The patient is being sued as the result of an accident ... 2

(d) Litigation is pending or workmen's compensation case with a
lawyer involved ... 3

XIV **If you had three wishes for anything in the world, what would
you wish for?**

(a) "Get rid of the pain" is the only wish ... 0

(b) "Get rid of the pain" is one of the three wishes ... 1

(c) Doesn't mention getting rid of the pain, but has specific wishes
usually of a personal nature such as for more money, a better

	relationship with spouse or children, and so forth	2
(d)	Does not mention pain, but offers general, nonpersonal wishes such as for world peace	3

XV Have you ever been depressed or thought of suicide?

(a)	Admits to depression; or has a history of depression secondary to pain and associated with crying spells and thoughts of suicide	0
(b)	Admits to depression, guilt, and anger secondary to the pain	1
(c)	Prior history of depression before the pain or a financial or personal loss prior to the pain; now admits to some depression	2
(d)	Denies depression, crying spells, or "feeling blue"	3
(e)	History of a suicide attempt prior to the onset of pain	4

POINT TOTAL

KEY TO HENDLER SCREENING TEST FOR CHRONIC BACK PAIN

A score of 18 points or less suggests that the patient is an objective pain patient and is reporting a normal response to chronic pain. One may proceed surgically if indicated, and usually finds the patient quite willing to participate in all modalities of therapy, including exercise and psychotherapy. Occasionally, a person with conversion reaction or post-traumatic neurosis will score less than 18 points; this is because subjective distress is being experienced on an unconscious level. Persons scoring 14 points or less can be considered objective pain patients with more certainty than those at the upper range (14-18) of this group.

A score of 15-20 points suggests that the patient has features of an objective pain patient as well as of an exaggerating pain patient. This implies that a person with a poor premorbid adjustment has an organic lesion that has produced the normal response to pain; however, because of the person's poor pre-pain adjustment, the chronic pain produces a more extreme response than would otherwise occur.

A score of 19-31 points suggests that the patient is an exaggerating pain patient. Surgical or other interventions may be carried out with caution. This type of patient usually has a premorbid (pre-pain) personality that may increase his/her likelihood of using or benefiting from the complaint of chronic pain. The patient may show improvement after treatment in a chronic pain treatment center, where the main emphasis is placed on an attitude change toward the chronic pain.

A score of 32 points or more suggests that a psychiatric consultation is needed. These patients freely admit to a great many pre-pain problems, and show considerable difficulty in coping with the chronic pain they now experience. Surgical or other interventions should not be carried out without prior approval of a psychiatric consultant. Severe depression, suicide, and psychosis are potential problems in this group of affective pain patients.

PLEASE NOTE: The Hendler Screening Test for Chronic Back Pain Patients is copyrighted by Nelson Hendler, M.D., M.S., and any commercial use without permission is prohibited. Anyone wishing to collect data with the instrument should contact Dr. Hendler so that information regarding utilization and updated norms can be exchanged.

COMPETENCY TO STAND TRIAL ASSESSMENT INSTRUMENT *

Paul D. Lipsitt and David Lelos

This instrument was designed to improve communication between the behavioral science disciplines (particularly psychiatry) and the law in an area of mutual responsibility - the determination of competency to stand trial. Prior attempts at such communication have suffered from the understandable tendency of each of these disciplines to adhere to the language and concepts of their own discipline. Thus, the findings of the clinician have not been delivered in a form and language which are appropriate to the needs of the court. Insofar as clinical opinion has been delivered to the courts in this area, it has tended to be global, conclusional, and not substantiated by relevant clinical data.

We sought, therefore, to develop an instrument which delivered clinical opinion to the court in language, form, and substance sufficiently common to the disciplines involved to provide a basis for adequate and relevant communication. The purpose of the instrument is to standardize, objectify, and quantify the relevant criteria for competency to stand trial.

THE INSTRUMENT

The instrument may be described as a series of thirteen functions related to an accused's ability to cope with the trial process in an adequately self-protective fashion. These functions or items were culled from appellate cases, the legal literature, and our clinical and courtroom experience. The total series is intended to cover all possible grounds for a finding of incompetency. The weight which the court may be expected to assign to one or another of the items will not be equal, nor is it intended to be. Neither will the weight assigned to a given item by the court in reaching a finding on competency for a particular defendant necessarily apply to the next defendant. For example, in the court's view, it may be far more critical to the defense of a particular defendant that he or she be able to "testify relevantly" than for another defendant whose attorney does not intend to put him or her on the stand. Considerations of the weight to be assigned a given item in the case of a particular defendant goes beyond the scope of what should be expected of the examining clinician. The task for the clinician is the providing of objective data, the import of which is the responsibility of the court.

This instrument is designed to reflect the competency status of a defendant at the time of examination. It is not a predictive instrument. Our experience indicates that with the passage of time and variations in clinical status, even from day to day, a given defendant will vary in the scores attained. This is particularly true of patient-defendants recovering from an acute psychosis.

It is important to note at the onset that the inability to function indicated by low scores on this instrument must arise from mental illness and/or mental retardation and not, for example, from ideological motivation. When there is doubt as to its connection with abnormal and mental processes, the item should not be scored and it should be indicated that the opinion does not reach reasonable clinical certainty on the particular item.

At the very least, individual items which are scored at one or two (out of a scale of five) should be substantiated by diagnostic and clinical data of adequate richness to establish a serious degree of mental illness or retardation and the manner in which such disability relates to the low degree of functioning in the particular item.

It should be noted that defendants with mental disability of a serious degree, including psychosis and moderate mental retardation, frequently are quite competent and may achieve high scores on any or all of the items. Mental disability is relevant to a competency determination only insofar as it is manifested by malfunctioning in one or more of the specific items of the instrument.

In the scoring of this instrument, a basic assumption is that the accused will be adequately aided by counsel. A second basic assumption is that the professional who is using this instrument has at least a basic understanding of and experience in the realities of the criminal justice system.

Each item in the instrument is scaled from 1 to 5 ranging from "total incapacity" at one to "no incapacity" at five. If the instrument is used for outpatient or incourt screening purposes, a majority or a substantial accumulation of scores of three or lower in the thirteen items could be regarded as grounds for a period of inpatient observation and more intensive workup.

In our experience with patient-defendants who are in good contact, the examination and scoring, using this instrument, usually does not require more than one hour. Grossly psychotic or passive, concrete and under-responsive defendants obviously may require more extended examination. Care should be taken not to resort to leading questions. The device of offering two or three alternative choices to such defendants has been found to be useful.

In using this instrument interrater reliability can be significantly enhanced by frequent reference to the brief definitions of each item which follow. Expanded definitions, an interview protocol and brief clinical examples of defendants functioning at different levels of each of the thirteen items, and a summary of the studies of interrater reliability completed prior to the general dissemination of the instrument are available in the report, **COMPETENCY TO STAND TRIAL AND MENTAL ILLNESS,** prepared by the Harvard Medical School Laboratory of Community Psychiatry and available through the National Institute of Mental Health.

A score of **one** on the instrument indicates that for the item scored a close to or total lack of capacity to function exists of the order of a mute or incoherent person or a severe retardate.

A score of **two** indicates that for the item scored there is severely impaired functioning and a substantial question of adequacy for the particular function.

A score of **three** indicates that there is moderately impaired functioning and a question of adequacy for the particular function.

A score of **four** indicates that for the item scored there is mildly impaired functioning and little question of adequacy for the particular function. An individual can be mildly impaired on the basis of lack of experience in the legal process or sociocultural deprivation with or without attendant psychic pathology.

A score of **five** indicates that for the item scored there is no impairment and no question that the defendant can function adequately for the particular function.

A score of **six** indicates that the available data do not permit a rating which is within reasonable clinical certainty.

BRIEF DEFINITIONS

1. **Appraisal of available legal defenses:** This item calls for an assessment of the accused's awareness of the possible legal defenses and how consistent these are with the reality of his or her particular circumstances.

2. **Unmanageable behavior:** This item calls for an assessment of the appropriateness of the current motor and verbal behavior of the defendant and the degree to which this behavior would disrupt the conduct of a trial. Inappropriate or disruptive behavior must arise from a substantial degree of mental illness or mental retardation.

3. **Quality of relating to attorney:** This item calls for an assessment of the interpersonal capacity of the accused to relate to the average attorney. Involved are the ability to trust and to communicate relevantly.

4. **Planning of legal strategy including guilty pleas to lesser charges where pertinent:** This item calls for an assessment of the degree to which the accused can understand, participate, and cooperate with counsel in planning a strategy for the defense which is consistent with the reality of his or her circumstances.

5. **Appraisal of role of:**

    a. Defense counsel
    b. Prosecuting attorney
    c. Judge
    d. Jury

e. Defendant
f. Witnesses

This set of items calls for a minimal understanding of the adversary process by the accused. The accused should be able to identify prosecuting attorney and prosecution witnesses as foe, defense counsel as friend, the judge as neutral, and the jury as the determiners of guilt or innocence.

6. **Understanding of court procedure:** This item calls for an assessment of the degree to which the defendant understands the basic sequence of events in a trial and their import for him or her (e.g., the different purposes of direct and cross examination).

7. **Appreciation of charges:** This item calls for an assessment of the accused's understanding of the charges against him or her and, to a lesser extent, the seriousness of the charges.

8. **Appreciation of range and nature of possible penalties:** This item calls for an assessment of the accused's concrete understanding and appreciation of the conditions and restrictions which could be imposed and their possible duration.

9. **Appraisal of likely outcome:** This item calls for an assessment of how realistically the accused perceives the likely outcome and the degree to which impaired understanding contributes to a less adequate or inadequate participation in his or her defense. Without adequate information on the part of the examiner regarding the facts and circumstances of the alleged offense, this item would be unratable.

10. **Capacity to disclose to attorney available pertinent facts surrounding the offense including the defendant's movements, timing, mental state, and actions at the time of the offense:** This item calls for an assessment of the accused's capacity to give a basically consistent, rational, and relevant account of the motivational and external facts. Complex factors can enter into this determination. These include intelligence, memory, and honesty. The difficult area of the validity of an amnesia may be involved and may prove unresolvable for the examining clinician. It is important to be aware that there may be a disparity between what an accused is willing to share with a clinician as opposed to what he or she will share with the attorney, the latter being the more important.

11. **Capacity to realistically challenge prosecution witnesses:** This item calls for an assessment of the accused's capacity to recognize distortions in prosecution testimony. Relevant factors include attentiveness and memory. In addition, there is an element of initiative in that, if false testimony is given, the degree of activism with which the defendant will apprise his or her attorney of inaccuracies is of importance.

12. **Capacity to testify relevantly:** This item calls for an assessment of the accused's ability to testify with coherence, relevance, and independence of judgment.

13. **Self-defeating v. self-serving motivation (legal sense):** This item calls for an assessment of the accused's motivation to adequately protect himself or herself and appropriately utilize legal safeguards to this end. It is recognized that accused persons may appropriately be motivated to seek expiation and appropriate punishment in their trials. At issue here is the pathological seeking of punishment and the deliberate failure by the accused to avail himself or herself of appropriate legal protections. Passivity or indifference do not justify low scores on this item. Actively self-destructive manipulation of the legal process arising from mental pathology does justify low scores.

Paul D. Lipsitt, LL.B., Ph.D., is currently Director of the Mental Health-Law Program, Erich Lindemann Mental Health Center, Director of the East Boston Court Clinic, Lecturer on Psychology in the Department of Psychiatry, Harvard Medical School, and Clinical Associate, Boston University Student Mental Health Clinic. He is a Diplomate and Founding Director of the American Board of Forensic Psychology. Dr. Lipsitt may be contacted at 322 Franklin Street, Newton, MA 02158.

David Lelos, M.A., is currently Chief Psychologist, Boston Municipal Court Clinic. He was formerly a research psychologist at the Laboratory of Community Psychiatry, Harvard Medical School. Mr. Lelos may be contacted at 322 Franklin Street, Newton, MA 02158.

COMPETENCY TO STAND TRIAL ASSESSMENT INSTRUMENT

		Total	Severe	Degree of Incapacity Moderate	Mild	None	Unratable
1.	Appraisal of available legal defenses	1	2	3	4	5	6
2.	Unmanageable behavior	1	2	3	4	5	6
3.	Quality of relating to attorney	1	2	3	4	5	6
4.	Planning of legal strategy, including guilty plea to lesser charges where pertinent	1	2	3	4	5	6
5.	Appraisal of role of:						
	a. Defense counsel	1	2	3	4	5	6
	b. Prosecuting attorney	1	2	3	4	5	6
	c. Judge	1	2	3	4	5	6
	d. Jury	1	2	3	4	5	6
	e. Defendant	1	2	3	4	5	6
	f. Witnesses	1	2	3	4	5	6
6.	Understanding of court procedure	1	2	3	4	5	6
7.	Appreciation of charges	1	2	3	4	5	6
8.	Appreciation of range and nature of possible penalties	1	2	3	4	5	6
9.	Appraisal of likely outcome	1	2	3	4	5	6
10.	Capacity to disclose to attorney available pertinent facts surrounding the offense including the defendant's movements, timing, mental state, actions at the time of the offense	1	2	3	4	5	6
11.	Capacity to realistically challenge prosecution witnesses	1	2	3	4	5	6
12.	Capacity to testify relevantly	1	2	3	4	5	6
13.	Self-defeating v. self-serving motivation (legal sense)	1	2	3	4	5	6

Examinee_____ Examiner_____

Date_____

RESOURCES

Harvard Medical School Laboratory of Community Psychiatry. COMPETENCY TO STAND TRIAL AND MENTAL ILLNESS. (National Institute of Mental Health, DHEW Publication No. (ADM) 77-103). Washington, DC: U. S. Government Printing Office, 1973.

Gutheil, T. G. & Appelbaum, P. S. CLINICAL HANDBOOK OF PSYCHIATRY AND THE LAW. New York: McGraw-Hill, 1982.

Slovenko, R. The developing law on competency to stand trial. JOURNAL OF PSYCHIATRY AND LAW, 1977, **5**, 165-200.

EVALUATION OF SERVICE QUESTIONNAIRES

Peter A. Keller and J. Dennis Murray

In recent years it has generally been recognized that it is important for mental health clinicians to seek feedback from both clients and referral sources. Unfortunately, formal evaluation of services has been a task undertaken mainly in mental health centers where staff are assigned specifically to program evaluation. The program evaluation literature contains a considerable amount of information pertaining to the collection of data on patient satisfaction in such settings (e.g., Larsen, Attkisson, Hargreaves, & Nguyen, 1979; Sorenson, Kantor, Margolis, & Galano, 1979). With recognition of the fact that feedback is no less important for clinicians who practice outside of organizational settings, three service evaluation questionnaires are included here. The first questionnaire can be used to help assess the client's satisfaction and perception of progress in treatment. Its administration has the potential to stimulate discussion of resistance to change, priorities of therapy, and hidden agenda. The second questionnaire is designed to be given to clients to obtain feedback after treatment is terminated. Both questionnaires are brief and can be completed in less than five minutes. The third questionnaire is designed to be given to other professionals in the community to obtain their perceptions regarding a clinician's services.

Anyone using these informal questionnaires in their practice should be aware of several important limitations. First, these questionnaires were designed after reviewing a number of others and distilling them to obtain items we felt were best suited for noninstitutional practice. These are informal instruments designed only to provide users with subjective feedback. No reliability, validity, or factor analytic studies have been undertaken. Further, there are known to be a number of pitfalls in relying on client survey data. Perhaps the most interesting one is a consistent finding of high rates of satisfaction across applications of such surveys (e.g., Frank, Salzman, & Fergus, 1977). For example, satisfaction rates of 80% are not unusual. While there may be varied reasons for this finding, it is important for potential users to be aware of this phenomenon if they are to make meaningful interpretation of any data collected.

Peter A. Keller, Ph.D., is currently an Associate Professor and Psychology Graduate Coordinator at Mansfield University. He is also the Senior Editor of the Professional Resource Exchange, Inc. He holds a doctorate in clinical psychology. Dr. Keller may be contacted at P. O. Box 453, Mansfield, PA 16933.

J. Dennis Murray, Ph.D., is currently an Associate Professor of Psychology at Mansfield University and teaches in the Rural Community Psychology Program. He holds a doctorate in clinical psychology. He also serves as Associate Editor of Continuing Education for the Professional Resource Exchange, Inc. Dr. Murray may be contacted c/o the Department of Psychology, Mansfield University, Mansfield, PA 16933.

RESOURCES

Frank, R., Salzman, K., & Fergus, E. Correlates of consumer satisfaction with outpatient therapy assessed by postcards. COMMUNITY MENTAL HEALTH JOURNAL, 1977, **13**, 37-45.

Larsen, D. L., Attkisson, C. C., Hargreaves, W. A., & Nguyen, T. D. Assessment of client/patient satisfaction: Development of a general scale. EVALUATION AND PROGRAM PLANNING, 1979, **2**, 197-207.

Lebow, J. Consumer satisfaction with mental health treatment. PSYCHOLOGICAL BULLETIN, 1982, **91**, 244-259.

A comprehensive review of the literature on evaluation of consumer satisfaction with mental health treatment. Important methodological and practical problems are considered.

Sorenson, J. L., Kantor, L., Margolis, R. B., & Galano, J. The extent, nature and utility of evaluating consumer satisfaction in community mental health centers. AMERICAN JOURNAL OF COMMUNITY PSYCHOLOGY, 1979, **7**, 329-337.

ASSESSMENT OF THERAPY PROGRESS

Rate the degree to which you agree or disagree with each of the following statements by circling one number after each item. The results may be discussed during your therapy session. Remember, the value of this questionnaire depends upon your honesty in responding.

1. In general, I have been making good progress in therapy.

Strongly Agree	Agree	Unsure	Disagree	Strongly Disagree
(1)	(2)	(3)	(4)	(5)

2. My therapist seems to have a good understanding of my problems.

Strongly Agree	Agree	Unsure	Disagree	Strongly Disagree
(1)	(2)	(3)	(4)	(5)

3. My goals in therapy are clear.

Strongly Agree	Agree	Unsure	Disagree	Strongly Disagree
(1)	(2)	(3)	(4)	(5)

4. There are certain things which I have been afraid to share in therapy.

Strongly Agree	Agree	Unsure	Disagree	Strongly Disagree
(1)	(2)	(3)	(4)	(5)

5. My therapist seems genuinely interested in my problems and progress.

Strongly Agree	Agree	Unsure	Disagree	Strongly Disagree
(1)	(2)	(3)	(4)	(5)

6. In general I am satisfied with therapy.

Strongly Agree	Agree	Unsure	Disagree	Strongly Disagree
(1)	(2)	(3)	(4)	(5)

7. I am handling things better now than when I started therapy.

Strongly Agree	Agree	Unsure	Disagree	Strongly Disagree
(1)	(2)	(3)	(4)	(5)

CLIENT SATISFACTION SURVEY

Please take a few minutes to complete this anonymous questionnaire. It will be very helpful to me in evaluating the quality of services I provide. For each question, circle the response which best indicates your answer. Write in any additional comments you wish to make on the back of this page. Your honest responses will help me to provide my clients with the best possible care.

1. How many times were you seen for psychotherapy?

    5 or less   6 to 15   16 to 25   More than 25
      (1)   (2)   (3)   (4)

2. Did your therapist have a good understanding of your problems?

    Very Poor   Poor   Fair   Good   Very Good
      (1)   (2)   (3)   (4)   (5)

3. Have your problems changed for the better or worse as a result of therapy?

    Much Worse   Worse   No Change   Better   Much Better
      (1)   (2)   (3)   (4)   (5)

4. How well are you coping with your problems now, compared to when you began therapy?

    Much Worse   Worse   No Change   Better   Much Better
      (1)   (2)   (3)   (4)   (5)

5. Over all, how would you rate your therapist?

    Very Poor   Poor   Fair   Good   Very Good
      (1)   (2)   (3)   (4)   (5)

6. Over all, how would you rate the services you received?

    Very Poor   Poor   Fair   Good   Very Good
      (1)   (2)   (3)   (4)   (5)

7. If you had other personal or family problems, would you return here again for services?

    Definitely Not   Probably Not   Maybe   Probably   Definitely
        (1)   (2)   (3)   (4)   (5)

8. If you had any concerns about therapy or dissatisfactions with your therapist, did you feel your therapist was open to discussing them with you?

    Very Open   Open   Don't Know   Closed   Very Closed
      (1)   (2)   (3)   (4)   (5)

COMMENTS ABOUT THERAPY

Things about therapy that worked best for me:

Things that didn't work:

Concerns I have that were not resolved in therapy:

Office or therapy procedures that were confusing or that I would change:

Other comments or suggestions:

Thank you for your feedback!

REFERRING PROFESSIONAL SATISFACTION SURVEY

Please take a few minutes to complete this questionnaire. Your honest responses will help improve the services we offer to the community. Your feedback is greatly appreciated.

1. How many clients have you referred to us in the past year?

    None   1-5   6-10   11 Or More
    (1)   (2)   (3)   (4)

If you answered "None," skip the numbered questions and go directly to the comments section on the other side of this page.

2. How satisfied were you with the promptness of our response?

    Very Satisfied   Satisfied   Dissatisfied   Very Dissatisfied
        (1)   (2)   (3)   (4)   (5)

3. How well did we meet your expectations for treatment of your client(s)?

    Very Well   Fairly Well   Not Too Well   Not At All Well
       (1)   (2)   (3)   (4)   (5)

4. How satisfied were you with the level of feedback you received about the outcome of your referral(s)?

    Very Satisfied   Satisfied   Dissatisfied   Very Dissatisfied
        (1)   (2)   (3)   (4)   (5)

5. Over all, how satisfied are you with the care received by your referred client(s)?

    Very Satisfied   Satisfied   Dissatisfied   Very Dissatisfied
        (1)   (2)   (3)   (4)   (5)

6. How likely are you to send additional clients to us for services?

    Very Likely   Likely   Unlikely   Very Unlikely
       (1)   (2)   (3)   (4)   (5)

COMMENTS

Things you appreciate about our services:

Things you would like to see us change:

Needed clinical services you would like to see us develop for our community:

General comments or suggestions:

Your name and address (optional):

_____

_____

_____

Telephone: (____)_____

Thank you for your feedback!

MARITAL INTAKE FORM

Rhonda S. Keller

The marital intake form which follows grows out of my need for a brief, straightforward means of collecting information about couples and families in marital therapy. It is based on my review of several intake forms, inventories, and checklists designed for general use in clinical practice but which seemed inadequate for administration to couples presenting for marital therapy. Most of the forms I reviewed failed to allow couples to make note of common marital problems or information about previous marriages.

In addition to collecting basic information about each of the partners, the Marital Intake Form has a two-part checklist designed to identify common areas of marital difficulty. The first checklist contains concerns about children and may be filled out jointly. The second checklist requires partners to **separately** identify concerns about themselves or their partner. This permits the therapist to note areas of agreement and disagreement in the way couples view themselves and their problems. Also, I find couples are sometimes willing to identify a problem on paper before they feel ready to raise it in a session.

I am flexible in the way I use the form. Usually I have a couple complete the form at home after their initial visit to my office. In some instances when I have had an extended telephone conversation prior to the first session, I may mail the form to a couple and ask that it be completed prior to the office visit. If there are no children, the section which deals with children can obviously be omitted.

It should be emphasized that this is only a form for information collection. I have found it helpful in my own practice, but no studies have been done regarding its use. Readers who desire a more structured assessment of marital problems with normative data may wish to refer to Swensen and Fiore's "Scale of Marital Problems" in Volume I of **INNOVATIONS IN CLINICAL PRACTICE: A SOURCE BOOK**.

Rhonda S. Keller, ACSW, is a marriage and family therapist in private practice. She is a clinical member of the American Association for Marriage and Family Therapy. She may be contacted at P. O. Box 453, Mansfield, PA 16933.

MARITAL INFORMATION FORM

Your cooperation in completing this form will be very helpful in providing appropriate services. The first and second parts of the form should be completed jointly by you and your partner if possible. The third part should be completed by you independently; however, your therapist may wish to discuss the answers with you together.

PART I. GENERAL PERSONAL AND FAMILY BACKGROUND

Name_____ Birthdate_____ Age_____
    first   middle   last

Name_____ Birthdate_____ Age_____
    first   middle   last

Home Telephone Number(___)_____ Best Phone Number to Contact You(___)_____

Address_____

_____ Zip Code_____

EMPLOYMENT

Husband's Place of Employment_____Phone(___)_____

Wife's Place of Employment_____Phone(___)_____

MARITAL STATUS (Check As Appropriate)

Married & Live Together____ Separated____ Divorced____ Other____ Explain: _____

_____

Were either of you married before? Yes___ No___ If yes, please answer the following:

                              Husband   Wife

Date(s) of Previous Marriage(s)_____

Date(s) Previous Marriage(s) Ended_____

Reason(s) Previous Marriage(s) Ended_____

_____

Name(s) of Previous Partner(s)_____

EDUCATION

Husband: ____Grade School ____High School ____College ____Graduate Study

Wife: ____Grade School ____High School ____College ____Graduate Study

RELIGION

Husband: _____   Active_____   Inactive_____

Wife: _____   Active_____   Inactive_____

Children: _____   Active_____   Inactive_____

FAMILY MEMBERS

Identify all persons who are your children, for whom you assume personal or family
responsibility, or who live in your home.

NAME	RELATIONSHIP	AGE	BIRTHDATE	RESIDENCE

HEALTH CARE INFORMATION

Your Primary Physicians: When Last Seen/Reason for Visit

Husband:_____   _____

Wife:_____   _____

Children:_____   _____

          _____   _____

List Any Current Health Problems: List All Current Medications:

Husband:_____   _____

Wife:_____   _____

Children:_____   _____

          _____   _____

List Major Hospitalizations of Family Members in Last Five Years:

NAME	DATE	HOSPITAL	REASON

List All Previous Professional Help You Have Received for Personal, Marital, or Family Concerns:

NAME	DATE	THERAPIST	REASON

Name of Person Who Referred You Here_____

Fees Associated with Treatment Will Be Paid By:

Name_____Phone(___)_____

Address (If Different)_____

Signature(s) of Client(s) Completing this Form:

_____   Date_____

_____   Date_____

PART II. CHILDREN (Go to Part III if you have no children.)

This section is optional and should be completed only if you have children and only if the children represent a concern to be addressed in treatment. Identify with a check mark any of the following which concern you **or** your partner regarding one or more of your children. If only one of you is concerned about the issue or sees it as a problem, put that person's initials after the check mark.

____Bad Dreams   ____Moods   ____Health Problems

____Hyperactivity   ____Worrying   ____Relations with Step Children

____Fighting   ____Fears   ____Interference of Ex-spouse

____Temper Tantrums   ____Arguing   ____Visitation Arrangements

____Jealousy   ____Unhappiness   ____School Performance

____Sleep   ____Anger   ____Shyness

____Physical or Sexual Abuse   ____Stealing   ____Impulsiveness

____Friendships   ____Complaining   ____Disobedience

____Running Away   ____Depression   ____Drug or Alcohol Use

____Allergies   ____Bedwetting   ____Lying

____Sexual Concerns   ____Immaturity   ____Other:_____

____School Work   ____Attentiveness   ____Other:_____

On a separate page, describe in more detail any concerns you have about your children.

PART III. MARITAL AND PERSONAL CONCERNS

One copy of this section should be filled out **separately** by each partner. There are
two lists: The first deals primarily with individual concerns, the second with
relationship issues. Use initials to mark the items which apply to you or your
partner as individuals, or which apply to both of you. For example, if in your
opinion both of you are concerned about **arguing,** you would mark this item with both of
your initials. If you think that an item just applies to your partner, you would only
list his or her initials, or your initials if the item just applies to you.

_____

Individual Items:

____Nerves   ____Depression   ____Fears

____Shyness   ____Suicidal Thoughts   ____Finances

____Drug Use   ____Alcohol Use   ____Friends

____Anger   ____Sleep   ____Self-Control

____Stress   ____Work   ____Relaxation

____Headaches   ____Tiredness   ____Legal Matters

____Memory   ____Ambition   ____Making Decisions

____Loneliness   ____Inferiority Feelings   ____Concentration

____Education   ____Career Choices   ____Health Problems

____Temper   ____Dreams   ____Appetite or Weight

____Bowel Troubles   ____Thoughts   ____Stomach Troubles

Relationship Items:

____Closeness   ____Sexual Desire   ____Affection

____Sexual Performance   ____In-laws   ____Conflicting Schedules

____Communication   ____Relatives   ____Finances

____Friendships   ____Use of Time   ____Jealousy

____Infidelity/Affairs   ____Verbal Fighting   ____Physical Fighting

____Recreation   ____Housing   ____Common Interests

____Spouse's Cleanliness   ____Showing Appreciation   ____Agreeing on Chores

____Common Goals   ____Trusting Each Other   ____Having Fun Together

____Flirting Behavior   ____Parenting   ____Solving Problems Together

____Holding Other Down   ____Other:_____

Why did you seek help at this time? (Attach additional sheets if necessary)

Signature_____   Date_____

LEVEL OF FUNCTIONING SCALES: THEIR USE IN CLINICAL PRACTICE*

Frederick L. Newman

How is the client functioning now? Do you expect therapy to improve a client's ability to function in the next three months? At what level can the client with this diagnosis function in his or her ordinary community setting? If the client were to move to his or her own apartment, how would the move influence his or her overall ability to function now and six months from now? Do my colleagues' perceptions of this client's functioning match my perceptions? What treatments (treatment durations or amounts) are recommended to raise the client to a more satisfactory level of functioning?

A level of functioning scale, when used properly, can provide a systematic, reliable, and efficient frame of reference for formulating and communicating responses to these questions. This systematic frame of reference would be useful for communicating among colleagues who are working with the same client. It would also be useful when communicating with third-party payors about a client's capability to function in his or her ordinary community setting, and describing how therapy might support the client's movement to a more satisfactory level.

A level of functioning scale is seen as a complement to, rather than a substitute for a diagnostic system, or for symptom or problem scales. While diagnostic systems and symptom scales are useful to identify the nature of a client's disorder and symptoms, a level of functioning scale can be useful to describe the client's ability to function at one point in time and over time. Usually a level of functioning scale is applied to describe the client's ability to function over a short period of time(e.g., from one day on an inpatient unit to one or two weeks on an outpatient basis). The exception is the fifth axis of the American Psychiatric Association's Diagnostic System Manual, third edition (DSM-III), which requires a rating of the client's highest "Level of Adaptive Functioning During the Past Year (Spitzer, 1980)." The averaging of functioning over a several month period during the past year on the Adaptive Functioning Scale of the DSM-III does not lend itself to communication about the client's community functioning "now" and "over time." This is unfortunate, since the greatest potential of the level of functioning scales is their use in communication about the client's current, past, and future functioning.

*The research discussed in this chapter was supported by NIMH grant MH-37038.

A level of functioning scale is typically designed to provide a holistic view of the client, one which includes considerations of the client's social supports and temporal situations, as well as the symptoms and history involved in the formulation of a diagnosis. A level of functioning scale score describes the client's ability to function at the present time, and would most likely fluctuate over time as the client's ability to function in his or her ordinary community setting fluctuates. Most diagnostic systems refer to the suitability of the diagnosis at a particular point in time or label the diagnosis as being "in remission." Thus, a level of functioning scale can serve as a useful adjunct to a diagnostic system or to a symptom or problem scale.

Level of functioning scales are in popular use by both private and public mental health programs because of their relative ease in adoption and their face validity in providing a holistic description of a client's functioning over time. The scales can be used to describe the outcome of services designed to improve a client's functioning during a clinical episode. The changes in the client's functioning ratings over the course of the clinical episode can be described, along with the costs of services provided during the episode. This outcome and service cost information would be particularly helpful in evaluating the fees which need to be charged to cover the costs of services that have been typically associated with desirable patterns of client functional level outcomes. For example, these data could be used to justify a fee schedule in a contract with an employee assistance program for a private corporation.

Level of functioning scales typically avoid jargon and attempt to describe the client's ability to function in a fashion which is understandable to the lay person as well as to professionals. This feature is particularly useful when attempting to communicate with other practitioners in related health and social service professions.

There was a time when the private practitioner did not have to be concerned about providing a systematic means of communicating about the client's ability to function. But this is becoming less true now. Systematic communication about a client's functioning is often needed in justifying third party payor claims. Reliable communication is also needed in communicating with other professionals who may also be working with the client. Moreover, it is needed to maintain a permanent record on the client for later referral or in situations where there is legal involvement.

THE CHARACTERISTICS OF LEVEL OF FUNCTIONING SCALES

The label "level of functioning" has been associated with a group of scales which attempt to integrate multiple considerations about a client into a global description of the client's ability for community functioning. Level of functioning scales usually require the rater to integrate a number of facets about the client into a holistic description. Factors which are most often considered in the integrated judgment of functioning are (a) the client's cognitive and social abilities to perform expected role functions (e.g., that of a developing child, that of a working adult and/or provider, that of a husband, a wife, or a friend), (b) the client's self-care skills and problems (e.g., psychological signs and symptoms, stressors), and (c) the

TABLE 1: MAJOR LEVEL OF FUNCTIONING SCALES IN USE

SCALE	HISTORY	REFERENCES	DIMENSIONS
Menninger Health-Sickness Scale (H-S)	Influenced by first President's commission on Mental Health and developed within psychodynamic framework.	Luborsky, 1962; Luborsky & Bachrach, 1974.	(1) Functioning ability, (2) Symptom severity (3) Degree of discomfort (4) Effect of environment (5) Utilization of abilities (6) Interpersonal relations (7) Interests
Global Assessment Scale (G.A.S.)	Influenced by Health-Sickness Scale, but attempted to have more behavioral anchors	Endicott, Spitzer, Fleiss, & Cohen, 1976.	(1) Subjective distress (2) Behavioral disturbance (3) Reality testing (4) Summary role
Level of Functioning (LOF), Adaptations for local programs and populations	Influenced by Health-Sickness Scale and the community mental health movement.	Carter & Newman, 1976; Newman & Rinkus, 1978; Newman, 1980.	As adapted by local programs: Institute of Psychiatry of Northwestern Memorial Hosp.: (1) Physical functioning (2) Interpersonal relations (3) Social role performance (4) Psychological signs and symptoms
Index of Well-being (W-B)	Developed to provide an index of patient movement for planning and evaluating health care services.	Kaplan, Bush, & Berry, 1976.	(1) Mobility (2) Physical activity (3) Social activity (4) Symptom/problem

*Adapted from Newman (1980).

client's social and family supports and interactions. It should be noted that these three areas (abilities, problems, and supports) are not necessarily independent considerations when the clinician formulates the client's overall level of functioning. They are considered as an integral part of the whole picture. In fact, from research data my colleagues and I are currently analyzing, we are finding that there appears to be a "global functioning" factor which is highly correlated with separate ratings of clients' overall emotional symptom severity, vocational-task skill level, and social-interpersonal abilities.

One can select or adapt a level of functioning scale from a set of scales which have a fairly good history of reliable and valid application. The scales typically differ on what they emphasize in their focus on community functioning. Table 1 gives a summary of the major global functioning scales currently in use. The table outlines the antecedents which influenced the scale's development, the principal literature references, and the major dimensions which are integrated in formulating the global level of functioning rating.

It should be noted that the discussion in this contribution focuses on global level of functioning scales and not on scales that contain a number of subscales which, when combined, provide an overall level of functioning rating. Global level of functioning scales are typically used in conjunction with multifacet symptom or problem lists which are used to describe the pieces that contribute to the whole person. Thus, the level of functioning scales under discussion here are not seen as substitutes for multifaceted scales, but rather as a complement to these scales. The level of functioning scale provides a means of describing how the various components come together to influence the person's overall functioning in their ordinary community setting.

The first scale to be used in a variety of settings was the Menninger Health-Sickness scale (Luborsky, 1962). The Global Assessment Scale and the Level of Functioning scales trace their origins to the Health-Sickness scale. The Health-Sickness scale was developed in support of the first President's Commission on Mental Health which recommended that an overall goal of mental health services was to help mentally distressed and disabled citizens achieve their highest level of functioning. Luborsky led a panel of professionals in the development of the scale so that it would reflect that status of the client relative to the goal of autonomous functioning in the community. The scale contains eight ordered paragraphs describing a person's capability to function at that level in terms of the characteristics of the seven dimensions given in the last column of Table 1. Each paragraph represents a point on an interval scale from 0 to 100. Then, 34 examples of brief case vignettes are offered to describe points along the continuum, with the examples ranging in ratings from level 5 to level 95. Each of the case vignettes provides information on all seven factors. One problem cited with the Health-Sickness scale is that the language of the eight anchor points uses some of the language of the APA Diagnostic System (e.g., neuroses, schizophrenics). A desire for more descriptive language led to the development of other scales.

The Global Assessment Scale (GAS) and the Level of Functioning (LOF) scales are probably the most popular scales in use today. The GAS is reproduced in Table 2, and an LOF scale is reproduced in Table 3. The GAS is the scale with the greatest popularity (e.g., all of the programs in Arizona use the GAS, and

TABLE 2: GLOBAL ASSESSMENT SCALE (GAS)*

Rate the subject's lowest level of functioning in the last week by selecting the lowest range which describes his functioning on a hypothetical continuum of mental health illness. For example, a subject whose "behavior is considerably influenced by delusions" (range 21-30) should be given a rating in that range even though he has "major impairment in several areas" (range 31-40). Use intermediate levels when appropriate (e.g., 35, 58, 63). Rate actual functioning independent of whether or not subject is receiving and may be helped by medication or some other form of treatment.

91-100	No symptoms, superior functioning in a wide range of activities, life's problems never seem to get out of hand, is sought ought by others because of warmth and integrity.
81-90	Transient symptoms may occur, but good functioning of all areas, interested and involved in a wide range of activities, socially effective, generally satisfied with life, "everyday" worries that only occasionally get out of hand.
71-80	Minimal symptoms may be present but no more than slight impairment in functioning, varying degrees of "everyday" worries and problems that sometimes get out of hand.
61-70	Some mild symptoms (e.g., depressive mood and mild insomnia) OR some difficulty in several areas of functioning, but generally functioning pretty well, has some meaningful interpersonal relationships most untrained people would not consider him "sick."
51-60	Moderate symptoms or generally functioning with some difficulty (e.g., few friends and flat affect, depressed mood and pathological self-doubt, euphoric mood and pressure of speech, moderately severe antisocial behavior).
41-50	Any serious symptomatology or impairment in functioning that most clinicians would think obviously requires treatment or attention (e.g., suicide preoccupation or gesture, severe obsessional rituals, frequent anxiety attacks, serious antisocial behavior, compulsive drinking).
31-40	Major impairment in several areas, such as work, family relations, judgment, thinking, or mood (e.g., depressed woman avoids friends, neglects family, unable to do housework) OR some impairment in reality testing or communication (e.g., speech is at times obscure, illogical, or irrelevant), OR single serious suicide attempt.
21-30	Unable to function in almost all areas (e.g., stays in bed all day) OR behavior is considerably influenced by either delusions or hallucinations OR serious impairment in communication (e.g., sometimes incoherent or unresponsive) or judgment (e.g., acts grossly inappropriately).
11-20	Needs some supervision to prevent hurting self or others, or to maintain minimal personal hygiene (e.g., repeated suicide attempts, frequently violent, manic excitement, smears feces), OR gross impairment in communication (e.g., largely incoherent or mute).
1-10	Needs constant supervision for several days to prevent hurting self or others, or makes no attempt to maintain minimal personal hygiene.

---

*GAS by R. L. Spitzer, M. Gibon, and J. Endicott. Reprinted from Hargreaves, Attkisson, Siegel, McIntyre, and Sorensen, 1977, in the public domain.

TABLE 3: LEVEL OF FUNCTIONING SCALE*

Using the four problem areas (physical functioning, interpersonal relationships, social role performance, and psychological signs and symptoms) rate the person's ability to function autonomously in the community by circling the level which most nearly applies.

If the following criteria do not apply to the person (e.g., ability to work or go to school, and ability to live with family and friends) disregard them in your rating.

LEVEL 0:   Unknown.

LEVEL 1:   Dysfunctional in all four areas and almost totally dependent upon others to provide supportive, protective environment.

LEVEL 2:   Not working or going to school; family/friends cannot or will not tolerate the person; can perform minimal self-care functions but cannot assume most responsibilities or tolerate social encounters beyond restrictive settings (e.g., in group, play, or occupational therapy).

LEVEL 3:   Not working or going to school; living and/or getting along with family or friends but not without considerable strain on the patient and/or others. Symptoms are such that movement in the community should be restricted or supervised.

LEVEL 4:   Not working or going to school, although may be capable of doing either in a very restrictive setting. Person BARELY able to live or get along satisfactorily with family/friend/others. Can assume responsibility for all personal self-care.

LEVEL 5:   Emotional stability and stress tolerance is low. Person MARGINALLY capable of going to work or school in a nonprotective setting. Marginally able to live and/or get along satisfactorily with family/friend/others.

LEVEL 6:   Interpersonal relationships and social role performance are stable. Person CAPABLE of going to work or school in a nonprotective setting; able to live and/or get along with family/friend/others. The presence of psychological symptoms and their severity, however, are probably sufficient to be both noticeable and somewhat disconcerting to the person and/or others.

LEVEL 7:   Functioning well; however, psychological signs and symptoms are present to the degree that regular therapeutic intervention is needed even though these symptoms are not disconcerting to family/friends/others.

LEVEL 8:   Functioning well in all four areas with little evidence of distress present. However, a history of symptom reoccurrence suggests the need for periodic contact.

LEVEL 9:   Functioning well in all areas and does not need further services.

---

*LOF from the Institute of Psychiatry, Northwestern Memorial Hospital, Northwestern Community Mental Health Center. Reprinted by permission.

California mental health programs use an adaptation of the GAS called the Global Impairment Scale. The reliability of the GAS in Arizona has been found to be above .70 when accompanied by training. When training was not extensively deployed and when the scale was not used regularly, except as information recorded on a form, reliability decreased (Green, Nguyen, & Attkisson, 1979; Newman & Rinkus, 1978).

The Community Mental Health Center and Institute of Psychiatry of Northwestern Memorial Hospital (Chicago) adapted an LOF scale to complement severity ratings of client physical functioning, interpersonal relationships, social role performance, and psychological signs and symptoms. Here the LOF is part of an automated clinical record system and is used as part of regular feedback in the clinical record for supervision and review. After training in the use of the scale, reliability was found to be .90. Without training, the reliability was .56.

The validity of the GAS and LOF scales have been established by studies which correlated the scores on these scales with measures of psychological distress, symptom-problem severity, interpersonal relations and adaptive social functioning, and vocational and educational role skills. Statistically significant correlations between GAS and LOF ratings and these measures have been found in studies with adequate research designs. The results of the validity and reliability studies conducted up to the middle of 1980 are reviewed in Newman (1980). As I will describe in the next section, if a scale is properly selected and used you can expect it to provide a reliable and valid means of communicating your clients' levels of functioning.

SELECTION AND USE OF LEVEL OF FUNCTIONING SCALES

SCALE SELECTION

There are three general suggestions for selecting a level of functioning scale. The first is to define what you want of a scale (i.e., to identify the general characteristics of the client target population whose functioning level you wish to describe, along with the general goals of treatment in terms of impact on client functioning). The second suggestion is that the language of the scale should be easy for you to use when communicating with colleagues about clients. The third suggestion is that the scale you adopt or adapt should have a good record of reliable and valid usage.

The first suggestion, defining the client target population and the service goals, can be best understood by example:

ADULT MENTAL HEALTH SERVICES

> To provide services for the purpose of helping clients attain the highest level of psychosocial functioning in their ordinary community setting.

CHILDREN'S MENTAL HEALTH SERVICES

> To provide services which help children achieve optimal functioning and growth, relative to their developmental stage, in their ordinary family, community, and educational setting.

GERIATRIC MENTAL HEALTH SERVICES

To provide services which help older adults function and adapt to the physical and social changes which accompany the aging process.

ALCOHOL AND DRUG ABUSE

To provide services which help those abusing alcohol or drugs to reduce the risk (frequency) of such abuse, and to increase their ability to function in their ordinary community setting.

DEVELOPMENTAL DISABILITIES

To provide services which help developmentally disabled citizens operate in an environment and in a fashion which utilizes the fullest potential of their skills and available resources.

Once the overall target population goal statement is spelled out, it is also wise to identify the major subsets (domains) of functioning you expect the global level of functioning scale to cover. These subsets usually cover the three areas of personal, interpersonal, and community functioning.

The second and third suggestions, together, require four steps: (1) get your hands on a number of scales which have been used by others; (2) identify the reliability and validity of the scales which look most appropriate for your use (also note the conditions under which high reliability and validity were obtained); (3) select a set of two or more scales which can qualify for use on the basis of scale reliability with interrater correlation coefficients greater than .70 and validity suggested by statistically significant correlations between the level of functioning scale and the major areas of functioning identified under service goals; and (4) have a small group of colleagues, with whom you wish to frequently communicate, rate the scales in terms of how comfortable they are in using them for communication purposes. Usually a simple rank order voting procedure works well here. This procedure will provide a measure of consensus on each of the scales being considered.

While minor changes in the scale may be needed to obtain group consensus, drastic changes should be avoided unless the group is willing to run a study on the reliability and validity of the newly derived scale. This would involve having a group of clinicians rate a common set of cases, using the adapted level of functioning scale, plus an established multifaceted scale such as the Brief Psychiatric Rating Scale (Overall & Gorham, 1962, found elsewhere in this volume) or the Psychiatric Status Schedule (Spitzer, Endicott, Fleiss, & Cohen, 1970). Then, correlations of ratings across clinicians will describe inter-rater reliability. The correlations of the level of functioning ratings with subscales of the established multifaceted scale will describe the scale's validity. While reliability studies can be performed easily with two or more clinical raters independently rating 10 to 20 cases, validity studies are considerably more difficult. Validity studies usually require a large sample size. For example, a set of five clinicians would need to rate as many as 20 cases each to obtain sufficient power to perform such validity studies. Thus, I am recommending that you adopt a scale with an established record, invoking only minor changes, if any at all. From a psychometric point of view, it is preferable not to change the original scale at all. On the other hand, group consensus and support for scale use is equally important; thus minor changes in scale wording may be required.

PREPARATION FOR APPLICATIONS

Once a scale or scales have been selected, it is relatively easy to implement and use the scale if certain precautions are taken. Maintaining the scale's reliability, validity, and credibility requires training and relatively frequent use in clinical communication with colleagues who are also using the language of the scale. If the private practitioner decides that a level of functioning scale would be useful, then it is typically easy to arrange for inexpensive preparation to take place.

Training is the first requisite. Without proper training the scale's reliability tends to deteriorate. Fortunately, training in the use of a level of functioning scale is relatively simple. Simple, that is, if two prerequisites are satisfied. First, we will assume that the clinician has three or more colleagues with whom she or he wishes to communicate with fairly regular frequency. Second, we will assume that a level of functioning scale, mutually agreed upon, should be used to provide a common frame of reference in such communication.

The training involves scheduling a three hour session for the group to independently rate and discuss a set of cases which represents the majority of those cases the group has in common. The simplest procedure is to have each clinician provide a summary of a few cases as at a staffing conference. The presenting clinician should not make a judgment of the client's level of functioning until after the others have independently rated the case. Then the group would compare and discuss their ratings, attempting to resolve any differences in their perceptions of the client's level of functioning.

There are also several variations on the theme of these training sessions. For example, the clinicians could rate, in addition to the client's current level of functioning, the principal and secondary presenting problems and the severity of these problems, the probable level of the client's community functioning six weeks or six months from now, the services or techniques which might be needed to maintain or move the client's functioning level a given amount (e.g., one level on a nine point scale), and the adequacy of the information provided to formulate the level of functioning rating. Another training exercise might be to have the participants describe what changes in the client's behavior they would want to observe before they would agree the client has moved a certain number of steps on the scale.

Finally, if the level of functioning scale is to have content validity it is important that the clinician have some observable facts in the clinical record which substantiate the rated level of functioning. This substantiation can be a brief narrative note or a multifaceted problem or behavioral checklist which is recorded at intake and at termination.

The need for this substantiation raises the question of why one should have a level of functioning scale if more substantiation is required anyway. There are two reasons. One reason for selecting the level of functioning scale is that you may not want to use the detailed information to communicate with others (e.g., third party payors or colleagues in social or health agencies). Second, it is more expensive to communicate the more extensive information about clients. Thus, the level of functioning scale can provide a reliable and valid summary of the client's status during and as a result of treatment. However, if the level of functioning information is to remain credible to others, care must be exerted to assure its reliability and validity.

Frederick L. Newman, Ph.D., is currently Director of Clinical Research at the Institute of Psychiatry of Northwestern University, Department of Psychiatry and Behavioral Sciences. He is the former director of the Systems Research Unit of the Eastern Pennsylvania Psychiatric Institute and was affiliated with the Medical College of Pennsylvania and the University of Pennsylvania. His research interests are in clinical decision making and in mental health cost outcome studies. Dr. Newman may be contacted at the Department of Psychiatry and Behavioral Sciences, 320 East Huron (4th Floor), Chicago, IL 60611.

RESOURCES

Carter, D. E. & Newman, F. L. A CLIENT ORIENTED SYSTEM OF MENTAL HEALTH SERVICE DELIVER AND PROGRAM MANAGEMENT: A WORKBOOK AND GUIDE (2nd ed.). (Formerly Series C, No. 12, 1976, DHHS publication No. (ADM) 80-307). Washington, DC: U. S. Government Printing Office, 1980.

Endicott, J., Spitzer, R. L., Fleiss, J. L., & Cohen, J. The Global Assessment Scale: A procedure for measuring overall severity of psychiatric disturbance. ARCHIVES OF GENERAL PSYCHIATRY, 1976, **33**, 766-771.

Green, R. S., Nguyen, T. D., & Attkisson, C. C. Harnessing the reliability of outcome measures. EVALUATION AND PROGRAM PLANNING, 1979, **2**, 137-142.

Hargreaves, W. A., Attkisson, C. C., Siegel, L. M., McIntyre, M. H., & Sorensen, J. E. RESOURCE MATERIALS FOR COMMUNITY MENTAL HEALTH PROGRAM EVALUATION (2nd ed.). (NIMH, DHEW Publication No. (ADM) 75-222). Washington, DC: U. S. Government Printing Office, 1977.

Kaplan, R. M., Bush, J. W., & Berry, C. C. Health status: Types of validity and an index of well-being. HEALTH SERVICES RESEARCH, 1976, **11**, 486-488.

Luborsky, L. Clinician judgments of mental health: A proposed scale. ARCHIVES OF GENERAL PSYCHIATRY, 1962, **7**, 407-412.

Luborsky, L. & Bachrach, H. M. Factors influencing clinician's judgments of mental health: Eighteen experiences with the Health-Sickness Rating Scale. ARCHIVES OF GENERAL PSYCHIATRY, 1974, **31**, 319-334.

Newman, F. L. Global scales: Uses and problems of global scales as an evaluation instrument. EVALUATION AND PROGRAM PLANNING, 1980, **3**, 257-268.

Newman, F. L. & Rinkus, A. J. Level of functioning, clinical judgment, and mental health service evaluation. EVALUATION AND THE HEALTH PROFESSIONS, 1978, **1**, 175-194.

Overall, J. E. & Gorham, D. R. The Brief Psychiatric Rating Scale. PSYCHOLOGICAL REPORTS, 1962, **10**, 799-812.

Spitzer, R. L. (Ed.). DIAGNOSTIC AND STATISTICAL MANUAL OF MENTAL DISORDERS (3RD ED.). Washington, DC: American Psychiatric Association, 1980.

Spitzer, R. L., Endicott, J., Fleiss, J. L., & Cohen, J. The Psychiatric Status Schedule: A technique for evaluating psychopathology and impairment in role functioning. ARCHIVES OF GENERAL PSYCHIATRY, 1970, **23**, 41-55.

BRIEF PSYCHIATRIC RATING SCALE AND BRIEF PSYCHIATRIC HISTORY FORM

John E. Overall

The Brief Psychiatric Rating Scale (BPRS) was developed in 1962 to provide a quick and efficient description of the major dimensions of manifest psychopathology (Overall & Gorham, 1962). The initial use of this brief multidimensional rating scale was in the evaluation of treatment response in clinical psychopharmacology research; however, investigations soon extended to questions of diagnosis and classification. Those investigations prompted the addition, in 1966, of two other rating constructs to better delineate the excited states and organic brain syndromes. The BPRS that is widely used in clinical research today consists of 18 symptom rating constructs, each of which is rated on a seven-point scale of severity ranging from "not present" to "extremely severe." The symptom constructs, together with brief definitions, can be presented in a one-page format, as shown at the end of this chapter.

The BPRS is said to be a "construct" rating scale, as contrasted with molecular behavior rating scales. The aim in development of the BPRS was to provide experienced clinicians with an instrument for recording judgments about psychopathology at a level of abstraction that is consistent with ordinary clinical conceptualization. The alternative molecular approach, as represented in several lengthier rating scales, involves recording observations concerned with more basic units of behavior. Factor scores, which are assumed to represent the higher-level clinical constructs, are then produced by summing the molecular observations.

The symptom constructs that are rated on the BPRS were chosen to directly represent clinical concepts, such as anxiety and depressive mood, most of which correspond to primary factors identified in earlier analyses of larger item pools. The experienced clinician is accepted as a superior organizer and interpreter of the psychiatric significance of molecular observations. Because clinicians normally organize their observations around somewhat abstract constructs, it is most natural for them to record judgments about the severity of manifest psychopathology in those same terms. Psychiatrists and clinical psychologists have most often served as raters; however, the BPRS has been used successfully by nurses and by specially trained research assistants.

Although the BPRS is designed for recording the kinds of judgments about psychopathology that should be a natural consequence of any good clinical interview, for more formal research, a brief semistructured interview of 18 to

20 minutes duration similar to that described by Overall and Gorham (1962), is recommended. Attention is called to the fact that a majority of the rating constructs in the BPRS relate to behavior or manner of verbalization, and do not depend on the specific content that is discussed. Ratings of emotional withdrawal, tension, mannerisms and posturing, motor retardation, uncooperativeness, blunted affect, and excitement depend almost entirely on observation of the behavior of the patient during the interview. Conceptual disorganization is a construct that pertains to the logic and syntax of what is said, rather than the specific topics discussed. Thus, approximately two-thirds of the brief interview can be consumed by nondirective discussion of the patient's problems as he or she conceives them. The completion of a research interview may require further probing on specific issues that were avoided or which were not otherwise clarified in the nondirective portion.

FACTOR STRUCTURE AND SCORING

For numerical analysis, individual BPRS ratings should be scored 0 through 6 for severity levels of "not present" to "extremely severe." The location of the zero-point is important for mathematical operations such as multiplication, division, or the calculation of ratios. Not present is a meaningful natural origin, or zero-point, for a scale of symptom severity.

Numerous factor analyses have been accomplished on intercorrelations among items of the BPRS. A summary of these, as well as results pertaining to reliability and validity, is provided in an excellent review by Hedlund and Vieweg (1980). Five factors representing major symptom constellations have been rather uniformly reported, although the factor scoring proposed by different authors on the basis of those results has differed somewhat, due primarily to the size of factor loadings that the particular author considered significant.

The factor scoring that the present author recommends as being consistent with the results from most factor analyses of the 18-item BPRS involves summing of the ratings on the following subsets of items:

Thinking Disturbance
    Conceptual Disorganization
    Hallucinatory Behavior
    Unusual Thought Content

Anxious Depression
    Anxiety
    Guilt Feelings
    Depressive Mood

Withdrawal Retardation
    Emotional Withdrawal
    Motor Retardation
    Blunted Affect

Hostile Suspiciousness
    Hostility
    Suspiciousness
    Uncooperativeness

Agitation Excitement
    Tension
    Excitement

Although the suggested factor scoring does not utilize four of the BPRS symptom ratings, it has the advantage of being balanced insofar as an equal number of ratings define each of the first four factors. Earlier factor analyses were accomplished on the original 16-item version of the BPRS, and the first four factors were consistently identified in those analyses also.

The agitation excitement dyad appears only in analyses that were accomplished after addition of the excitement scale in 1966.

PHENOMENOLOGICAL CLASSIFICATION

Cluster analysis and related numerical taxonomy methods have been used to identify naturally occurring, phenomenologically homogeneous subgroups within the general adult psychiatric population. Many different profile patterns can be recorded on the BPRS, but some patterns occur more frequently than others. It is safe to say that some never occur. Cluster analysis methods can be used to identify the profile patterns that occur frequently in highly similar form. Patients who share a common symptom profile pattern are said to constitute a phenomenological type. Each phenomenological type can be represented by a prototype pattern, and the individuals belonging to the phenomenological type can be adequately characterized by saying that they are similar to the prototype.

Over the years, repeated investigations have gradually developed and solidified typologic concepts from large BPRS data bases. Eight distinct profile configurations have been found to account for most individual differences in BPRS profile patterns within the general adult psychiatric population (Overall, 1974). A large data base was recently acquired from the National Institute of Mental Health and used to refine the typology (Overall & Rhoades, 1982). Mean BPRS profiles for patients classified into the eight groups are presented in Figures 1 and 2. Four of the eight phenomenological

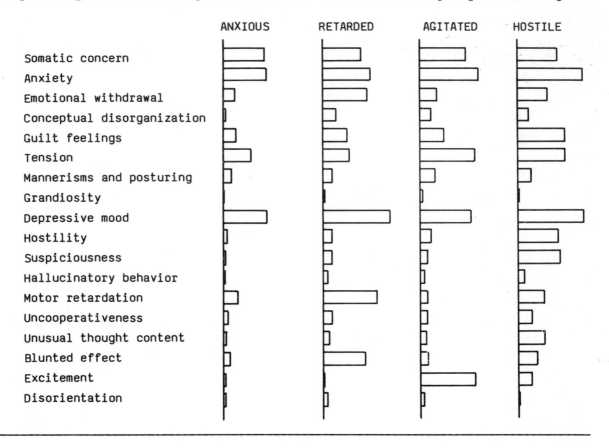

Figure 1.

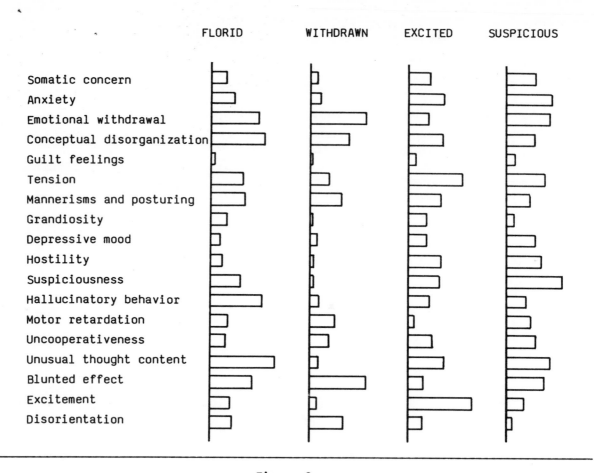

Figure 2.

types are considered to be subtypes of depressive disorder, and the remaining four are thought disorder and agitation/excitement syndromes. The phenomenological types have been described in detail in the referenced publications, as well as in an article by Overall and Hollister (1982) which also presents objective methods for assigning individual patients among the eight classes. Utility of phenomenological classification based on BPRS symptom profiles is considered by Overall and Rhoades (1982). I believe phenomenological classification to be a missing axis in the current Diagnostic and Statistical Manual (DSM III) (Overall, 1983).

A flow sheet that can be adapted for clinical use in classifying patients among the phenomenological types is shown in Figure 3. The subscripts identify particular BPRS symptom ratings by the numbers associated with them in the rating scale (e.g., X_5 = guilt feelings). One can frequently identify by inspection the pair of symptoms that received the highest average rating. When that is not possible, or when two or more pairs have equal average severity ratings, the sums for indicated pairs of symptoms can be entered on the right in a worksheet similar to that shown in Figure 3. The priority in case of ties is established by the order in the flow sheet. This is, of course, a very simple heuristic for phenomenological classification similar to "code typing" MMPI profiles. If one desires to consider more of the information present in the complete BPRS, numerical profile analysis methods discussed by Overall and Hollister (1982) can be used.

Innovations In Clinical Practice: A Source Book

FLOW SHEET FOR PHENOMENOLOGICAL CLASSIFICATION OF
BRIEF PSYCHIATRIC RATING SCALE (BPRS) PROFILE

A. Hostile Suspiciousness

$$X_{10} + X_{11} + 1.0$$
$$X_{10} + X_{14} + 1.0$$
$$X_{11} + X_{14} + 1.0$$

_____
_____
_____

B. Florid Thinking Disorder

$$X_4 + X_{12}$$
$$X_4 + X_{15}$$
$$X_{12} + X_{15}$$
$$X_{11} + X_{15}$$

_____
_____
_____
_____

C. Withdrawn Disorganized

$$X_3 + X_4$$
$$X_3 + X_{16}$$
$$X_4 + X_{16}$$

_____
_____
_____

D. Retarded Depression

$$X_3 + X_9$$
$$X_9 + X_{13}$$

_____
_____

E. Agitated Depression

$$X_9 + X_{17}$$

_____

F. Hostile Depression

$$X_9 + X_{10}$$

_____

G. Anxious Depression

$$X_2 + X_9 - 1.0$$

_____

H. Agitation-Excitement

$$X_6 + X_{17}$$

_____

Sum ratings for pairs of symptoms as indicated. Add 1.0 to the sum of pairs in frame A, and subtract 1.0 from the sum of the pair in frame G. Consider the resulting sums in order from A to H. If any sum is equal to or greater than the sums for all pairs of symptoms listed below it in the ordering, assign the patient to the indicated category.

___

Figure 3.

DIAGNOSTIC CONSIDERATIONS

The BPRS has been used to examine diagnostic concepts of clinicians and to provide actuarial norms for diagnostic classification based on actual clinical practices. Although the recent development by the American Psychiatric Association of more objective criteria for determining proper diagnoses has the commendable aim of establishing greater uniformity, the rather arbitrary criteria are the work of a committee. An alternative approach, which this author believes superior, is to capture, in a statistical sense, the central tendency of clinical practice among more numerous experienced clinicians.

The BPRS was first used to investigate clinical concepts of diagnostic entities within the United States and then to compare diagnostic concepts between several countries. That work had the incidental value of revealing the diagnostic distinctions to which the BPRS is sensitive or insensitive. In general, the distinctions between major diagnostic entities, such as depressive disorders versus schizophrenias, are quite clearly represented by the BPRS. Paranoid, schizoaffective, and core schizophrenia profiles differ, but within the schizophrenia domain other distinctions (if useful) are not provided by the BPRS. As an illustrative of the distinctions that are clearly made, the mean profiles for actual patient samples from four major diagnostic groups are shown in Figure 4.

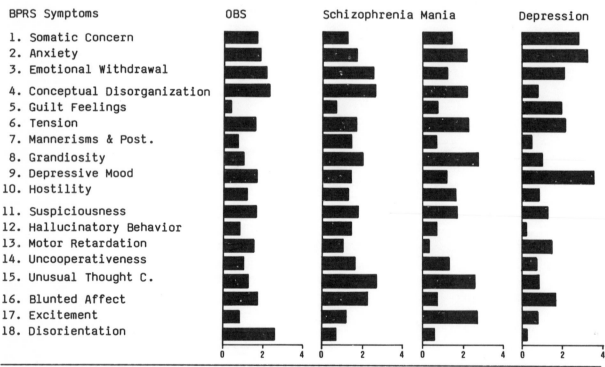

Figure 4.

As large data bases accumulated, an effort was made to develop a statistical model that corresponded to clinical practice more closely than do the narrow, somewhat arbitrary, research diagnostic criteria. The so-called Texas Actuarial Criteria have the aim of defining schizophrenia and depression consistent in nature and number with treatment practices (Overall, 1981). This statistical approach utilized empirically defined weights to combine BPRS symptom ratings with selected demographic indicators to obtain numerical indices for schizophrenia, depression, and other disorders. The "other" classification is meaningful as an exclusion for schizophrenia and depression.

The Texas Actuarial Criteria consider more information than do other narrow research diagnostic criteria and, hence, acquire the reliability advantage of a "longer test." Research diagnostic criteria that rely on a very few indicators are more affected by a single error in perception or judgment. In a study of 100 consecutive inpatient admissions, two psychologist research assistants independently recorded the BPRS ratings based on a joint interview, and the Texas Actuarial Criteria were scored from their separate ratings. The kappa coefficient was 0.96 for agreement on a diagnosis of schizophrenia and 0.80 for agreement on a diagnosis of depressive disorder. This level of agreement was higher than the corresponding values for several research diagnostic criteria that rely on less information (Overall, Cobb, & Click, 1982). The scoring for Texas Actuarial Criteria is described in this report and the previously referenced chapter (Overall, 1981).

THE BRIEF PSYCHIATRIC HISTORY FORM

A complete psychiatric data base must recognize the importance of history and background information in addition to symptom manifestations. In our own use, the BPRS is accompanied by the Brief Psychiatric History Form (BPHF), found at the end of this chapter. The BPHF is a condensed checklist data form that can be printed on the reverse side of the BPRS symptom rating form to minimize the amount of paper that needs to be included in a patient's record. The recording of both background data and symptom description on a single form has the advantage of insuring that the two types of information remain together.

Because of interest in its brevity, the BPHF does not contain all items that an individual clinician or investigator may desire for specific purposes. The items that are included have been identified repeatedly as being predictive of differences in manifest psychopathology. Several have been verified to relate to treatment outcome, although the relationship to treatment outcome differs as a function of type of syndrome and mode of treatment. The history and background variables that have most consistently been found to distinguish between major diagnostic groups include age, sex, marital status, work level, alcohol abuse, drug abuse, sleep difficulties, history of previous psychiatric hospitalizations, and positive family history. It is no coincidence that those variables, which can be abstracted from the BPHF, are included with BPRS symptom ratings in scoring of the Texas Actuarial Criteria which were described in the preceding section.

The BPHF has the advantage of having been used in numerous previous clinical investigations and convenient references for it are included elsewhere (Overall, 1981). Apart from diagnostic significance, items from the BPHF are almost necessary as control variables in the analysis of clinical research data. In the development of psychiatric data bases, some specific questions may be posed at the outset; however, the data base concept makes feasible numerous post hoc analyses for which a proven pool of core data is useful. In our own treatment setting, the BPRS and BPHF are completed for each new patient. Those data are acquired primarily as a foundation for specific research projects that may involve additional data (e.g., biochemical markers) on selected subsets of patients.

BRIEF PSYCHIATRIC RATING SCALE

J. E. Overall and D. R. Gorham

Directions: Place an X in the appropriate box to represent level of severity of each symptom.

PATIENT_____

RATER_____

NO._____

DATE_____

	Not Present	Very Mild	Mild	Moderate	Mod. Severe	Severe	Extremely Severe
1. SOMATIC CONCERN - preoccupation with physical health, fear of physical illness, hypochondriasis.	☐	☐	☐	☐	☐	☐	☐
2. ANXIETY - worry, fear, overconcern for present or future.	☐	☐	☐	☐	☐	☐	☐
3. EMOTIONAL WITHDRAWAL - lack of spontaneous inter-action, isolation, deficiency in relating to others.	☐	☐	☐	☐	☐	☐	☐
4. CONCEPTUAL DISORGANIZATION - thought processes con-fused, disconnected, disorganized, disrupted.	☐	☐	☐	☐	☐	☐	☐
5. GUILT FEELINGS - self-blame, shame, remorse for past behavior.	☐	☐	☐	☐	☐	☐	☐
6. TENSION - physical and motor manifestations or nervousness, overactivation, tension.	☐	☐	☐	☐	☐	☐	☐
7. MANNERISMS AND POSTURING - peculiar, bizarre, un-natural motor behavior (not including tic).	☐	☐	☐	☐	☐	☐	☐
8. GRANDIOSITY - exaggerated self-opinion, arrogance, conviction of unusual power or abilities.	☐	☐	☐	☐	☐	☐	☐
9. DEPRESSIVE MOOD - sorrow, sadness, despondency, pessimism.	☐	☐	☐	☐	☐	☐	☐
10. HOSTILITY - animosity, contempt, belligerence, disdain for others.	☐	☐	☐	☐	☐	☐	☐
11. SUSPICIOUSNESS - mistrust, belief others harbor malicious or discriminatory intent.	☐	☐	☐	☐	☐	☐	☐
12. HALLUCINATORY BEHAVIOR - preceptions without normal external stimulus correspondence.	☐	☐	☐	☐	☐	☐	☐
13. MOTOR RETARDATION - slowed, weakened movements or speech; reduced body tone.	☐	☐	☐	☐	☐	☐	☐
14. UNCOOPERATIVENESS - resistance, guardedness, rejection of authority.	☐	☐	☐	☐	☐	☐	☐
15. UNUSUAL THOUGHT CONTENT - unusual, odd, strange, bizarre thought content.	☐	☐	☐	☐	☐	☐	☐
16. BLUNTED AFFECT - reduced emotional tone, re-duction in normal intensity of feelings, flatness.	☐	☐	☐	☐	☐	☐	☐
17. EXCITEMENT - heightened emotional tone, agitation, increased reactivity.	☐	☐	☐	☐	☐	☐	☐
18. DISORIENTATION - confusion or lack of proper associ-ation for person, place, or time.	☐	☐	☐	☐	☐	☐	☐

Drugs Continued:_____New Drugs:_____

Patient_____   Date_____

Patient Present Age

____Below 15
____15-19
____20-24
____25-29
____30-39
____40-49
____50-59
____60 or Above

Ethnicity

____White
____Black
____Mexican-American
____Other Minority

Sex

____Male
____Female

Education (Level)

____0-7 Years
____8-11 Years
____12 Years
____13-15 Years
____16 Years
____More Than 16 Years

Work Level (When Working)

____Never Worked
____Housewife
____Unskilled
____Skilled
____Clerical
____Sales or Business
____Profession or
    Managerial
____Student

Work Attitude

____Negative
____Indifferent
____Normal Interest
____Excess Involvement
____Retired

Current Marital Status

____Single
____Married
____Separated
____Divorced
____Widowed

Marital History

____No Previous Divorces
____One Previous Divorce
____Two Previous Divorces
____Multiple Divorces
____Widowed Remarried

Children of Patient

____No Children
____One Child
____Two to Four Children
____More Than Four

Alcohol

____Abstain
____Moderate
____Frequent
____Problem Drinking

Criminal Record

____Person Crimes
____Person Violent Crimes
____Property Crimes
____Social Code Violations
____Other

Religious Attitude

____Atheist
____Agnostic (Doubting)
____Indifferent
____Moderate Positive
____Strong Positive
    or Fanatic

Precipitating Factors

____Marital Conflict
____Separation or Divorce
____Death of Loved One
____Criminal Victimization
____Criminal Apprehension
____Work Problems
____Financial Problems
____Alcohol Abuse
____Drug Abuse
____Physical Illness
____Organic CNS Involvement
____Other
____None

Major Problem Areas

____Marital Problems
____Social Interpersonal
____Antisocial Behavior
____Work Interference
____Sexual Inadequacy
____Poor Impulse Control
____Alcohol Abuse
____Drug Abuse
____Sleep Problems
____Physical Problems
____CNS Dysfunction
____Other

**Problems in Parental Home
Before Age 12**

____Severe Discord
____Divorce
____Death of Parent
____Death of Sibling
____Severe Economic
____Other Stress

Father's Education

____Less Than High School
____High School Graduate
____Some College

Mother's Education

____Less Than High School
____High School Graduate
____Some College

Duration This Episode

____Less Than 1 Month
____1-6 Months
____6-12 Months
____1-2 Years
____More Than 2 Years

Course of Illness

____Chronic Stable
____Slow Decline
____Recurrent Acute Episodes
____First Episode

**Previous Psychiatric
Hospitalization**

____No Previous Admission
____Single Previous Admission
____Multiple Previous Admissions

**Previous Outpatient Psychiatric
Treatment**

____None
____Nonpsychiatric Rx
____Psychiatrist
____Psychologist

Nature of Previous Episodes

____None
____Depression
____Agitation-Excitement
____Thinking Disturbance
____Other

Family Psychiatric History

____Father
____Mother
____Siblings
____Other Relatives

Patient Perception of Problem

____Mental
____Mood
____Character
____Physical
____Interpersonal Adjustment
____No Problem (Denial)
____Other

```
Phenomenological Type

____Simple Anxiety
____Anxious Depression
____Hostile Depression
____Retarded Depression
____Agitated Depression
____Florid Thinking Disorder
____Withdrawn-Disorganized
    Thinking
____Hostile Suspiciousness
    Syndrome
____Agitation-Excitement
    Syndrome
____Confusion-Disorientation
____No Overt Psychopathology

DIAGNOSIS (APA)

(1)_____

(2)_____
```

John E. Overall, Ph.D., is currently Professor in the Department of Psychiatry and Behavioral Sciences at the University of Texas Medical School at Houston. He was formerly an Associate Professor, Department of Psychology, at Kansas State University and Chief, Criterion Development, Veterans Administration Central Neuropsychiatric Laboratory, where he collaborated with Donald R. Gorham, Ph.D., in the development of the Brief Psychiatric Rating Scale (BPRS). Dr. Overall may be contacted at University of Texas Medical School, P. O. Box 20708, Houston, TX 77025.

RESOURCES

Hedlund, J. L. & Vieweg, B. W. The brief psychiatric rating scale (BPRS): A comprehensive review. JOURNAL OF OPERATIONAL PSYCHIATRY, 1980, 11, 48–65.

Overall, J. E. The brief psychiatric rating scale in psychopharmacology research. In P. Pichot & R. Oliver-Martin (Eds.), PSYCHOLOGICAL MEASUREMENTS IN PSYCHOPHARMACOLOGY: MODERN PROBLEMS IN PHARMACOPSYCHIATRY. Basel: Karger, 1974.

Overall, J. E. Criteria for the selection of subjects for research in biological psychiatry. In H. M. Van Praag, M. H. Lader, O. J. Rafaelsen, & E. G. Sachar (Eds.), HANDBOOK OF BIOLOGICAL PSYCHIATRY, PART VI, PRACTICAL APPLICATIONS OF PSYCHOTROPIC DRUGS AND OTHER BIOLOGICAL TREATMENTS. Basel: Marcel Dekker, 1981.

Overall, J. E. Phenomenological heterogeneity of depressive disorders. In J. Maas & J. E. Davis (Eds.), AFFECTIVE DISORDERS. Washington, DC: American Psychiatric Press, Inc., 1983.

Overall, J. E., Cobb, J. C., & Click, M. A., Jr. The reliability of psychiatric diagnoses based on alternative research criteria. JOURNAL OF PSYCHIATRIC TREATMENT & EVALUATION, 1982, 4, 209–220.

Overall, J. E. & Gorham, D. R. The brief psychiatric rating scale. PSYCHOLOGICAL REPORTS, 1962, 10, 799–812.

Overall, J. E. & Hollister, L. E. Decision rules for phenomenological classification of psychiatric patients. JOURNAL OF CONSULTING & CLINICAL PSYCHOLOGY, 1982, 50, 535–545.

Overall, J. E. & Rhoades, H. M. Refinement of phenomenological classification in clinical psychopharmacology research. PSYCHOPHARMACOLOGY, 1982, 77, 24–30.

INTRODUCTION TO SECTION IV: COMMUNITY INTERVENTIONS

In this section we have included a group of articles which address nontraditional functions for the practitioner. This section has been included in the volume because of our belief that clinicians have often selected narrowly defined roles which unnecessarily limit their impact on the community. By including this section, we hope to stimulate readers' thinking about innovative interventions which might have impact on a larger number of people or be more preventive in outcome. Only through such interventions in the community will broad changes that reduce distress and enhance adjustment result.

COMMUNITY INTERVENTIONS as we have defined them include a wide range of activities, often requiring special skills for successful implementation. Haas begins the section by discussing a number of important ethical issues the consultant must address. These are often somewhat different than the concerns faced by practitioners in traditional roles. The contribution by Bouhoutsos on work with the media also addresses a number of important ethical concerns clinicians must face when seeking to extend their influence through this important avenue.

The remaining contributions consider consultant roles in three different settings. Goodstein and Cooke skillfully describe organization development using analogies to the traditional clinical setting. Fitzhugh discusses the growing role of behavioral science consultants with the police and provides examples of several developing areas of intervention. Ingersoll and Geboy discuss the rapidly growing interface between mental health clinicians and dentists and offer concrete examples of how such work can be initiated. In each instance, the authors offer specific suggestions for the reader who wishes to follow up on the area of intervention.

COMMUNITY INTERVENTIONS

ETHICAL ISSUES IN CONSULTATION

Leonard J. Haas

This contribution is aimed at the practitioner who provides consultation services, or who is considering offering such services. It is an attempt to identify the common features of the incredibly diverse range of activities known as consultation, to consider the ways in which the general issues of professional ethics apply to consulting activities, and to develop some rules of thumb that may help the consultant to resolve or, ideally, prevent common ethical problems.

Consider first the range of services classified as consultative. Mental health and psychological consultants work in school systems, industry, public service, police departments, courts, nursing homes, libraries, media, and religious institutions (Manninno, MacClennan, & Shore, 1975). This diversity of activities has been classified according to the focus of the process (e.g., Caplan, 1970), the institutional setting of the consultation (e.g., Goodstein, 1978), the underlying theory of the consultant (e.g., Woody, 1975), and the type of intervention (e.g., Blake & Mouton, 1976). Are there common threads that run through this range of activities and theories?

At the risk of blurring some important distinctions, certain common elements can be identified. At the minimum, consultation involves a system or institution utilizing the services of an expert, who is not ordinarily part of the work team, in order to improve some aspect of the functioning of that team. Therefore, a key feature of consultation which distinguishes it from other mental health activities (e.g., therapy, testing, teaching, and research) is that the consultant provides services to individuals in an organizational context. This means that consultees are both consumers of the consultant's services and holders of particular roles in the host organization (and they may have other roles as well). This fact has important implications for a consideration of ethics in consultation, and will be elaborated on further.

A second feature of consultation is that, typically, the receivers of the consultation (consultees) use their new knowledge and skills to affect the lives of others (clients). For example, pupils' lives are affected by their teachers' use of consultation. This fact also has important implications for an ethical analysis of consultation.

A third feature of consultation is the often ambiguous nature of the activity. Any psychological service involves some ambiguity; diagnoses change with new information, objectives shift as treatment goes on. Consultants, though, must also cope with the often unrealistic ideas consultees have about the process. As Caplan (1970) clearly points out, consultation is different from therapy, supervision, education, and collaboration. Consultees, however, typically identify the consultant with his or her profession, and identify the activity with some familiar aspect of that role. For example, it is likely that the university faculty member providing consultation to the staff of a correctional facility will be seen as a teacher, and the clinician consulting to a nursing home as a therapist. Again, this fact has implications for the development of consultation ethics.

Regardless of the special features of consultation, it is valuable for the consultant to think through the ethical implications of his or her activities **before** problems arise. Ethics are highly context-dependent; there is no set of rules that, blindly followed, will result in ethical behavior. Rather, the ethical practitioner applies a set of principles to specific situations, with results often unique to that situation. In what follows, some of these general principles will be identified, and their specific applications in certain consulting situations will be discussed. There will undoubtedly be disagreement with some of the recommendations, and questions about areas that cannot be completely covered. Nonetheless, it is important to stimulate the process of thinking through some of these issues in advance.

In summary, the present purposes are first, to highlight some features of consultation that make the development of ethical practice somewhat different from other professional activities, second, to highlight specific problems that emerge regularly in many forms of consultation, third, to provide some rules of thumb for the prevention and resolution of ethical dilemmas, and fourth, to identify, at least in passing, some of the legal issues in consultation (although a full treatment of that area is beyond the present scope).

SOME USEFUL DISTINCTIONS IN PROFESSIONAL ETHICS

Ethical behavior is often made to seem synonymous with "right" behavior; there are several senses in which behavior may be considered right (or wrong), and it is helpful to distinguish among them. This section distinguishes ethical from prudent or polite behavior, distinguishes private from professional ethics, and distinguishes technical from ethical problems.

ETHICS, PRUDENCE, AND POLITENESS

Codes of ethics, guidelines for self-protection, and rules of conventional propriety are all means to regulate behavior so that individuals "act right." Unethical behavior, at least for the purposes of the present analysis, is behavior which causes some harm or violates some principle, without being justifiable on the basis of producing some good or upholding some other principle. Ethical behavior should be based on ethical reasoning (in fact, there is some question whether behavior can actually be considered ethical if it was done for reasons of prudence or politeness). Ethical reasoning, in turn, involves the application of principles to one's actions and consideration of the consequences of those actions. This point may be clarified by contrasting ethical with prudent or "polite" behavior.

Prudence is self-interest. While it is possible to argue that the preservation of one's personal well-being is ethical, it is generally considered nonethical reasoning to decide to act on the basis of the likelihood of one's being caught or punished. Thus, the therapist who refrains from sexual contact with a desirable patient because he or she might be sued is acting prudently, but without further information it is impossible to say if he or she is acting on ethical grounds.

Politeness is conventionality. Many actions are judged wrong (or right) on the basis of "normal" behavior. Thus, a therapist who makes house calls may be considered to act unusually, but without further information it would be impossible to say that such behavior is unethical.

Note that these standards are orthogonal. It is possible for an act to be at the same time ethical, prudent, and "polite," but it is equally possible for an ethical act to be both impolite and imprudent, or to be unethical but prudent, and so on.

PRIVATE VERSUS PROFESSIONAL MORALITY

It was noted previously that consultees are both autonomous individuals and the holders of roles in particular contexts. This point is also true of consultants, who are simultaneously individuals and members of a profession. This fact adds another dimension to the ethical reasoning of consultants. First, their actions affect not only themselves but other holders of the same professional role; second, their actions are based on an implicit promise to their clients and to society.

Specifically, the benefits bestowed upon professionals (e.g., licensure, economic rewards, prestige) are based in part on the expectation that they use scientifically valid procedures and knowledge to benefit their clients. In addition, there is the implicit expectation that professionals use their power and skill in ways that benefit society. Commentators on this state of affairs have sometimes decried it because it makes mental health professionals into agents of social control (cf. Halleck, 1971). Other commentators claim that responsibilities of the professional provide a suitable "repayment" to society (cf. Strupp & Hadley, 1977). While perhaps not numerous, there are certainly instances in which the demands of the professional role call for actions the individual considers morally objectionable. This sort of dilemma is not resolved easily with rules such as "your professional ethics come before your personal ethics" or vice versa. Rather, careful deliberation, and perhaps consultation with peers and colleagues, is necessary.

TECHNICAL VERSUS ETHICAL ISSUES

There is another sense in which actions can be judged right or wrong: the technical sense. For example, the therapist who attempts to change the behavior of an abusive parent by lecturing on the evils of his or her actions may be said to be acting badly, but only in the sense of "making a mistake" rather than "acting unethically." Ethical considerations may sometimes involve questions of whether a particular goal has been accomplished, but more often they concern questions about the goal itself. It is certainly true that many apparent conflicts of ethical principles can be resolved by creative technical means; it is also true that the search for technical solutions, as MacIntyre (1979) has pointed out, can disguise the nature of the ethical questions.

THREE MAJOR ISSUES IN PROFESSIONAL ETHICS

This contribution is obviously not a substitute for a thorough understanding of the **ETHICAL PRINCIPLES OF PSYCHOLOGISTS** (American Psychological Association, 1981), the **NASW CODE OF ETHICS** (National Association of Social Workers, 1980), the **PRINCIPLES OF MEDICAL ETHICS** (American Psychiatric Association, 1981), or other professional codes; it is nonetheless useful to consider three concepts that seem to be fundamental to professional morality regardless of the specialty field. These principles are responsibility, integrity, and competence.

RESPONSIBILITY

The autonomy granted to (or at least claimed by) mental health professionals carries with it the assumption of responsibility. That is, the professional is assumed to be the author of his or her actions and the causal agent in the results of those actions. Put differently, this principle means that professionals cannot take refuge in the fact that they were ordered to act in particular ways, or that they were not being paid to consider the longer range effects of their behavior.

Applying this principle to consultation implies that the consultant must consider the impact of the service on consultees and on those whom they serve. It also means that consultants have a duty to play an active part in the decision to utilize consultation in the first place (rather than to assume that sponsors' willingness to pay for it means it should go on).

Ironically, this notion conflicts with a widely-held view that consultants must not "take responsibility" for consultees and increase their dependency. The apparent contradiction dissolves, however, when it is realized that responsibility multiplies as the number of actors in a situation increases. Thus, the consultant who trains a manager to run T-group sessions, and discovers that these sessions are destructive to the manager's employees, is as responsible as the manager for the results of the consultation.

INTEGRITY

The notion of integrity suggests that the professional have a clear awareness of his or her values and the ways in which they affect professional practice. At bottom, it has to do with honesty, towards oneself if not toward one's consultees. It is no longer possible to argue that any field of practice is value-free. Rather, the issue becomes one of identifying the value stances that underly professional practice, and to be able to articulate these values in ways that allow consumers of services to freely choose to be influenced by them. The other component of integrity has to do with the particular value of beneficence (Beauchamp & Childress, 1979). This concept, represented in slightly different ways in each of the mental health professions' ethical standards, implies that the overriding concern of the practitioner is the enhancement of client well-being, and that exploitation of the consultation for the consultant's personal needs is unethical.

COMPETENCE

A third component of professional ethics concerns competence. The professional context can be contrasted here with the commercial context. In the latter, the principle of **caveat emptor** ("let the buyer beware") is frequently invoked. It suggests that the consumer is competent to evaluate the service or product. In professional practice, the provider is assumed to possess skills or knowledge which the consumer may not be able to adequately evaluate. As a result, **caveat emptor** is not necessarily a useful principle in such cases. Rather, assurance of competent service must be the responsibility of the professional. However, if the professional (or the entire profession) must be the arbiter of competence, how is this to be judged? Even in the psychotherapy arena, competence is not easily judged. There is even more disagreement about what constitutes competence in consultation. This may require a reliance on relative competence, but is it really sufficient to claim that one provides services no worse than those offered by other sources? That one does no more harm than "no treatment?" The answers to these questions are by no means clear-cut, but they must be considered; they relate to informed consent issues, which are often central to the negotiation of an adequate consultation contract.

PRACTICAL ISSUES IN THE ETHICS OF CONSULTATION

This section details five issues that commonly arise when questions of providing ethically sound consultation are raised. They are: identifying the consultee; providing informed consent; clarifying information boundaries; handling power issues; and insuring competent consultation.

IDENTIFYING THE CONSULTEE

Questions regarding the identity of the "consumer" are not unique to consultation; they arise in every form of mental health service in which third parties pay for, sponsor, or direct the clinician's efforts (cf. Monahan, 1980). As noted above, in almost all consultative efforts, the consultee works with a client, giving the consultant impact on an unseen third party. In addition, as Bermant and Warwick (1978) note, often the sponsor of a consultation is not the target of the consultative effort. For example, the management of a library may hire the consultant to provide communications training to the staff (who may in turn use these skills with patrons). This calls into question the idea proposed by Caplan (1970) among others, that consultees are free to reject the consultant's advice (or perhaps even the service itself). In organizational contexts, the advocacy of consultation by higher echelons is a clear message that the service must be used.

At the minimum, the consultant has a duty to become familiar with the organizational context in which the services are being provided. What voice have the targets of the work had in the decision to use consultation? What voice have they had in the design of the consultative effort? What consequences might follow from their decisions to accept or resist consultative input? And what are the various objectives of the sponsor(s), target(s), and client(s)? Once these questions are answered, the consultant is in a better position to identify the consultee, and perhaps to make an informed choice about who the consultee should be. It may be worthwhile to note that the self-definition of the consultant is closely connected to this decision. For example, the consultant who defines himself or herself as an agent of social change would likely decide that the consultee in an organizational consultation to a juvenile justice system is different than would a consultant who had the self-definition of a process observer.

PROVIDING INFORMED CONSENT

The idea of informed consent suggests that those impacted by a consultation should be provided with sufficient understandable information that they can freely choose to participate in the enterprise. While there are a variety of influences that determined the emergence of this principle (cf. Beauchamp & Childress, 1979), from an ethical perspective it can readily be seen that informed consent rests on the idea that consumers ought to be treated as autonomous individuals capable of making free choices. This contrasts with paternalistic action, in which things are done for people because it is good for them. In consultation, the questions concern who should be able to consent, and how they should be informed.

Consider the case in which a fifth-grade teacher asks for consultation on issues of bereavement because one child in her class has just lost a parent through death and another child's parents are divorcing. From whom should the ethical consultant obtain consent?

The teacher should certainly be provided enough information to make an informed decision about engaging in the process; that is, the teacher should be informed about the usual procedures of consultation in such a case, the potential outcomes, the possible costs of obtaining consultation (e.g., time, money, effort, outside reading), and the possible costs and benefits of not receiving consultation (e.g., the children may improve on their own, they may be referred to a special group in the school, their parents may be counseled). If elements of the process are ambiguous at the outset, provisional consent may be obtained (e.g., the teacher may agree to a certain number of sessions to see how the process works, and then agree or not agree to pursue matters further).

Should the children give their consent? This is a harder question, because allowing the children to give consent to the teacher's consultation in effect gives them veto power over the teacher's desire to improve her skills. This is a case in which the consultant must determine the possible changes in the relationship between the teacher and the pupils, and decide whether obtaining informed consent is warranted. If the consultation results simply in the teacher having more empathy for the bereaved children, it would be difficult to distinguish this from the ordinary course of events in which the students had no control over what the teacher chose to learn. On the other hand, if the consultation results in the teacher learning how to conduct a support group for bereaved children, the potential group members should certainly be given the chance to consent to being included.

The consent of parents may be necessary as well, since legally they are the guardians of the childrens' welfare. Must they be provided with information about the consultation, or is it sufficient to argue that they have implicitly consented to the provision of whatever effective classroom management the school thinks necessary? Could the oversight function of such representative groups as the PTA be considered a form of proxy consent by representatives of the parents' interests? Questions such as these can help the prospective consultant clarify what elements of the process are likely to be problematic, and can also help to generate creative technical solutions to the problem of obtaining consent.

The question of how much detail is necessary for informed consent is also sometimes vexing. It may seem to the consultant that honesty and effectiveness do not mix. For example, if a manager is being given information about a potential team-building consultation, too much detail might result in an increase of defensiveness (or resistance) before the meetings. On the other hand, too little information could be seen as deceptive or coercive.

To summarize the elements of informed consent: Consultees should know from whom they are receiving services (i.e., they should know something about the qualifications of the consultant); they should know something about the consultant's values, and theory of change (i.e., what kinds of results the consultant considers desirable, and how he or she thinks they occur); they should know roughly how much time, money, and effort the proposed intervention will require and the possible risks, if any; they should also know the same facts about alternatives to consultation. This last may be difficult for consultants to provide, but they should at least acknowledge that other solutions beside consultation exist (cf. Cherniss, 1976, for a discussion of this issue).

The vehicle for insuring informed consent is frequently the consultation contract. The contract, which may be written or verbal, should specify the statement of the problem as the consultant understands it, should identify the relevant actors (sponsors, targets, clients) in the intervention and their responsibilities, and should indicate the responsibilities of the consultant, sponsors, and targets. The contract should further specify who has access to what information and should indicate at what point an evaluation of the intervention will take place.

CLARIFYING INFORMATION BOUNDARIES

The consultant's primary resource is information, and questions about who provides it, what is provided, and who gets access to it are serious ones indeed. The following elements are important: What will be done with the information? What did the initial contract specify? What will be the likely consequences of breaking or adhering to the contract?

Consider the following cases: The consultant to a nursing home discovers that substandard care is being provided; the consultant to a business is asked if a particular candidate for promotion is capable of handling increased responsibility; a consultant to a research firm discovers that a particular staff member may be committing industrial sabotage; the consultant to a school system discovers that the principal of one of the elementary schools is an alcoholic.

These situations have several features in common. First, they were not dealt with in the initial contract; second, they involve questions about confidentiality; third, the principles of confidentiality and welfare of the consumer apparently conflict; fourth, it is unclear what alternatives to disclosure exist and what benefits they would offer. In such circumstances, the ethical consultant tries to find alternatives to disclosure. For example, the consultant could inform the affected parties about the conflict and encourage them to disclose voluntarily. The consultant could also obtain the permission of the affected parties to disclose. The consultant may also choose to breach confidentiality, if the consequences of keeping silent are felt to be so serious that to uphold the ethical standard of confidentiality would be to undermine the ethical standard of beneficence. However, it must be recognized that in such cases, the consultant is likely to sacrifice future effectiveness with this particular consultee system.

An additional problem is created by consultant disclosure. Initial disclosure gives later nondisclosure new meaning. Consider the following example: The manager of a research and development unit asks the unit's consultant for an evaluation of a particular worker's capacity for advancement. The consultant thinks the worker is particularly able, and asks the worker if disclosure to the manager may be made. The worker agrees, and the consultant provides an assessment. What happens in the future when the information is not beneficial? The manager may assume that "no news is bad news." The better process would be to remove oneself from the middle of such situations.

HANDLING POWER ISSUES

It should be clear from the discussion above that in order to provide competent service, and in order to avoid becoming embroiled in internal struggles within the system, the consultant must be constantly aware of power issues. There is first of all the power of the sponsors of the consultation to terminate the consultant's contract. Second, there is the power the upper echelons have over the lower ones. Third, there is the independent power (or range of alternative resources) possessed by particular units in the organization. There is also the theoretical orientation of the consultant, which may dictate his or her stance in regard to the use of organizational power. As Mirvis and Seashore (1979) point out, a reality of organizational life is that power is used to accomplish things. To deny this fact, or to help consultees engage in actions that ultimately are detrimental to them for the sake of a theoretical position, may be ethically questionable, especially if the consultees have not been given the opportunity for informed consent. In fact, they may assume that higher management has implicitly given permission for the actions recommended by the consultant when this is not the case.

The consultant must also be aware of the ways in which he or she is directly a source of power, and may be manipulated for that end. For example, if the consultant is used to "help a demotee accept his fate" (Kelman & Warwick, 1978) he or she is perhaps being used as part of a power-oriented change.

INSURING COMPETENT CONSULTATION

As noted previously, there is much disagreement about what constitutes competence. It may be tempting (and often is effective consultative strategy) to take a functional approach to defining competence and ask, "Competent to do what?" In most cases, the answer will be something fairly specific, such as, "teach my nursing home staff to handle psychiatric emergencies," or, "help our community board reach consensus on the mental health center's priorities." In such cases, the question then becomes whether the consultant can help the consultees effectively in reaching their goals. The ethical consultant treads a fine line between being too cautious in describing the possible benefits he or she may be able to help produce, and being too grand in making promises (this will primarily result in the consultees' distrust of the entire process). A sensible solution is technical; build in periodic review points at which progress toward the agreed-on goals can be jointly assessed by consultant, sponsors, and target groups. The ethical consultant must resist the urge to live up to the omnipotent image often held by admiring consultees. Consultants must constantly remind themselves that the consultees bear a major share of the responsibility in affecting changes.

One additional point bears mention in regard to competence. One way to define competence is in relation to a particular content; a second way is to define it in terms of problem-solving processes. Thus, as Bloom (1977) notes, there are consultation theorists who claim that being expert in group process and relationship-building in itself is grounds to claim competence as a consultant. Others maintain that consultants must have some content expertise. Research findings are somewhat sparse in this area. Robbins, Spencer, and Frank (1970), in one of the few studies to address this question, found that consultants perceived as interested and open were more effective than those with content expertise in relevant areas. On the other hand, Laue and Cormick (1978), in a case analysis of a consultation failure, note that consultants' lack of awareness of various issues specific to that setting contributed to their lack of effectiveness.

An additional issue in the assessment of competence is that of self-awareness. The ethical consultant must have a sort of meta-awareness, or ability to know when he or she does **not** know. This results in an improved ability to know when one is being asked to do the impossible, when another consultant should perhaps be involved, and when a reassessment of the progress of the consultation should be held with the sponsors. This is also, interestingly, a good example of living one's theory, since it is an axiom of consultation practice that asking for help is an adaptive behavior.

As in other forms of professional practice, it is sometimes felt that competence improves with experience. From this perspective, the ethical consultant should have had experience consulting under supervision in a system like the one currently requesting consultation.

Clearly, in these areas, the ethical issues overlap broadly with the technical ones.

LEGAL ISSUES

The consideration of legal issues in consultation is largely beyond the scope of this paper. On one hand, legal issues are rarely a problem in consultation, as the consultees give up many fewer prerogatives than institutionalized individuals, research subjects, psychotherapy patients, or testing subjects. On the other hand, the consultant, especially in systems in which organized labor or legally-mandated rights are at issue, must be cognizant of the legal realities. Excellent resource material for consultants interested in the general issues touched upon in this section can be found in Schwitzgebel and Schwitzgebel (1980) and in Cohen (1979). In the following discussion, only the barest outline of legal issues will be presented.

LICENSURE AND PRIVILEGED COMMUNICATIONS

Since the practice of consultation is not licensed, but rather takes place in the context of the professional's licensure (if he or she belongs to a licensed profession), there is little to be said about the legal regulation of consultants by the state. The considerations relevant to all licensed professionals apply, and concerned consultants should be familiar with the licensure laws of their particular state.

Unlike psychotherapists, who in most states are legally permitted to refuse to divulge in court information shared in the professional relationship, consultants are unlikely to be able to claim privileged communication (cf. Cohen, 1979; Schwitzgebel & Schwitzgebel, 1980). Consultees should be made aware of this if there is any question of consultants or their records being subpoenaed.

LIABILITY

The general issue of professional liability is usually expressed as "malpractice" (e.g., Wright, 1981). That is, the consultant is legally liable if negligent or otherwise improper consultation results in damages to the consultee. Since identifying standards of proper practice involves the issue of defining competence as previously noted, it is typically claimed that "usual and customary practices" of the profession are sufficient to determine appropriateness of behavior. In addition, in order for malpractice to be proven (not alleged) a professional relationship must have existed, the professional must have acted in an inappropriate manner, and damages from that inappropriate action must have resulted (cf. Cohen, 1979; Wright, 1981).

RIGHTS

As more consultants practice in settings in which there are legal judgments about the rights of various groups, it is important that they have accurate knowledge of these rights. For example, public employees have certain rights to privacy and protection against punishment that might be infringed by consultation. Similarly, organized labor may have rights and prerogatives that conflict with ideas of participatory decision making and conflict resolution proposed by the consultant. In addition to consulting the references noted in this area, the concerned consultant should obtain legal advice from an attorney with experience in the relevant area. It is rarely the case that legal action will be taken against a consultant (rather, it is taken against those who hired the consultant), but it is not impossible.

RECOMMENDATIONS

After prolonged discussions of complicated, sometimes unresolvable issues, the provision of a set of recommendations may seem presumptuous. Nonetheless, these "rules of thumb" are offered in hopes that they will serve as useful stimuli for thinking through potential ethical problems in consultation (cf. Pfeiffer & Jones, 1977, for additional rules of this sort).

1. **Know Who Your Client Is.** As previously noted, this means knowing what impact your consultation will have on whom, clarifying relationships within the system, and knowing your own theoretical and value positions.

2. Know the Law. This means knowing the law(s) regulating your practice as a professional, the law(s) protecting your consultees, and the law(s) protecting their clients.

3. Know the Code of Ethics. This means reading the appropriate ethical standards (as well as other work on professional ethics that might help to explicate them).

4. Know Your Own Values. This means knowing what you value as outcomes, as process, what areas you are willing to compromise in, and where your sympathies are likely to lie.

5. Involve the Relevant Stakeholders. This means finding out who they are, and being assertive and politically astute enough to find a way for them to get a voice. The voice (as noted) may be either direct or indirect.

6. Be Candid. In part, this means resisting the temptation to disguise your uncertainty about ability from sponsors, but at the same time resisting the temptation to shift the responsibility to sponsors or consultees by claiming inadequacy. It also means resisting the temptation to try to please the sponsors at all costs by apparent willingness to give them what they want even when this conflicts with deeply held values of your own.

7. Develop a Clear Contract. This is simply another way to state the candor guideline; the contract should be accurate, clear, meaningful, and preferably written.

8. Build Re-evaluation Points into the Process. This once again is a technical point, but one which bears repeating. The assumption of responsibility does not mean that only the consultant is responsible; it does mean that collaboration with sponsors and consultees (and perhaps even clients) is vital to effective consultation.

9. Consult with Senior Colleagues, Sponsors, and Peers As Needed. This is simply a version of "practicing what you preach," since having consultants of your own is as good a way to improve consultation effectiveness (and maintain ethical awareness) as having consultants for clients is to improve system effectiveness.

Leonard J. Haas, Ph.D., is currently coordinator of field training for the Clinical Psychology Training Program at the University of Utah. His professional interests include community psychology, social networks, and family therapy. He has written numerous articles on professional ethics, as well as presented the topic in other formats. Dr. Haas may be reached at the Department of Psychology, University of Utah, Salt Lake City, UT 84112.

RESOURCES

American Psychiatric Association. PRINCIPLES OF MEDICAL ETHICS. Washington, DC: Author, 1981.

American Psychological Association. ETHICAL STANDARDS OF PSYCHOLOGISTS. Washington, DC: Author, 1981.

Beauchamp, T. & Childress, J. PRINCIPLES OF BIOMEDICAL ETHICS. New York: Oxford, 1979.

Bermant, G. & Warwick, D. P. The ethics of social intervention: Power, freedom and accountability. In G. Bermant, H. C. Kelman, & D. P. Warwick (Eds.), THE ETHICS OF SOCIAL INTERVENTION. New York: Hemisphere, 1978.

Blake, R. R. & Mouton, J. S. CONSULTATION. Reading, MA: Addison-Wesley, 1976.

Bloom, B. L. COMMUNITY MENTAL HEALTH: A GENERAL INTRODUCTION. Monterey: Brooks/Cole, 1977.

Caplan, G. L. THE THEORY AND PRACTICE OF MENTAL HEALTH CONSULTATION. New York: Basic Books, 1970.

Cherniss, C. Preentry issues in consultation. AMERICAN JOURNAL OF COMMUNITY PSYCHOLOGY, 1976, 4, 13-21.

Cohen, R. MALPRACTICE: A GUIDE FOR MENTAL HEALTH PROFESSIONALS. New York: Free Press, 1979.

Goodstein, L. CONSULTING WITH HUMAN SERVICE SYSTEMS. Reading, MA: Addison-Wesley, 1978.

Halleck, S. L. THE POLITICS OF THERAPY. New York: Science House, 1971.

Kelman, H. C. & Warwick, D. P. The ethics of social intervention: Goals, means, and consequences. In G. Bermant, H. C. Kelman, & D. P. Warwick (Eds.), THE ETHICS OF SOCIAL INTERVENTION. New York: Hemisphere, 1978.

Laue, J. & Cormick, G. The ethics of intervention in community disputes. In G. Bermant, H. C. Kelman, & D. P. Warwick (Eds.), THE ETHICS OF SOCIAL INTERVENTION. New York: Hemisphere, 1978.

MacIntyre, A. Utilitarianism and cost/benefit analysis: An essay on the relevance of moral philosophy to bureacratic theory. In T. Beauchamp & J. Bowie, ETHICAL THEORY AND BUSINESS. Englewood, NJ: Prentice-Hall, 1979.

Manninno, F. W., MacClennan, B. W., & Shore, M. F. THE PRACTICE OF MENTAL HEALTH CONSULTATION. New York: Gardner, 1975.

Mirvis, P. & Seashore, S. Being ethical in organizational research. AMERICAN PSYCHOLOGIST, 1979, 34, 766-780.

Monahan, J. (Ed.). WHO IS THE CLIENT? THE ETHICS OF PSYCHOLOGICAL INTERVENTION IN THE CRIMINAL JUSTICE SYSTEM. Washington, DC: APA, 1980.

National Association of Social Workers. CODE OF ETHICS. Silver Spring, MD: Author, 1980.

Pfeiffer, J. W. & Jones, J. E. Ethical considerations in consulting. In J. W. Pfeiffer & J. E. Jones (Eds.), 1977 ANNUAL HANDBOOK FOR GROUP FACILITATORS. San Diego: University Associates, 1977.

Robbins, P., Spencer, E. C., & Frank, D. A. Some factors influencing the outcome of consultation. AMERICAN JOURNAL OF PUBLIC HEALTH, 1970, 60, 524-532.

Schwitzgebel, R. L. & Schwitzgebel, R. K. LAW AND PSYCHOLOGICAL PRACTICE. New York: Wiley, 1980.

Strupp, H. & Hadley, S. A tripartite model of mental health and therapeutic outcomes: With special reference to negative effects in psychotherapy. AMERICAN PSYCHOLOGIST, 1977, 32, 187-196.

Woody, R. H. Process and behavioral consultation. AMERICAN JOURNAL OF COMMUNITY PSYCHOLOGY, 1975, 3, 277.

Wright, R. H. Psychologists and professional liability (malpractice) insurance: A retrospective review. AMERICAN PSYCHOLOGIST, 1981, 36, 1485-1493.

CONSULTATION WITH DENTISTS: INNOVATIVE ROLES FOR THE CLINICIAN

Barbara D. Ingersoll and Michael J. Geboy

Dentistry has often been described as a highly stressful profession. It is so stressful, in fact, that some studies have placed the suicide rate of dentists at twice that of the national average for adult males and among the highest of any professional group (Blachly, Osterud, & Josslin, 1963; American Dental Association, 1975). The longevity of dentists is lower than for the average male population (Howard, Cunningham, Rechnitzer, & Goode, 1976) and coronary disease and hypertension, both stress-related disorders, are 25% more prevalent among dentists (Nielsen & Polakoff, 1975). There are also indications that dentists have a disproportionate incidence of substance abuse, marital problems, and depression (Sword, 1977).

Why is dentistry such a stressful profession? Although the nature of the work demands great precision and attention to detail, it is not, apparently, the technical aspects of dentistry that are perceived as the major source of job-related stress. Rather, it is in the areas of patient and staff management that difficulties are most often encountered. Godwin and colleagues (Godwin, Stark, Green, & Koran, 1981) reported that patient management problems were the most frequently identified source of stress in practice, cited by 73% of respondents to an open-ended questionnaire. Staff management problems were cited by 33% of respondents.

Our own research (Ingersoll, Ingersoll, Seime, & McCutcheon, 1978; Ingersoll, McCutcheon, & Seime, 1979) has focused on precise identification of specific problems within these categories. We sampled 589 dentists, who reported the patient and staff management problems presented in Table 1.

How well prepared is the average dentist to cope with the problems listed in Table 1? While there has been a marked trend toward increasing the number of behavioral science courses in the dental school curriculum, these courses typically provide little more than an introduction to the behavioral aspects of dentistry. Dental students seldom receive the supervised practice necessary to develop skill in managing human behavior problems. Certainly, the fact that these problems are so widespread suggests that, in general, dentists have not really developed effective methods for resolving them.

APPLICATIONS OF PSYCHOLOGY IN THE DENTAL SETTING

Many of the problems described in the preceding section are of a sort familiar to clinical psychologists and other mental health practitioners. In fact,

TABLE 1: PATIENT AND STAFF MANAGEMENT PROBLEMS*

PROBLEM	% REPORTING PROBLEM
(Patient Management)	
Fear	87
Broken, cancelled, late appointments	76
Not motivated for oral hygiene	76
Do not follow treatment instruction	75
Disruptive or uncooperative children	59
Parents	39
(Staff Management)	
Interacting with patients	53
Poor motivation	52
Personality conflict	47
Training or retraining	46

*As reported by a national sample of practicing dentists. From Ingersoll, Ingersoll, McCutcheon, and Seime, 1979.

psychologists have recently begun to apply the methods developed and employed in mental health settings to problems in the dental setting, with promising results. Topics which have received particular attention are the reduction of dental fear and avoidance in adult patients, reduction of anxiety and uncooperative behavior in child patients, correction of oral habit disorders, and treatment of various chronic facial pain syndromes.

ASSESSMENT AND TREATMENT OF DENTAL FEAR IN ADULTS

Fear of dentistry has long been known to be a major factor in neglect of oral health. Early informal surveys indicated that approximately 5-6% of the population avoid dental treatment due to fear, but more recent studies place this figure closer to 12% (Gatchel, Ingersoll, Bowman, Robertson, & Walker, 1982).

Dental fear poses significant problems for the dentist, because fearful patients are three times more likely than nonfearful patients to fail appointments (Kleinknecht & Bernstein, 1978). In addition, they require as much as 20% more chair time than less anxious patients, even for routine procedures (Filewich, Jackson, & Shore, 1981).

Assessment of Dental Fear. Although in the popular view the anxious patient can be recognized easily by such overt behaviors as trembling, moaning, sweating, and flushing, recent research (Kleinknecht & Bernstein, 1979) casts doubt on the value of behavioral observations and measures of physiological reactivity in assessing dental fear. Instead, these investigators conclude, the combination of patient self-report and records of dental care obtained appear to be the most sensitive and meaningful measures of dental fear.

The most commonly employed self-report measures for assessing dental fear are the Dental Anxiety Scale (Corah, 1969) and the Dental Fear Survey (Kleinknecht, Klepac, & Alexander, 1973). Both have been shown to be valid and reliable and both are suitable for routine office use.

The Dental Anxiety Scale (Figure 1) is scored by assigning one point for each "a" choice, two points for each "b" choice, and so on. Points are added to yield a single summary score. According to the authors, a score of 13 or 14 "should make the dentist suspicious that he or she is dealing with an anxious patient," and patients who earn a score of 15 or more are almost always highly anxious (Corah, Gale, & Illig, 1979).

DENTAL ANXIETY SCALE

1. If you had to go the dentist tomorrow, how would you feel about it?

    a. I would look forward to it as a reasonably enjoyable experience.
    b. I wouldn't care one way or the other.
    c. I would be a little uneasy about it.
    d. I would be afraid that it would be unpleasant and painful.
    e. I would be very frightened of what the dentist might do.

2. When you are waiting in the dentist's office for your turn in the chair, how do you feel?

    a. relaxed
    b. a little uneasy
    c. tense
    d. anxious
    e. so anxious that I sometimes break out in a sweat or almost feel physically sick

3. When you are in the dentist's chair waiting while he gets his drill ready to begin working on your teeth, how do you feel?

    a. relaxed
    b. a little uneasy
    c. tense
    d. anxious
    e. so anxious that I sometimes break out in a sweat or almost feel physically sick

4. You are in the dentist's chair to have your teeth cleaned. While you are waiting and the dentist is getting out the instruments which he will use to scrape your teeth around the gum, how do you feel?

    a. relaxed
    b. a little uneasy
    c. tense
    d. anxious
    e. so anxious that I sometimes break out in a sweat or almost feel physically sick

---

Figure 1. From N. L. Corah, "Development of a Dental Anxiety Scale," JOURNAL OF DENTAL RESEARCH, **48**, 596. Copyright 1969 by the American Association for Dental Research. Reprinted by permission.

Treatment of Dental Fear. Behavioral approaches have emerged as especially promising in the treatment of dental fear and avoidance. Among the methods which have been employed are systematic desensitization, modeling, and training patients to use coping strategies during dental treatment.

The effectiveness of systematic desensitization has been demonstrated in several case studies. Gale and Ayer (1969), for example, reported the successful treatment of an intensely fearful patient who had avoided dental treatment since childhood. Treatment consisted of nine 1-hour sessions, during which the patient was trained in relaxation and presented with hierarchy items (Figure 2).

PATIENT'S HIERARCHY*

1. Thinking about going to the dentist
2. Getting in your car to go to the dentist
3. Calling for an appointment with the dentist
4. Sitting in the waiting room of the dentist's office
5. Having the nurse tell you it's your turn
6. Getting in the dentist's chair
7a. Seeing the dentist lay out his instruments, one of which is a probe
7b. Seeing the dentist lay out his instruments, one of which is pliers that are used to pull teeth
8. Having a probe held in front of you while you look at it
9. Having a probe placed on the side of a tooth
10. Having a probe placed in a cavity
11. Getting an injection in your gums on one side
12a. Having your teeth drilled and worrying that the anesthetic will wear off
12b. Having a tooth pulled
13a. Getting an injection on each side
13b. Hearing the crunching sounds as your tooth is being pulled

---

*Figure 2. From "Treatment of Dental Phobias" by E. N. Gale and W. A. Ayer, JOURNAL OF THE AMERICAN DENTAL ASSOCIATION, 1969, **78**, 1306. Copyright 1969 by the American Dental Association. Reprinted by permission.

Controlled investigations (cf. Bernstein & Kleinknecht, 1979) have also supported the usefulness of systematic desensitization in reducing dental fear, but success rates reported are lower than those obtained with patients suffering other types of phobias (probably because dental fear is not altogether "irrational" since some discomfort accompanies virtually all dental treatment). Typically, success rates average about 55-60% with individuals whose fear is so intense that they cannot even enter a dental operatory. With less intensely fearful patients, we would expect a higher rate of successful outcomes.

When systematic desensitization is combined with modeling (i.e., when patients are taught relaxation and are then shown films of patients undergoing dental treatment) success rates rise to about 78% (Shaw & Thoreson, 1974; Wroblewski, Jacob, & Rehm, 1977). A minor drawback of this method is that access to videotape equipment is necessary, although a slide-tape program might be substituted.

A less costly alternative available for use with mildly to moderately fearful patients is to give patients a "take-home" audiotape cassette containing

Innovations In Clinical Practice: A Source Book

relaxation instructions and scenes from a standard dental fear hierarchy. An even simpler approach is to have patients listen through headphones to tape-recorded relaxation instructions during dental treatment (Corah, Gale, Pace, & Seyrek, 1981).

Gatchel's (1980) work suggests that a dental fear reduction program should include teaching patients to use coping strategies during dental treatment. When information about basic dental procedures was combined with group discussion of specific coping skills, 100% success was obtained with fearful dental avoiders. Coping skills taught included raising a hand to signal the dentist to stop and asking for additional anesthetic, if necessary. An interesting aspect of this study was that Gatchel trained two dentists to administer the fear-reduction programs to the subjects.

Investigating the use of biofeedback in the dental setting, dentist-psychologist Richard Hirschman has obtained favorable results with a technique known as "paced respiration" (Clark & Hirschman, 1980). With this method, patients are taught to pace their respiration at a slower-than-normal rate by listening to a tape recording with the word "inhale" spaced at intervals of 7.5-seconds. This simple but effective method has the effect of inducing relaxation, focusing the patient's attention on a task, and muffling the frightening sounds of the drill.

BEHAVIOR MANAGEMENT IN PEDIATRIC DENTISTRY

Approximately one-third of grade school children and adolescents report some fear of dentistry and 16-17% describe themselves as very fearful (Morgan, Wright, Ingersoll, & Seime, 1980; Stricker & Howitt, 1965). Fearful children tend to be uncooperative during dental treatment and, in fact, dentists in general practice describe management problems with one to two children per week (Weinstein, Getz, Ratener, & Domoto, 1982). (Pedodontists would probably report a higher incidence, as children who present management problems are often referred to the pedodontist by the general practitioner.)

Predicting and Assessing Anxiety and Uncooperative Behavior. The child's age, socioeconomic status, behavior during medical visits, and the mother's anxiety about the visit are all correlated with behavior at the first dental visit (Ingersoll, 1982; 1983). Questionnaires which tap these variables are useful in predicting how the child will behave at the initial visit (Figure 3).

Valuable information can also be obtained from the child. The Venham Picture Test (Venham & Gaulin-Kremer, 1979), for example, is a self-report device that has been used with children ages 2 to 14 years to predict behavior and to assess response to intervention. Another useful self-report measure is Melamed's modification of a children's fear survey schedule (Melamed, Hawes, Heiby, & Glick, 1975; Melamed, Weinstein, Hawes, & Borland, 1975).

Reducing Anxiety and Uncooperative Behavior. A preparatory letter to the parents and a special note to the child help in preparing the inexperienced youngster to accept dental treatment (Ingersoll, 1982; 1983). A familiarization visit at which no dental treatment is provided does **not** appear to yield special benefits. However, before the child enters the operatory for the first time, a get-acquainted period of 15 minutes or so with the dental assistant in a non-clinic room does appear to reduce anxiety and disruptive behavior.

MATERNAL QUESTIONNAIRE

Please circle the answer which most closely applies

1. How do you think your child has reacted in the past to dental and medical procedures?*

   a. Very poor   c. Moderately good

   b. Moderately poor   d. Very good

2. How do you think your child will react to this procedure?*

   a. Very poor   c. Moderately good

   b. Moderately poor   d. Very good

3. How would you rate your own anxiety at this moment?[+]

   a. High   c. Moderately low

   b. Moderately high   d. Low

4. Does your child think there is anything wrong with his (her) teeth such as a chipped tooth, decayed tooth, gumboil, etc.?[+]

   a. Yes   b. No

5. During the past year has your child been in contact with anyone who has had an unpleasant dental experience?

   a. Yes   b. No

6. In the last two years my child's contacts with medical doctors have been....[+]

   a. Always enjoyable   c. Usually unpleasant

   b. Usually enjoyable   d. Always unpleasant

7. In the past two years my child usually looked forward to contacts with medical people....[+]

   a. With much fear   c. With no fear

   b. With little fear

8. In the last two years my child has experienced actual physical pain in connection with medical procedures....[+]

   a. Quite often (three or more times)   c. None

   b. Occationally (once or twice)

Figure 3. *From "Relationship of Maternal Anxiety of the Behavior of Young Children Undergoing Dental Extraction" by R. Johnson and D. C. Baldwin, JOURNAL OF DENTAL RESEARCH, 1968, 47, 801. Copyright 1968 by the American Association for Dental Research. Reprinted by permission.
[+]From "Variables Influencing Children's Cooperative Behavior at the First Dental Visit" by G. Z. Wright and G. D. Alpern, JOURNAL OF DENTISTRY FOR CHILDREN, 1971, 33, 124. Copyright 1971 by American Society of Dentistry for Children. Reprinted by permission.

Inconsistent results have been reported with systematic desensitization approaches and, in general, this method appears to be only moderately useful. There are even indications that approaches which focus on fearful procedures and equipment can sensitize inexperienced children, resulting, in some cases, in increases in anxiety and disruptive behavior.

On the other hand, modeling has consistently emerged as an effective method (Melamed, Hawes, Heiby, & Glick, 1975; Melamed, Weinstein, Hawes, & Borland, 1975; Melamed, Yurcheson, Fleece, Hutcherson, & Hawes, 1978). The beneficial effects of filmed modeling are maximized by having the patient view a child similar to himself or herself in age and race and by using longer (10 minutes) instead of shorter (4 minute) films. The use of live models is also an alternative. As models, older siblings of the patient and confederates of the investigator have been used successfully. An approach which appears particularly effective as well as simple to implement is to have uncooperative children not only observe other children but, in turn, be observed themselves. This method, described by Williams, Hurst, and Stokes (1982), appears to produce excellent results, regardless of whether the child observes another child behaving cooperatively or uncooperatively.

Like anxious adults, children also benefit from using coping skills during dental treatment. Ayer (1973), for example, taught three phobic children to use visual imagery by imagining themselves playing with their loudly barking dogs. Siegel and Peterson (1980) trained 3-1/2 to 5 year old children to use general body relaxation, deep breathing, and pairing of positive cue words to reduce stress during dental treatment.

Operant shaping approaches, employed during dental treatment or at between-visit training sessions, also appear to have merit. Kohlenberg, Greenberg, Reymore, and Hass (1972) used fruit juice squirted into the mouth to teach retarded children to sit back in the chair and hold their mouths open. In our laboratory, we have obtained good results with contingent presentation and removal of videotaped cartoons, displayed on a ceiling-mounted monitor. Currently, we are evaluating contingent use of audiotaped songs and stories, presented through headphones.

ORAL HABIT PROBLEMS

During the last two decades, the number of patients seeking treatment for oral habit problems has increased steadily. These disorders, many of which are responsive to behavioral interventions, include thumbsucking, lip- and cheek-biting, and bruxism.

Thumbsucking. Thumbsucking is common among children and probably affects almost half of all children sometime between birth and 16 years (Traisman & Traisman, 1958). It is generally unlikely to result in permanent damage to dentition if terminated by age 4 or 5, but the likelihood of harmful effects increases if the habit persists beyond this age (Popovich & Thompson, 1973). Thumbsucking is also socially undesirable, especially in the school-aged child.

To treat thumbsucking, dentists often use fixed (cemented to the teeth) or removable stainless steel bars inserted in the child's mouth to prevent sucking. These devices often effectively eliminate thumbsucking, but they are aesthetically unpleasant and side effects include disruption of speech and swallowing and increased susceptibility to caries.

Although behavioral approaches have been found effective in treating thumbsucking, these approaches currently are not widely utilized by dentists. Generally, behavioral approaches have focused on reinforcing thumb-out-of-mouth behavior and token economy programs such as that described by DeLaCruz and Geboy (1982) are often quite successful. A habit-reversal procedure, consisting of awareness training and instruction in positive corrective actions, has also been found effective (Azrin, Nunn, & Frantz, 1980).

Lip-Biting and Related Behaviors. The incidence of such destructive oral habits as biting, sucking, or chewing the lips, tongue, or cheeks in the adult population is unknown. However, among children aged 6 to 12 years, Lapouse and Monk (1959) reported an 11% incidence.

Negative practice has been advocated as a means of treating a variety of oral habit problems. While modest success has been reported with this method, the habit reversal procedure developed by Azrin's group (c.f. Azrin, Nunn, & Frantz-Renshaw, 1982) appears to be much more effective. According to the authors, this approach can be implemented in a single, 2 hour training session.

Bruxism. Nocturnal bruxism (clenching and grinding the teeth during sleep) is estimated to occur in about 20% of the population (Meklas, 1971). Of this number, a small percent exhibit the behavior to such an extent that damage to oral structures and pain result.

To one unfamiliar with bruxism, this habit might appear deceptively simple to diagnose and treat. However, as several reviewers (c.f. Bailey & Rugh, 1979; Klepac, 1977) have discussed, diagnosis and assessment are problematic, due to lack of definitive diagnostic methods and means of quantifying the behavior. The situation is further complicated by the fact that bruxism appears to be a cyclical, stress-related problem (Glaros & Rao, 1977). As Rugh and Robbins (1982) observe, "Patients usually report for help when the symptoms are at a peak. Anything done is likely to be followed by a reduction in symptoms" (p. 198).

This, of course, complicates attempts to evaluate the effectiveness of various treatment methods. Negative practice, for example, was earlier hailed with enthusiasm, but closer scrutiny has not verified the clinical effectiveness of this technique. Currently, EMG biofeedback appears promising for temporary relief of bruxism.

Bear in mind, however, should you decide to work with bruxers, that no treatment has been found to stop nocturnal bruxism permanently. To quote Rugh and Robbins (1982) again, "Nocturnal bruxism is seldom cured; rather, the problem must be continuously 'managed'" (p. 195). These authors suggest that long-term management of bruxism might, in some cases, require implementation of a more encompassing stress-control program designed to help the patient alter his or her lifestyle. (For useful discussions of bruxism, see Glaros & Rao, 1977, and Rugh & Robbins, 1982.)

Myofascial Pain-Dysfunction Syndrome (MPD). MPD, also termed temporomandibular joint pain-dysfunction syndrome (TMJ), is a chronic condition characterized by several symptoms including pain in the muscles of mastication, limitation of mandibular movement, deviation of the mandible upon opening, and clicking or crepetus in the joint (Gessel & Alderman, 1971). Estimates suggest that it occurs in about 20% of all dental patients and is more commonly reported in women than in men.

The etiology of MPD is disputed. The position traditionally held in dentistry is that poorly meeting teeth require continuous muscle tension in compensation, eventually leading to pain and other symptoms characteristic of the syndrome. More recent formulations suggest that psychological stress results in muscle hyperactivity which, in turn, leads to fatigue and the development of symptoms.

A useful assessment instrument for MPD is an hourly pain record which the patient uses for self-monitoring. It requires the patient to rate the severity of his or her pain at 2-hour intervals during the day on a scale ranging from 0 (pain absent) to 10 (extreme pain) (Rugh & Robbins, 1982). Completion of the record for a two-week period provides clues to the etiology and makes it easier to demonstrate to the patient the relationship between stress and onset or exacerbation of symptoms.

Preferred treatment methods, of course, depend upon one's view of etiology and numerous treatments for MPD have been attempted, with mixed results. Traditional dental treatments include applications of moist heat, spraying with ethyl chloride, direct injections of local anesthetic, use of muscle relaxants such as meprobamate, and occlusal adjustments (Seltzer, 1978).

Psychologically-based treatment approaches have focused on relaxation training, using progressive relaxation (Reading & Raw, 1976; Stenn, Mothersill, & Brooke, 1979) and EMG feedback (Budzynski & Stoyva, 1973; Gale, 1979; Gessel, 1975). Although both approaches appear to have some merit, they seem most effective when used with patients who are self-directed and task-oriented (Gessel & Alderman, 1971). In contrast, they are less effective with individuals who are depressed or have significant emotional conflicts.

PATIENT COMPLIANCE

It is generally agreed that dental caries and periodontal disease can be prevented if individuals comply with home-care instructions for brushing and flossing. Unfortunately, noncompliance is often a significant problem for the dentist, whose training seldom includes the skills necessary to effect changes in patient behavior.

Contingency management procedures have been used successfully to establish sound oral health habits (cf. Greenberg, 1977; Price & Kiyak, 1981) and to obtain patient compliance with the more complex demands of orthodontic treatment (White, 1974). Iwata and Becksfort (1981) describe an ingenious program in which patients had a portion of their fees refunded contingent upon improvement in oral cleanliness scores. As the authors explain, this approach appears to be economically feasible and might be of particular interest to dentists whose practice is largely preventive (i.e., periodontists).

Of course, it is not likely that patients would accept a referral to a mental health professional for help with a compliance problem. Instead, your skills might be used in a consulting role, training dental assistants and dental hygienists to employ contingency management procedures. As a useful adjunct in such a training program, we recommend the excellent text by Weinstein and Getz (1978).

WORKING WITH DENTISTS

INTERACTION STRATEGIES

As can be seen from this chapter, mental health professionals do possess numerous skills which would be of benefit to dentists and their patients. To what extent can we say that dentists recognize the potential benefits of a working relationship with a mental health professional?

To explore this question, we conducted a small (N=50) survey of general practice dentists in a major metropolitan area. Although few of our respondents reported ever having referred a patient to a mental health professional, when asked if they would consider using the services of a professional with expertise in dental-related problems, most responded affirmatively concerning at least some of the problems listed on the questionnaire. (Problems included: fear; bruxism; MPD; thumbsucking/lip-biting; uncooperative child; compliance problem; fainting; and gagging.)

We also asked our respondents to comment on three types of working relationships between dentists and mental health professionals. These interaction styles and our respondents' reactions to each are described in the following sections.

Referral Strategy. With this arrangement, the dentist identifies patients with specific problems and refers the patient to the mental health professional for treatment. This strategy has the advantage of requiring little effort on the part of the mental health professional beyond introducing himself or herself to local dentists (see next section).

A major drawback is that the dentist has little incentive to refer patients. In fact, as some of our respondents noted, some patients might be offended at the suggestion that they seek a mental health professional. Further, even if the dentist were to make a referral, the patient might not follow up on it. In general, however, this was the strategy that seemed most acceptable to the majority of our respondents.

Consultant Strategy. Dentists do make use of practice management consultants for advice on such matters as billing, bookkeeping, inventory, and utilization of space, so the idea of a consultant is not new or strange. Survey responses to this approach were generally rather positive, although the economic viability of the approach was questioned. As our respondents observed, it is more profitable for the dentist to spend his or her time providing dental treatment than developing behavior change programs for patients.

On the other hand, some dentists expressed interest in expanding their knowledge and skills to include management of the problem patient. Others, as well, might be interested in employing a consultant to train the dental staff (dental assistant, hygienist) to manage such problems as excessive fear and uncooperative child behavior.

Associate Strategy. With this arrangement, the mental health professional actually works with the dentist's patients in the dental office during hours when the dentist is not treating patients. The patient pays for this service (many will have third-party coverage, as problems such as phobias and habit disorders are legitimate mental health problems), and the mental health professional pays the dentist a fee to cover the latter's overhead expenses.

This strategy has the advantage that the patient is not referred out-of-office, but can receive all dental-related care in a setting with which he or she is already familiar. In addition, the dentist receives income for use of the office during off-hours.

Some of our respondents wondered if a single practice could support such an endeavor. In an established solo practice, this would almost certainly be a problem. However, a large group practice might yield enough problem patients to make this strategy feasible, especially if the professional community and potential patients were made aware of the availability of these services. This idea might have particular appeal to the young dentist struggling to build a practice, as the availability of such special services might serve to attract new patients.

MAKING DENTAL CONTACTS

Implementation of any of the interaction strategies described above requires that you first develop contacts with dental professionals. The following suggestions are intended to help you make these contacts:

1. **Send a letter and a curriculum vitae to area dentists.** Describe yourself and your practice as it relates to dentistry (see Figure 4). This approach is particularly suited to developing a referral arrangement with members of the local dental community.

SAMPLE LETTER OF INTRODUCTION TO AREA DENTISTS

Dear Colleague:

I am writing to call to your attention my psychological practice as it relates to dentistry. I am prepared to offer treatment for a number of dentally-related conditions, including myofascial pain dysfunction syndrome, oral-habit problems such as thumbsucking and lip-biting, and fear of dental treatment. I am also available for the treatment of other psychological conditions, such as depression, that you might encounter in your practice.

The type of treatment I employ depends upon the particular condition. Treatment of MPD focuses on the use of relaxation training to control pain and stress-management training for long-term change. Dental fear is treated through the use of systematic desensitization and cognitive restructuring to help the patient learn to cope successfully. Bruxism and thumbsucking are treated by means of a variety of behavior management techniques. Treatment of all dental conditions is undertaken in collaboration with the patient's dentist.

Please feel free to call me if you would like to discuss or refer a patient.

Sincerely,

Figure 4.

2. **Offer to speak at local dental society meetings.** All states and some

2. **Offer to speak at local dental society meetings.** All states and some cities and regions have dental societies which hold monthly meetings. Some also hold yearly meetings of 1 or 2 days' duration. If your own dentist is a member, he or she might be an initial contact. Topics we have been invited to discuss at such meetings include stress management for the dentist, interpersonal communication, and the relationship between dentistry and the behavioral sciences. There is also growing interest in personnel management and performance appraisal.

3. **Teach at a dental school.** Part-time teaching can be an excellent way to make dental contacts and to familiarize yourself with dentistry. Although interest in the behavioral sciences in dental education is increasing, there are often too few faculty with relevant backgrounds to teach these subjects effectively. Your own dentist might serve as an initial contact: Since most dental schools have large adjunct clinical faculties, he or she might be a part-time faculty member. Otherwise, contact the dean of the school. A word of caution: As most dental schools are experiencing cut-backs in federal funding and declining student enrollment, they are operating on reduced budgets. Therefore, do no expect to be highly paid for your services as an instructor.

FAMILIARIZING YOURSELF WITH DENTISTRY

Before embarking on consultation with dentists, it is important to familiarize yourself with the profession. Some familiarity with dental training and the practice of dentistry will facilitate your interactions with dentists, regardless of the interaction strategy you utilize.

Many dentists are sensitive to the public's perception of dentistry. Some even avoid telling new acquaintances their profession. Similarly, dentists are sensitive about comparisons between dentistry and medicine. It is wise, for example, to say "dentists and physicians," instead of "dentists and doctors." The latter can elicit defensiveness, as dentists quickly (and correctly) point out that they are "doctors," too.

DENTAL EDUCATION

Currently there are 59 accredited dental schools in the United States. Most have 4 year programs, although some offer 3 year programs.

During the first 2 years, dental students receive substantial instruction in the basic sciences, including such subjects as gross and microscopic anatomy, biochemistry, pathology, and physiology. Because dentists, like physicians, are licensed to prescribe medication, students also receive instruction in pharmacology. The first 2 years also include laboratory courses in which students study dental materials, techniques, and procedures.

During the third and fourth years, the majority of time is spent practicing skills in restoring teeth, making dentures, and the like. Students also receive training in radiology and anesthesiology: Again, in common with physicians, dentists are licensed to use x-ray equipment and to use local and general anesthesia.

After graduation, the student must pass national and regional or state board examinations and is then licensed to practice dentistry. Increasingly, however, students elect to continue their education, either in 1 year general practice residency programs which provide additional experience in the diagnosis and treatment of oral disease or in 1 year or 2 year specialty training programs.

Currently, dental education is undergoing a period of change. A decline in federal support has led to substantial increases in tuition and the average indebtedness of the new graduate has risen to $23,000 (Blendon & Rogers, 1981). This has led, in turn, to decreases in dental school enrollment.

From our perspective, the most significant change has been the previously mentioned increased emphasis on the behavioral sciences. This, we think, has probably made today's generation of practitioners more aware than previous generations of the roles mental health professionals can play in maintaining oral health.

DENTAL PRACTICE

The pattern of dental practice is also changing. The majority of dentists practice alone but, because start-up costs are so high, only a small percent of new dentists immediately open their own offices today. Most join established dentists in partnerships or groups.

Another development is the emergence of "retail store dentistry": dental clinics located in department stores. The first such clinic was started only a few years ago and growth has been very rapid. With walk-in convenience and generally lower fees, these clinics offer significant competition to the private practitioner.

Other factors which have increased competition include increases in the number of practicing dentists, a significantly reduced incidence of caries due to fluoridated water, and difficult economic times which lessen patients' ability to pay for dental care. In some regions of the country, dentists also face competition from denturists. There is even a small but vocal group advocating independent practice for dental hygienists.

Increased competition and the easing of restrictions on advertising for professional services has resulted in a new emphasis on marketing in dentistry. It is likely that dentists will be increasingly interested in reaching that segment of the population that does not now utilize dental services. Of course, at least some of these potential patients (especially dental phobics) might be candidates for psychological intervention either prior to or concomitant with dental treatment.

Barbara Ingersoll, Ph.D., is currently Associate Professor in the Departments of Behavioral Medicine and Psychiatry and Community Dentistry at the West Virginia University Schools of Medicine and Dentistry. She holds clinical appointments at Georgetown University School of Dentistry and University of Maryland School of Medicine. She has authored numerous texts and articles on behavioral dentistry and is currently doing research in the area of behavioral methods of pediatric dentistry. Dr. Ingersoll may be contacted at 4838 Park Avenue, Bethesda, MD 20816.

Michael J. Geboy, Ph.D., is currently Director, Division of Behavioral Science and Dental Education, and Professorial Lecturer, Department of Community Dentistry, Georgetown University School of Dentistry. He has authored numerous articles and conducted continuing education workshops for dental practitioners on behavioral dentistry. Dr. Geboy may be reached at Georgetown University School of Dentistry, 3900 Reservoir Road, Washington, D.C. 20007.

RESOURCES

ASSOCIATIONS

American Dental Association, 211 E. Chicago Avenue, Chicago, IL 60611. The ADA produces a variety of materials concerning the dental profession. Of particular interest are publications produced by the Bureau of Economic and Behavioral Research.

PUBLISHED RESOURCES

American Dental Association, Bureau of Economic Research and Statistics. Mortality of dentists. JOURNAL OF THE AMERICAN DENTAL ASSOCIATION, 1975, **90**, 195-198.

Ayer, W. Use of visual imagery in needle phobic children. JOURNAL OF DENTISTRY FOR CHILDREN, 1973, **40**, 125-127.

Azrin, N. H., Nunn, R. G., & Frantz, S. E. Habit reversal vs. negative practice treatment of nervous tics. BEHAVIOR THERAPY, 1980, **11**, 169-178.

Azrin, N. H., Nunn, R. G., & Frantz-Renshaw, S. E. Habit reversal vs. negative practice treatment of self-destructive oral habits. JOURNAL OF BEHAVIOR THERAPY AND EXPERIMENTAL PSYCHIATRY, 1982, **13**, 49-54.

Bailey, J. O. & Rugh, J. D. Behavioral management of functional oral disorders. In P. Bryant, E. Gale, & J. Rugh (Eds.), ORAL MOTOR BEHAVIORS AND ORAL DISORDERS. Washington, DC: U. S. Government Printing Office, 1979.

Bernstein, D. A. & Kleinknecht, R. A. Comparative evaluation of three social learning approaches to the reduction of dental fear. In B. Ingersoll & W. McCutcheon (Eds.), PROCEEDINGS OF THE SECOND NATIONAL CONFERENCE ON BEHAVIORAL DENTISTRY: CLINICAL RESEARCH IN BEHAVIORAL DENTISTRY. Morgantown, WV: West Virginia University, 1979.

Blachly, P. H., Osterud, H. T., & Josslin, R. Suicide in professional groups. NEW ENGLAND JOURNAL OF MEDICINE, 1963, **268**, 1278-1282.

Blendon, R. J. & Rogers, D. E. Dental education: Preparing for the 1980's. JOURNAL OF DENTAL EDUCATION, 1981, **49**, 559-566.

Bryant, P., Gale, E., & Rugh, J. (Eds.). ORAL MOTOR BEHAVIORS AND ORAL DISORDERS. Washington, DC: U. S. Government Printing Office, 1979. Proceedings of a recent state-of-the-art conference.

Budzynski, T. & Stoyva, J. An electromyographic feedback technique for teaching voluntary relaxation of the masseter muscle. JOURNAL OF DENTAL RESEARCH, 1973, **52**, 116-119.

Clark, M. & Hirschman, R. Effects of paced respiration on affective responses during dental stress. JOURNAL OF DENTAL RESEARCH, 1980, **59**, 1533.

Corah, N. L. Development of a dental anxiety scale. JOURNAL OF DENTAL RESEARCH, 1969, **48**, 596.

Corah, N. L., Gale, E. N., & Illig, S. J. Assessment of a dental anxiety scale. JOURNAL OF THE AMERICAN DENTAL ASSOCIATION, 1978, **97**, 816-819.

Corah, N. L., Gale, E. N., Pace, L. F., & Seyrek, S. K. Relaxation and musical programming as means of reducing psychological stress during dental procedures. JOURNAL OF THE AMERICAN DENTAL ASSOCIATION, 1981, **103**, 232-234.

DeLaCruz, M. & Geboy, M. J. Elimination of thumbsucking through contingency management. JOURNAL OF DENTISTRY FOR CHILDREN, 1983, **50**, 39-41.

Filewich, R. J., Jackson, E., & Shore, H. EFFECTS OF DENTAL FEAR ON EFFICIENCY OF ROUTINE DENTAL PROCEDURES. Paper presented at the meeting of the International Association for Dental Research, Chicago, March 1981.

Gale, E. N. Biofeedback for TMJ pain. In B. Ingersoll & W. McCutcheon (Eds.), PROCEEDINGS OF THE SECOND NATIONAL CONFERENCE ON BEHAVIORAL DENTISTRY: CLINICAL RESEARCH IN BEHAVIORAL DENTISTRY. Morgantown, WV: West Virginia University, 1979.

Gale, E. N. & Ayer, W. Treatment of dental phobias. JOURNAL OF THE AMERICAN DENTAL ASSOCIATION, 1969, **98**, 1304-1307.

Gatchel, R. J. Effectiveness of two procedures for reducing dental fear: Group-administered desensitization and group education and discussion. JOURNAL OF THE AMERICAN DENTAL ASSOCIATION, 1980, **101**, 634-637.

Gatchel, R. J., Ingersoll, B. D., Bowman, L., Robertson, C., & Walker, C. THE PREVALENCE OF DENTAL FEAR AND AVOIDANCE: A RECENT SURVEY. Unpublished manuscript, University of Texas Health Science Center at Dallas, 1982.

Gessel, A. H. Electromyographic biofeedback and tricyclic antidepressants in myofascial pain dysfunction syndrome: Psychological predictors of outcome. JOURNAL OF THE AMERICAN DENTAL ASSOCIATION, 1975, **91**, 1048-1052.

Gessel, A. H. & Alderman, M. M. Management of myofascial pain dysfunction syndrome of the temporomandibular joint by tension control training. PSYCHOSOMATICS, 1971, **12**, 302-309.

Glaros, A. G. & Rao, S. M. Bruxism: A critical review. PSYCHOLOGICAL BULLETIN, 1977, **84**, 767-782.

Godwin, W. C., Stark, D. D., Green, T. G., & Koran, A. Identification of sources of stress in practice by recent dental graduates. JOURNAL OF DENTAL EDUCATION, 1981, **45**, 220-221.

Greenburg, J. S. A study of behavior modificatio applied to dental health. JOURNAL OF SCHOOL HEALTH, 1977, **47**, 594-596.

Howard, J. H., Cunningham, D. A., Rechnitzer, P. A., & Goode, R. C. Stress in the job and career of a dentist. JOURNAL OF THE AMERICAN DENTAL ASSOCIATION, 1976, **93**, 630-636.

Ingersoll, B. D. Behavior management in pediatric dentistry. In A. Baum & J. Singer (Eds.), HANDBOOK OF PSYCHOLOGY AND HEALTH, VOL. 2: ISSUES IN CHILD AND ADOLESCENT HEALTH. New Jersey: Lawrence Erlbaum, 1983.

Ingersoll, B. D. BEHAVIORAL ASPECTS IN DENTISTRY. New York: Appleton-Century-Crofts, 1982. Written primarily as a textbook for dental students, this volume reviews current work in all areas of application of psychology to dentistry.

Ingersoll, B. D., Ingersoll, T. G., McCutcheon, W. R., & Seime, R. J. BEHAVIORAL DIMENSIONS OF DENTAL PRACTICE: A NATIONAL SURVEY. Unpublished manuscript, West Virginia University School of Dentistry, 1979.

Ingersoll, T. G., Ingersoll, B. D., Seime, R. J., & McCutcheon, W. R. A survey of patient and auxiliary problems as they relate to behavioral dentistry curricula. JOURNAL OF DENTAL EDUCATION, 1978, **42**, 260-263.

Iwata, B. A. & Becksfort, C. M. Behavioral research in preventive dentistry: Educational and contingency management approaches to the problem of patient compliance. JOURNAL OF APPLIED BEHAVIOR ANALYSIS, 1981, **14**, 111-120.

Kleinknecht, R. A. & Bernstein, D. A. The assessment of dental fear. BEHAVIOR THERAPY, 1978, **9**, 626-634.

Kleinknecht, R. A., Klepac, R. K., & Alexander, L. D. Origins and characteristics of fear of dentistry. JOURNAL OF THE AMERICAN DENTAL ASSOCIATION, 1973, **86**, 842-848.

Klepac, R. K. Behavioral treatment of bruxism. In B. Ingersoll, R. Seime, & W. McCutcheon (Eds.), BEHAVIORAL DENTISTRY: PROCEEDINGS OF THE FIRST NATIONAL CONFERENCE. Morgantown, WV: West Virginia University, 1977.

Kohlenberg, R., Greenberg, D., Reymore, I., & Hass, G. Behavior modification and the management of mentally retarded dental patients. JOURNAL OF DENTISTRY FOR CHILDREN, 1972, **39**, 61-67.

Lapouse, R. & Monk, M. A. Fears and worries in a representative sample of children. AMERICAN JOURNAL OF ORTHOPSYCHIATRY, 1969, **29**, 803-818.

Melamed, B., Hawes, R., Heiby, E., & Glick, J. The use of filmed modeling to reduce uncooperative behavior of children during dental treatment. JOURNAL OF DENTAL RESEARCH, 1975, **54**, 797-801.

Melamed, B. G. & Siegel, L. J. BEHAVIORAL MEDICINE. New York: Springer Publishing Co., 1980. This text is oriented toward the treatment of medical conditions, but it contains a chapter on behavioral management of dentally related disorders.

Melamed, B., Weinstein, P., Hawes, R., & Borland, M. Reduction of fear-related dental management problems using filmed modeling. JOURNAL OF THE AMERICAN DENTAL ASSOCIATION, 1975, **90**, 822-826.

Melamed, B., Yurcheson, R., Fleece, L., Hutcherson, S., & Hawes, R. Effects of film modeling on the reduction of anxiety-related behaviors in individuals varying in level of previous experience in the stress situation. JOURNAL OF CONSULTING AND CLINICAL PSYCHOLOGY, 1978, **46**, 1357-1365.

Melkas, J. F. Bruxism: Diagnosis and treatment. JOURNAL OF THE ACADEMY OF GENERAL DENTISTRY, 1971, **19**, 31-36.

Morgan, P., Wright, L., Ingersoll, B., & Seime, R. Children's perceptions of the dental experience. JOURNAL OF DENTISTRY FOR CHILDREN, 1980, **47**, 243-245.

Nielson, N. & Polakoff, P. It hurts the dentist too. JOB SAFETY AND HEALTH, 1975, **3**, 21-25.

Popovich, F. & Thompson, G. W. Thumb and finger sucking: Its relation to malocclusion. AMERICAN JOURNAL OF ORTHODONTICS, 1973, **63**, 148-155.

Price, S. C. & Kiyak, H. A. A behavioral approach to improving oral health among the elderly. SPECIAL CARE IN DENTISTRY, 1981, **1**, 267-274.

Reading, A. & Raw, M. The treatment of mandibular dysfunction: Possible application of psychological methods. BRITISH DENTAL JOURNAL, 1976, **140**, 201-205.

Rugh, J. D. & Robbins, J. W. Oral habit disorders. In B. Ingersoll (Ed.), BEHAVIORAL ASPECTS IN DENTISTRY. New York: Appleton-Century-Crofts, 1982.

Seltzer, S. PAIN CONTROL IN DENTISTRY. Philadelphia: J. B. Lippincott, 1978.

Shaw, D. W. & Thoreson, C. E. Effects of modeling and desensitization in reducing dental phobia. JOURNAL OF COUNSELING PSYCHOLOGY, 1974, **20**, 415-420.

Siegel, L. J. & Peterson, L. Stress reduction in young dental patients through coping skills and sensory information. JOURNAL OF CONSULTING AND CLINICAL PSYCHOLOGY, 1980, **48**, 785-787.

Stenn, P. G., Motherkill, K. J., & Brooke, R. I. Biofeedback and a cognitive behavioral approach to treatment of myofascial pain-dysfunction syndrome. BEHAVIOR THERAPY, 1979, **10**, 29-36.

Stricker, G. & Howitt, J. Physiological recording during simulated dental appointments. NEW YORK STATE DENTAL JOURNAL, 1965, **31**, 204-206.

Sword, R. O. Stress and suicide among dentists. DENTAL SURVEY, March 1977, 12-18; April 1977, 10-16. (Two-part series)

Traisman, A. S. & Traisman, H. S. Thumb- and finger-sucking: A study of 2,650 infants and children. JOURNAL OF PEDIATRICS, 1958, **52**, 566-572.

Venham, L. & Gaulin-Kremer, E. A self-report measure of situational anxiety for young children. JOURNAL OF PEDIATRIC DENTISTRY, 1979, **1**, 91-96.

Weinstein, P. & Getz, T. CHANGING HUMAN BEHAVIOR: STRATEGIES FOR PREVENTIVE DENTISTRY. Chicago, SRA, 1978. A useful introduction to the application of behavioral management techniques to the problem of preventive home care.

Weinstein, P., Getz, T., Ratener, P., & Domoto, P. The effect of dentists' behaviors on fear-related behaviors in children. JOURNAL OF THE AMERICAN DENTAL ASSOCIATION, 1982, **104**, 32-38.

White, L. Behavior modification of orthodontic patients. JOURNAL OF CLINICAL ORTHODONTICS, 1974, **3**, 501-505.

Williams, J. A., Hurst, M., & Stokes, T. F. Decreasing uncooperative behavior in young dental patients through the observation of and by peers. Article submitted for publication in 1982.

Wroblewski, P. F., Jacob, T., & Rehm, L. P. The contribution of relaxation to symbolic modeling in the modification of dental fears. BEHAVIOR RESEARCH AND THERAPY, 1977, **15**, 113-115.

THE CONCEPTS AND TECHNIQUES OF ORGANIZATION DEVELOPMENT: AN INTRODUCTION

Leonard D. Goodstein and Phyliss Cooke

Organizations, like individuals and families, frequently find themselves in need of professional help. Sometimes the need is for content experts – persons who can solve or propose solutions to fairly specific technical problems (e.g., how to do market research to determine the company's appropriate product mix or how to float a stock issue). These experts are in plentiful supply as a check with your Yellow Pages under "Consultants" will readily reveal.

Often, however, the organization problem is not easily identified. There are symptoms, to be sure. Low energy, indifferent morale, tardiness, high employee turnover, and poor followership are some typical symptoms of organizational distress, just as headaches, anxiety, and loss of appetite are often symptoms of personal distress. With such conditions, the need is to look beyond the symptoms in order to gain some understanding of the problem(s) reflected in the symptoms. Organization Development (OD) consultants are those persons brought in to help the client organization to do this. They both diagnose and modify the underlying circumstances that have led to the presenting complaints. OD consultants are the clinicians to business and industrial organizations.

DEFINING ORGANIZATION DEVELOPMENT

Organization development (OD) is an educational process by which human resources are continuously identified, allocated, and expanded in ways that make these resources more available to the organization, and therefore, improve the organization's problem-solving capabilities. (Sherwood, 1972, p. 183)

OD is typically characterized as a long-range effort to introduce planned change based on a diagnosis which is shared by the members of an organization, involving the entire organization or a coherent system or part of it. The goal is to increase organizational effectiveness and enhance organizational choice and self-renewal, using various strategies to intervene in the ongoing activities of the organization in a way which facilitates learning and making choices about alternative ways to proceed. The most general objective of OD is to develop self-renewing, self-correcting systems of people who can organize themselves in a variety of ways (depending on the nature of their tasks) and who continue to expand the choices available to the organization as it copes with the changing demands of a changing environment.

While organization development is typically characterized as a result of planned change efforts, we should not lose sight of the fact that organizations also develop as a natural consequence of the day-to-day interactions within. Organization development as a concept refers to both the natural, emergent dynamics and to the change that results from consciously set goals and planned interventions. The task facing the consultant is to be helpful in the process of establishing desired change directions and in developing the skills needed to stay on top of the natural forces for change inherent in the system and in the environment.

While OD activities focus on people and groups and the changed relations between and among them, the objective of OD is to aid the organization itself. That is, while long-term success of any OD effort is dependent upon developing positive collaborative attitudes and interdependent behaviors within the system, OD is not simply human relations training. OD efforts are designed to guide the human resources within the organization in their understanding and effective management of the growth and direction of the organization.

Most OD consultants would prefer to work with healthy organizations, aiming toward fuller actualization or growth, but finding them is rare. Just as most individuals seeking clinical psychological treatment are in some kind of personal pain, it has been our experience that most organizations seeking OD help are in some kind of organizational "pain" and they, too, are inclined to terminate treatment after simple pain reduction, rather than move to new levels of competence.

For the purpose of drawing comparisons to the concepts and techniques of OD, let us assume that the work of an OD consultant is similar to that of the clinician. The similarities are even clearer when applied to the work of a family therapist since the object of both is to improve the entire system rather than to focus on only a part of that system. For example, consider the case where the presenting problem for the family therapist includes a mother's report of unruly behavior on the part of a child, feelings of depression experienced by herself, and a report of lethargy in the father's reaction to family problems. Where does the clinician begin in the attempt to gather relevant data to assess the situation, to diagnose the problems, and to prescribe correct solutions? Should the disruptive behavior of the child be the focus? Should the client be assumed to be the mother since she is presenting the problem? In answering these and related questions, the consultant, like the clinician, must, from a variety of theories and concepts, select those that fit and which can serve as effective tools in daily work.

Our approach is a systems approach, one in which organizations are seen as being composed of a series of interrelated subsystems, held together by common goals and a structure intended to achieve these goals. Just as the family therapist operates on the assumption that the whole family, as an interactive system, must be the target, the OD consultant operates on the assumption that the organization, not the individuals in the organization, is the client. The consultant responds to the problems presented (e.g., low morale, requests for team building, or help with the performance appraisal system) in terms of various theories and concepts which have been formulated to guide him or her

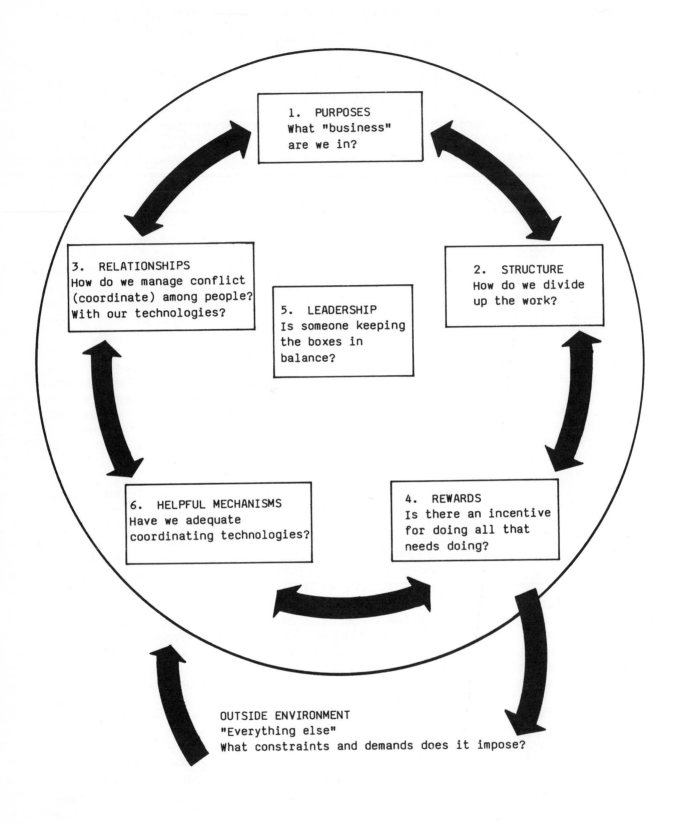

Figure 1. Weisbord's Six-box Model of Organizations

in attempting to assess, diagnose, and prescribe remedial measure for a given system.

MODELS OF ORGANIZATION DEVELOPMENT

The behavioral sciences, especially social psychology, offer a variety of general principles and organizing concepts from which we can describe and understand the functioning of organizations. By using some of these principles and concepts in their analysis, consultants can both evaluate the effectiveness of organizations in reaching their goals and the satisfaction level of members of the organization with their life in that system. These two concerns are the focus of much of what is termed organization development.

Conceptual models have been developed, primarily based upon open systems theory, which depict organizations as systems of interacting elements, and which identify both the explicit and implicit structures which produce organizational life. For example, Weisbord (1976, 1978) views organizations in terms of a Six-box Model (see Figure 1 on the preceding page) in which **leadership** is necessary to ensure that balance is achieved between and among the five other boxes, which include: the **purpose** of the organization which must be clearly identified and articulated; the **structure** which must allow for the optimal amount of work which is necessary to achieve the organization's purpose; the **rewards** for doing the work which need to be appropriate and sufficient; the **helpful mechanisms** needed to adequately coordinate work which need to be available and operating; and the **relationships** among people and groups which need to be managed appropriately to ensure high levels of satisfaction and productivity.

A somewhat more complete model, which should be more familiar to clinicians, is offered by Jones (1981) in his Organization Universe Model (see Figure 2 on the following page). It utilizes a series of concentric circles and places **values** at the core. Typical organizational values include respect and dignity in the treatment of people, cooperation, functional openness, interdependence, authenticity, and profitability. The next ring, **goals**, concerns how the values are articulated or operationalized. For example, if one of the values is respect for people, courtesy in all interpersonal interactions might be the operationalized goal. When people are treated discourteously, it can then be assumed that either the value of respect is simply espoused and not authentic or that the relationship between courteous behavior and the core value of respect is not clear to members of the organization or not explicit enough to guide the behavior of organization members.

Just as the values which affect the development of the family unit are often not clear to the family members, organizational values are often covert and difficult to clarify for organization members. Such clarification is one important function of the OD consultant, just as it is for the family therapist. Indeed, the identification of the core values and the determination of the clarity, congruence, and relevance of goals to these values is the central process of getting at the root causes of organizational distress.

The OD consultant must consider not only the organization's values and goals, but also how these goals will be implemented within the structure of the organization. Several structural elements must be reviewed by the consultant

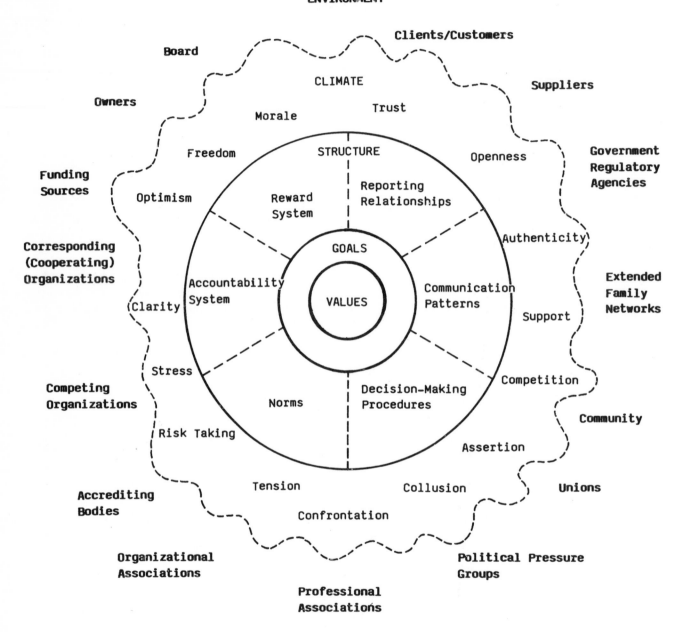

ENVIRONMENT

Clients/Customers

Board

CLIMATE

Suppliers

Owners

Morale   Trust

Freedom   STRUCTURE   Openness

Government
Regulatory
Agencies

Funding
Sources

Optimism   Reward   Reporting
                  System   Relationships

Authenticity

Corresponding
(Cooperating)
Organizations

GOALS

Extended
Family
Networks

Accountability   Communication
Clarity   System   VALUES   Patterns

Support

Competing
Organizations

Stress   Competition

Norms   Decision-Making
               Procedures

Community

Risk Taking

Assertion

Accrediting
Bodies

Tension   Collusion   Unions

Confrontation

Organizational
Associations

Political Pressure
Groups

Professional
Associations

Figure 2. Jones' Organization Universe Model

in order to adequately assess the functioning of an organization. Just as a therapist must be concerned with the various structural aspects of the family (living conditions, work schedules, finances, etc.), the OD consultant must examine the structural elements of the organization, how it is put together, and how well the structure is working. The examination must include both the formal structure (the organizational chart) and the informal structure (how things **really** work).

The functioning of the formal and informal structural systems need to be examined in several areas. These include: (a) accountability - the formal system established for evaluating individuals working within the structure as well as the individual latitude exercised and interpretations made of this dimension of organization life; (b) rewards - the tangible and intangible rewards given by the organization for work performed and the impact of the rewards on the quantity and quality of work done; (c) reporting relationships - the designated lines of authority and the demonstrated power to influence the behavior of others in a desired direction; (d) decision making procedures - the process through which problems are identified and solved and the individual preferences which guide the formal procedures are followed; (e) communication patterns - the formal and informal systems through which organization information is disseminated and meaning transferred within the organization; and (f) norms - the formal and informal rules of conduct, dress, and speech, as well as the actual observable behavior in these areas.

Organizational climate, the next ring of the model, is seen as a by-product of the interaction of the values guiding the organization, the goals, the structural elements, and the "goodness of fit" between these internal elements and the external environment in which the organization functions. Just as certain families feel "healthy" or "unhealthy," certain organizations feel right or troubled. But, just as the clinician knows that family climate indices are mainly symptomatic and offer little in the way of understanding the real causes of the problem, the OD consultant knows that these climate variables are little more than a surface description of the organization's distress, though these may be paramount concerns for the client. In both clinical work and OD consultation, little significant change can occur by addressing climate problems alone. As we noted earlier, the root causes are mainly to be found closer to the center of the Organization Universe.

ORGANIZATION ASSESSMENT AND DIAGNOSIS

A valid organization diagnosis involves a description of the root causes of the organization's malaise. For example, it may involve an analysis of how the organization's reward structure does not fit its stated value of achievement and has had little or no effect on its structure. Or, it may involve an analysis of how the constant dissention between various organizational groups together with a norm of smothering conflict has led to apathy and resignation. Such analyses, when supported by clear behavioral data, help both the consultant and the client understand what has happened to create the problem and what can be done to cure it.

There are several methods of data collection used by OD consultants which are similar to those used by clinicians. One method is that of direct observation, including using unobtrusive measures. Such observation begins when the consultant enters the waiting room of the client organization. How is the room decorated? How easily is entry gained? What is the attitude of the receptionist to the visitor? How are the offices arranged? The answers begin to provide data which can lead to a diagnosis, and the consultant continues to collect this direct observational data as contact is made with other aspects of the client system. Such additional data will either support or undermine the initial impression and the OD consultant, like the clinician, must be on guard that initial impressions do not cloud the real situation.

Another method of data collection is analyzing written records (e.g., reports, inter-office memoranda, news letters, appointment records, attendance at staff meetings, report distribution lists). Such data can provide a convenient source of information about patterns of communication and influence and the differences between the formal and informal structures of the organization, just as a family's correspondence, school records, and social calendar might provide useful data about the family.

The most general source of data, however, is the diagnostic interview, just as it is for the clinician. Who is interviewed and the content of the interview will largely be determined by the organizational model held by the consultant. The open systems model, explicit in both the Six-box and Organization Universe Models, concentrates on values, goals, and the supporting structures that articulate these central concerns. These models lead the consultant into examining the social psychology of the organization, how the various subsystems are bound together, and how effectively they operate. Weisbord (1978) has developed a semi-structured interview schedule for guiding the consultant in applying his or her diagnostic model to actual organizational life.

One other type of data collection includes a variety of paper-and-pencil inventories that can be used to tap such dimensions as morale, attitudes, and job satisfaction. This category includes such well-standardized instruments as the Survey of Organizations (Bowers & Franklin, 1977; Hausser, Pecorella, & Wissler, 1977), a host of semi-standardized instruments such as the Organizational Ideology Scale (Harrison, 1972), as well as those that are created specifically for an individual client by the consultant. The pros and cons of using such instruments are virtually the same as those involved in using such instruments with individuals, including the critical question of how to share the data collected.

Consultants vary considerably in their reliance upon different data sources, just as clinicians do. Like clinicians, some OD consultants prefer direct observation and interviews while others tend to rely more on formal assessment procedure. Also, the model of organizational life and views about organizational health and illness held by the consultant will very much affect the process of data collection, just as it does with the clinician.

ORANIZATION CHANGE THROUGH OD

Once the client and the consultant can agree upon the diagnosis of the organization's current difficulties, then attention can be turned to remediation. Among the intervention strategies typically used by OD consultants are training, coaching (individualized training), technostructural changes in the organization, role negotiation, formal (survey) feedback, participation in sensitivity training with other organization members, team building, and process consultation.

While it is beyond the scope of this paper to review each of these procedures in detail, a brief description of each is appropriate at this point. Training, especially training in communication skills, interpersonal relationships, management and supervisory practices, or performance appraisal can dramatically change the functioning of an organization. This is particularly true if the training programs are based upon remediating the root problems identified in the diagnosis and involve most of the relevant members of the organization. Of course, the training programs have to have some acceptance and impact if they are to be successful.

Coaching involves having the consultant spend a good bit of time with one or more key members of the organization, typically top managers, observing and reviewing their behavior and providing feedback to them about what has been observed. This strategy is particularly useful if the persons being coached have been identified as critical elements of the root problem. For example, if the president of the corporation espouses collaboration as a central value, but makes independent decisions on a regular basis, a consultant working regularly with this person can identify the behavior when it occurs and offer feedback on the discrepancy between espoused values and overt behavior. Such confrontation is expected to lead to change, just as it does in counseling or therapy.

Technostructural changes are those efforts which attempt to simultaneously change the way in which work is accomplished (the technology of work) and who does the work (the structure of the organization). To attempt to do either independently denies the close, natural interdependence of these two aspects of work. For example, consider the way in which psychiatric patients are managed in a typical mental hospital. The active treatment service is typically structurally removed from the outplacement and rehabilitation service. When patients make the transition from one to the other, too often there is little information passed on and patient care suffers, as does staff morale and competence. One possible resolution of this problem is to reorganize the patient care system so that one single system is responsible for the patient from entry through aftercare. But such a change in the technology of care often fails because the change neglects the structural issues, particularly those of territoriality, status, or interprofessional and interdisciplinary conflicts. Only when both the structural and technological issues are simultaneously addressed can successful organizational change occur.

In such a technostructural change, role negotiation is one critical substrategy. In such negotiations, the consultant attempts to help the various participants determine what they agree to do on the job and what they are willing to allow others to do. The overlaps and the gaps can then be identified and treated as problems to be solved rather than as ongoing, unspoken conflicts.

Formal (survey) feedback means collecting questionnaire data from all members of the organization, collating the data received, and making it available to the organization. Such data makes explicit the concerns which members identify and forces the organization to face up to the issues raised. The major problem, of course, is for the consultant to help the organization, particularly the several work groups, analyze their own data, accept or reject its validity, and successfully plan the steps to remedy the problems identified. The difficulties in accomplishing these steps in any organization should be readily apparent.

Team building, and sensitivity training as one vehicle for doing team development or team building, involves a simultaneous examination of the attitudes and skills of a work group or team to engage in the successful accomplishment of task and to maintain the cohesion and involvement of the members of the team (Goodstein, Cooke, & Goodstein, 1983). Teams have tasks to accomplish (plans to draw up, decisions to make, products to invent) and they need to be committed to such tasks and have the skills to accomplish them. Skills such as agenda building, identifying and utilizing the team's resources, and decision making are too often taken for granted in the creation of and assignment of tasks to work teams. Members of these teams will also differ in their attitudes toward group work (i.e., they will not agree on whether effective work can be done in teams, or on whether to temporarily suppress their own needs to get work done on the group level). They will also differ in their ability to get others involved in group activities and in their sensitivity to how others are feeling about what is happening. These skills are often unfamiliar to many members of teams. Team building involves the consultant in assessing the attitudes and skills of the various team members in both task and maintenance and then assisting the team to clarify its attitudes and acquire the necessary skills to be more effective.

In sensitivity training (an unstructured group therapy-like setting), the members of a work group are encouraged to explore their interpersonal relationships, especially those that have interfered with effective collaboration. The clinical skills of the consultant in such an intervention need to be exceptionally high, just as in any other type of therapy-like intervention. This is especially important since the issues raised in such work-group sensitivity-training sessions simply do not go away when the session is over, unlike such training with groups of persons who do not work together.

The unique OD consultation intervention, however, is process consultation (Burke & Goodstein, 1980). Process consultation, a term first introduced by Schein (1969), involves the examination of **how** things are done in an organization rather than what is done. Process consultation means examining the patterns of communication in an organization, how such patterns were developed, what such patterns mean about the distribution of power within the organization, and how it differs from the espoused values and goals that the organization believes it holds. The relationship of such process consultation to the interpretations of a therapist is a clear and direct one.

The OD consultant uses process consultation techniques in conjunction with any of the other techniques previously described. For example, while observing a staff meeting, the consultant might ask why no one ever seems to respond directly to the question asked by Fred, one of the members present, or why certain issues always seem to be so low on the agenda that they are never really addressed. By raising these questions, the consultant attempts to focus on the values and goals dilemmas, previously identified as core problems, as being at the root of the organization's distress. The role of the consultant here is to be counter normative, to ask why the Emperor is naked, even though all the others present seem to be pretending that his new clothes are quite elegant.

THE ROLE OF THE OD CONSULTANT

As in the case of clinical practice, the one element which the OD practitioner brings to every consultancy is himself or herself. Since the field of OD is still relatively undefined, atheoretical in practice, and relatively new as an area for applying the behavioral science, there are even fewer constraints on the individual OD consultant than there are on the clinician. However, checklists for monitoring one's interventions can be readily developed if common sense is applied to the task and if a professional orientation is desired. Once the consultant develops a clear understanding of his or her values, models, preferred modes of organizational functioning, and expectations about how people in organizations should interact, it is then easier to ask such value-based questions of the client. It is critical that the value-based questions have been first answered by the consultant. These include such critical questions as: What is an organization? What purpose(s) should organizations serve? For whom? What does the ideal organization look like? What should an organization do once it has met its major objectives? How should organizations balance their needs with the individual needs of their members? How do I understand the process of change on an organizational level? On a societal level? Since the personal answers by the consultant to these questions guide all phases of the professional's work, clarity and commitment to one's answers is a key aspect of OD consulting. And, since there are no easy or widely accepted answers to these questions, finding one's individual answers is a slow, developmental process.

Just as clinicians must understand their client's problems in terms of root causes before functional remedial efforts can be planned or executed, so must the OD consultant have an understanding of his or her client's problems in similar terms. Also, as with clinicians, consultants find these root causes in their models of organizations. Thus, as a clinician with a psychodynamic orientation will find the root cause in early childhood experience, the consultant with an open systems orientation will find the root cause in the failure of the system to adequately articulate its purpose and goals and the system will have gaps between the aspirations and the structures intended to accomplish them.

The role of the consultant in relating to the client system is another area that requires clarification. Since the client system must both generate the data necessary for a diagnosis and accept the consultant's diagnosis based upon such data, the typical medical model of expertness and distance rarely works. Even more importantly, the client system must accept full and direct responsibility for agreeing with and implementing the changes necessary to reach the desired state. While there may be initial receptivity towards hiring some kind of expert consultant to say what is wrong and how to fix it, organization development cannot occur if the organization itself does not undertake the task of improving its own functioning. Thus the most functional kind of relationship between consultant and client is one of collaboration and support in which the responsibility for both accepting and implementing any change is always the client's. Indeed, we might argue that this is exactly the same situation in which clinicians find themselves. Neither clinicians nor consultants can prescribe new behaviors to their clients with much certainty that the client will accept and implement such prescription. Only when the client "buys in" on the offered diagnosis and cure will there by any hope of change.

Despite our personal view that a collaborative style works best, there are other consultants who take a more directive style. This is typically a top-down approach in which what is to be done, to what standard, by whom, when, and in what manner is decided by the consultant. Many consultants who operate from an "expert" orientation utilize this directive style, but not exclusively. For example, a consultant operating from an expert orientation might still use a consultative approach where the final decision-making rested with the client. The expert would see his or her role as offering the client the best judgment about the potential consequences of various courses of action, but leave the choice up to the client, feeling that the full use of an organization's human resources to make the decision is more likely to produce commitment from those involved in the decision.

Still another style is the facilitative style in which all decision-making authority is turned back to the client system and the consultant avoids even the expert orientation. The consultant's focus is on identifying the key linking pins of the client system. Whatever information is necessary to make the decision can be found by these persons. The primary role of the consultant is to provide the support necessary to facilitate communication between the functioning units within the system. The efficacy of this approach is determined by the readiness of the system to participate in the change effort and by the resident problem-solving skills of the members. Obviously, this facilitative style is most useful when the energy of the organization for change is high and the skills level of organization members is well developed. Stepsis (1977) has provided a fuller exposition of these several consulting styles and how each might be best used. Also, the Consulting Skills workshops regularly offered by University Associates, Inc., provide participants with an opportunity to explore their preferred style and to receive feedback on how their style is experienced by others.

INTERNAL AND EXTERNAL CONSULTANTS

There are at least two major ways in which OD consultants work: as internal consultants (i.e., as full-time regular employees of the organization to which they provide help), and as external consultants (i.e., as outside specialists providing help on an irregular basis, either by retainer or per diem). One fascinating aspect of working as an OD consultant to organizations lies in the unique relationship that exists in those organizations where both an internal and external "agent of change" collaborate to bring about an OD effort. Internal consultants, sometimes called trainers, personnel administrators, employee relations specialists, program analysts, and others working within, have a different and fuller understanding of the organization. The staff can know levels of nuance and shades of meaning that no outsider can comprehend. On the other hand, the external consultant brings a freshness of approach to organizational issues which enables him or her to ask questions that simply would never occur to the internal person. Like everyone else who works in an organization, the internal person has agreed to agree that the Emperor's new suit is gorgeous. Such collusion blinds us all and only a fresh perspective can provide new awareness.

There is another element involved as well. The external consultant is, or at least should be, much more willing to take the risk of asking embarrassing questions, pointing out collusion, or saying the unspeakable. The external consultant should run the risk of losing the consultancy, which is a considerably smaller risk, both qualitatively and quantitatively than that run by the insider faced with loss of a job. This knowledge should be sufficient to give the external consultant the necessary courage to act. It is the subtle chemistry of an insider and an outsider that makes such relationships uniquely profitable for the organization.

In any event, the ultimate goal of the external consultant is to eliminate the need for his or her services. As the internal resources of the client system, including the internal change agents, develop the skills and with the perspective brought by the external consultant that are necessary to set and achieve organizational goals, the reliance and dependency upon external resources is diminished. Again, there is great similarity between the external OD consultant's movement out of a system and the clinician's gradual withdrawal from a client family's life.

SOME CONCLUDING COMMENTS

It was our intention to present a brief overview of organization development, to review some basic concepts involved in this process, and to present a sample of the techniques and issues facing the OD consultant. In addition, we wanted to provide a context for understanding the OD consulting process by identifying some obvious parallels which exist between the work of the family therapist and that of the OD consultant. We are satisfied if our intention has been recognized and that the motivated reader is adequately grounded to further explore this new application of the behavioral sciences.

Leonard D. Goodstein, Ph.D., is currently Chairman of the Board of University Associates, Inc., an international consulting and publishing organization. An ABPP diplomate in clinical psychology, he was formerly Chair and Professor of Psychology at Arizona State University, Director of Training in Professional Psychology at the University of Cincinnati, and Director of the Counseling Service and Professor of Psychology at the University of Iowa. He is the author of a number of books and articles in clinical and organizational psychology. Dr. Goodstein may be contacted at University Associates, 8517 Production Avenue, San Diego, CA 92121.

Phyliss Cooke, Ph.D., is currently the Director of Professional Services for University Associates, Inc. She is also Dean of the Intern training program and the Masters Degree program offered by University Associates. Her training is in clinical psychology and counselor education. She was formerly an Instructor at Kent State University and was Director of the Cleveland Institute for Rational Living in Ohio, where she also maintained a private clinical practice. Dr. Cooke may be contacted at University Associates, 8517 Production Avenue, San Diego, CA 92121.

RESOURCES

Bowers, D. G. & Franklin, J. L. SURVEY-GUIDED DEVELOPMENT I: DATA-BASED ORGANIZATIONAL CHANGE. San Diego, CA: University Associates, 1977.

Burke, W. W. & Goodstein, L. D. Organization development today: A retrospective applied to the present and the future. In W. W. Burke & L. D. Goodstein (Eds.), TRENDS AND ISSUES IN OD: CURRENT THEORY AND PRACTICE. San Diego, CA: University Associates, 1980.

Goodstein, L. D., Cooke, P., & Goodstein, J. T. The Team Orientation and Behavior Inventory (TOBI). In L. D. Goodstein & J. W. Pfeiffer (Eds.), THE 1983 ANNUAL FOR FACILITATORS, TRAINERS, AND CONSULTANTS. San Diego, CA: University Associates, 1983.

Harrison, R. Understanding your organization's character. HARVARD BUSINESS REVIEW, 1972, **50**, 119-128.

Hausser, D. L., Pecorella, P. A., & Wissler, A. L. SURVEY-GUIDED DEVELOPMENT DEVELOPMENT II: A MANUAL FOR CONSULTANTS. San Diego, CA: University Associates, 1977.

Jones, J. E. The organization universe. In J. E. Jones & S. W. Pfeiffer (Eds.), THE 1981 ANNUAL HANDBOOK FOR GROUP FACILITATORS. San Diego, CA: University Associates, 1981.

Schein, E. H. PROCESS CONSULTATION: ITS ROLE IN ORGANIZATION DEVELOPMENT. Reading, MA: Addison-Wesley, 1969.

Sherwood, J. J. An introduction to organization development. In J. W. Pfeiffer & J. E. Jones (Eds.), THE 1972 ANNUAL HANDBOOK FOR GROUP FACILITATORS. San Diego, CA: University Associates, 1972.

Stepsis, J. A. Structure as an integrative concept in management theory and practice. In J. E. Jones & J. W. Pfeiffer (Eds.), THE 1977 ANNUAL HANDBOOK FOR GROUP FACILITATORS. San Diego, CA: University Associates, 1977.

University Associates, Inc., 8517 Production Avenue, P. O. Box 26240, San Diego, CA 92126. University Associates is engaged in publishing, training, and consulting in the field of human resource development. Interested readers may wish to be placed on their mailing list.

Weisbord, M. R. ORGANIZATIONAL DIAGNOSIS: A WORKBOOK OF THEORY AND PRACTICE. Reading, MA: Addison-Wesley, 1978.

Weisbord, M. R. Organizational diagnosis: Six places to look for trouble with or without a theory. GROUP AND ORGANIZATION STUDIES, 1976, **1**, 430-447.

THE MENTAL HEALTH PROFESSIONS AND THE MEDIA

Jacqueline C. Bouhoutsos

Mental health professionals and the media have discovered each other and, for many, it's been love at first sight. Therapists are reaching vast audiences by serving as hosts for call-in shows, broadcasting their interviews with clients, appearing on news and features, serving as consultants for movies and television shows and writing self-help books and newspaper columns. The rapidly growing number of professionals eager to use media is matched by the opportunities for involvement in those media.

As early as the 1960's, George Miller (1969) urged American psychologists to give psychology away. It has taken us 20 years to realize that dissemination of information through mass media is probably the most effective way of accomplishing this, and the only way that major portions of the general population will obtain access to psychological information.

The time is right for such media activity by mental health professionals. Americans are experiencing a health care revolution brought on by the rising cost of services and by rediscovery of the old adage that "an ounce of prevention is worth a pound of cure." The resultant desire to prevent mental and physical disorders through self-help activities has created an increasing demand for information from clinicians by way of the media.

With increased opportunity for media use have come attendant problems for the mental health professions. Ethics Committees of the American Psychological and American Psychiatric Associations have appointed task forces to consider standards for ethical and responsible use of media (American Psychiatric Association, 1977; Larson, 1981). Concerns have arisen whether primacy of the welfare of the consumer can be maintained by media mental health professionals when they are confronted by the commercial demands of entertainment media. Also there is potential for unintentional harm to individual members of mass media audiences who might particularize general information or advice. Sensationalism, distortion and trivialization by the media have been viewed by some as antithetical to accurate presentation of scientific material (Keith-Spiegel & Koocher, in press).

Nonetheless, even the most ardent critics of media use by the mental health sciences and professions agree on the desirability of reaching mass audiences with psychological information. The controversy centers on type of material, the context, and by whom it is to be presented. This contribution will provide information about ways in which the various media have been used to date, the ethical and operational problems involved, and suggestions for future research and practice.

USE OF MASS MEDIA IN ACHIEVING BEHAVIOR CHANGE

Several recent studies have focused on the effectiveness of the mass media in preventing mental and physical disorders. In Finland, a television campaign was mounted to help people stop smoking. While only 1% of the targeted population were able to stop completely, it was demonstrated that each success was achieved at a cost of approximately $1.00 (McAlister, Puska, Koskela, Pallonen, & Maccoby, 1980; McCall, 1982). Stanford University has established a program designed to evaluate the use of mass media and face to face instruction in educating the public about ways to prevent heart disease. Information about diet, exercise, stress reduction, and other topics were provided by way of media in two counties of northern California and comparison was made with one county where no mass media information was provided. The results very clearly showed that mass media campaigns could be effective (NIMH, 1982).

In mental health, the State of California has undertaken a massive, three year campaign to promote "wellness," including establishment of community support groups to form social networks for combating isolation, recognized as one of the causative factors of both mental and physical diseases. Mental health professionals have been involved in all phases of these particular programs: the organization and planning aspects, the utilization of media to transmit the information, and the development of research designs and instruments to assess the effectiveness of the programs.

The role of mass media in less structured information transmission has been difficult to evaluate. For example, when the mastectomies of Betty Ford and Happy Rockefeller were announced on the air, examinations for breast cancer increased substantially according to informal physician reports. Broadcasts by radio stations with predominantly black audiences have been emphasizing the importance of attention to high blood pressure, one of the prime causes of premature death in black adults, and physicians have reported increased requests for blood pressure checks. These informal reports are heartening but have not provided quantifiable data.

In the area of mental health, preventive intervention becomes even more difficult to assess. An alternative methodology, although admittedly less scientifically defensible, is that of assessing changes in the demand for services on the part of the public. It might be noted that the media evaluate their effectiveness in terms of sales of products, audience counts, ratings, and readership.

THE PRINT MEDIUM

Sales of self-help books in the area of mental health have risen markedly. How-to primers on saying no without guilt, achieving orgasm, living with divorce, talking with teenagers, and other such subjects, find eager readers. Publishers are open to proposals from mental health professionals with new approaches to old topics, or new subjects not previously covered. General circulation magazines are also interested in receiving articles from mental health professionals and will often establish continuing columns if there is public approval of initial efforts. Concern by the American Psychological Association over unsubstantiated claims by self-help books led to creation of a Task Force on Self-Help Books. Its findings emphasized the necessity for scientific validation before the public is advised to follow specific programs or techniques (Rosen, 1981).

A new area which holds much promise is therapeutic journalism built on a community organization model (Joslyn-Scherer, 1980). News releases, newsletters, and newspapers are used to promote self-help, mutual aid, creation of group feeling, resource utilization and informed participation in mental health decision making. Scarce funding plus mass media disinterest in articles without broad readership appeal make self-publishing attractive for small publications addressed to groups with special needs. Entrepreneurial independence makes it possible to publish articles with appeal for particular readership and to involve "para-professionals" in the creative process, which may provide another benefit of therapeutic journalism.

TELEVISION

NEWS

Both radio and television news broadcasts have broadened their coverage in recent years to include segments not strictly "news" in that they do not meet the criterion of recency. Advice is provided on medicine, meteorology, dentistry, law, finance, consumer concerns and even veterinary medicine. Mental health professionals have become popular guests and frequently deliver 60 second to 5 minute "capsules" which address topics often related to current happenings, but more frequently are self-generated. Items of interest to the general public such as loneliness, depression, sexual functioning, stress reduction, and burn-out, to name just a few, are such topics.

"Talking heads" (i.e., reporting by individuals in the studio) is the usual format. However, it has become possible in the recently expanded programming of news for a mental health professional to act as producer and reporter and go on location with a camera crew. This greatly increases visual appeal and interest, but also necessitates more time commitment, since as much as a day can be spent filming what may appear as a 3 minute segment on the evening news. The advantage of on-site filming is the immediacy. Television is a visual medium, and talking about the effects of noise pollution in the studio is not as effective as using tapes of talking while surrounded by jack hammers clattering or airplanes taking off; discussing risk-taking behavior is not the same as carrying a camera while making a parachute jump. Obviously, this type of on-site reporting is not suitable for everyone, and ultimately station policy and finances determine the presentation format.

BEHIND THE SCENES

Far less stressful than on-site or on-camera appearances are activities performed as a consultant. Assessing programming for children, providing information on the impact of violent or sexual material, citing research material on learning or psychosocial development, poverty, racism, or women's issues, and consulting on production problems are all areas where psychological expertise may be helpful. Whether it is sought or used depends on the relationship built with station personnel and the perceived usefulness of the services provided.

THE ROLE OF "EXPERT"

A much more traditional role for those involved in mental health is that of guest. Television hosts on such programs as GOOD MORNING AMERICA, PHIL DONAHUE or the TODAY SHOW frequently interview behavioral scientists and professionals who have written books or whose research findings have been published in professional journals. Although often overlooked by media in the past, such material is now being publicized through press releases issued by public information offices of the various mental health disciplines or institutions where researchers work.

NEW DEVELOPMENTS

An example of a much more controversial use of television is a counseling program (featuring a psychiatrist) which currently airs twice a day in most major cities. Condensed from 2 to 3 hours of interviews, the half hour program, called COUPLES, may show same gender couples, a parent and child, two friends, or other combinations who are having problems for which they seek assistance on the air. The psychiatrist sees them separately first, then together, and subsequently comments to the audience on the nature of the difficulty. Letters from the audience are also read, and selected couples return to talk about what ensued after the initial visit.

This program, and several others now in the planning stage which will involve group therapy or audience members talking about their problems, raise serious questions about confidentiality as well as the impact of public self-disclosure. Since patients are on screen and readily identifiable, and tapings remain available for many years, it is possible that eventually, if not at the time of taping, material could be presented in reruns which would be detrimental to the individuals involved. Also, with the increasing number of video tape records, there is no control over who has copies of a particular tape or when it might be shown. It may be argued that informed consent is always obtained, but it is not always possible to know in advance the ramifications of, or motivations for, such appearances, and disclosure at one period in one's lifetime may be highly inappropriate at another. Longitudinal research is needed on these issues, and also on the impact of the condensation and editing process which may distort the nature of the interviews.

INTERACTIVE CABLE TELEVISION

The least developed television area of potential involvement for mental health professionals is that of cable. According to Gustave Hauser (Turkat, 1982), Chair of Warner Amex Cable Communications, 80% of all homes in the United States will have interactive cable television by 1990. Narrow-casting makes possible the targeting of certain interest groups, and such enterprises as Cable Health Network will be broadcasting programs 24 hours a day, transmitting information about mental and physical health. Many networks are already involved in production, and there is need for mental health professionals to provide program material or to appear on camera as hosts or panel members. There is potential for the delivery of mental health services to change drastically because of the interactive capacity. For example, clinicians may provide consultation and psychotherapeutic services from their offices to the client's home. Problems of confidentiality, privacy, intimacy, isolation, and socialization appear overwhelming. On the positive side, new research capabilities by way of cable promise immediate availability of national samples of specialized populations, simplified data collection, and immediate "publishing" through the medium.

MOTION PICTURES

Despite the inclusion of behavioral scientists on the Code and Rating Board (this author was the first, followed by Aaron Stern, a child psychologist/psychiatrist), entertainment motion pictures have not been receptive to involving mental health professionals in the creative process. The omission is not by design. Frequently, producers utilize clinicians to appear in, or consult on, educational films. Mental health professionals also write, produce, and distribute their own educational films, but few have been directly involved in the making of entertainment films.

Times have changed, however, from the era of Louis B. Mayer's classic injunction, "If you want to send a message, use Western Union." Sometimes, serendipitously, it is possible to bridge the gap between education and entertainment. In 1970, Dimension Films, an educational film company, set out to make a motion picture about a group of teenagers "rapping" to highlight concerns of adolescents. When the producers viewed their extensive footage, they found that 2 hours held together in a special way, telling the stories of four specific youngsters. This footage was marketed as SATURDAY MORNING, a full-length entertainment film. It did not make much money, but it was seen by a vast theater audience which learned a great deal about the way adolescents view the world. Historically, motion picture audiences have learned about mental health treatment and clinicians in such films as SPELLBOUND, THE THREE FACES OF EVE, DAVID AND LISA, the films of Woody Allen, such as ANNIE HALL and INTERIORS, FREUD (with Montgomery Clift), and ONE FLEW OVER THE CUCKOO'S NEST. Occasionally, real therapists have been used to portray movie therapists, such as the psychiatrist in BOB AND CAROL AND TED AND ALICE. A significant motion picture for the understanding of a mental health problem, based upon an incident which happened at the Los Angeles Suicide Prevention Center, was THE SILVER THREAD, with Anne Bancroft and Sidney Poitier.

Regardless of how well these themes were clarified or roles were played, the exposure of a mass audience to therapists and mental health problems was significant. Motion pictures also offer much potential for consultation by mental health professionals, but few clinicians have been able to enter the competitive arena of feature film-making.

RADIO

Currently, the most controversial area of media usage is "radio psychology." Programs have sprung up in most cities of the United States (not to mention Taiwan, Puerto Rico, Australia, and Germany), and local stations now have the choice of a local mental health professional or a network "star." Over 45 stations (the number changes rapidly as stations alter format and personnel) have opted for local clinicians, many of whom are on the air on weekends or late hours. The TONI GRANT SHOW, which, while originating in Los Angeles, has interactive capabilities across the nation, is now carried by 23 network affiliates.

THE PROS

Proponents of radio psychology point out that the size of the mass audience reached by these programs makes this medium the ideal instrument for the primary prevention of mental and emotional disorders. For example, information on stress, depression and isolation is provided to members of that huge audience who frequently would have no interest in, or access to, mental health professionals. Through such programs listeners or callers are informed that they are not unique, that others have similar problems. Validation is given to those who are insecure about mothering or dieting, or who are seeking to stop smoking. Talk radio can also provide alternatives. Discussion of problems frequently opens up possibilities not previously thought of by listeners. It may provide impetus for discussion between husbands and wives or parents and children where there was no prior communication. It demystifies psychology and destigmatizes psychotherapy, so that people are freer to seek help if they need it. Referrals are often made to community agencies, and this raises the consciousness of lawmakers and their constituencies about the need for funding such services. Radio call-in programs typically model ways to talk to one's family and friends, to listen rather than to judge, and to accept the inevitability of error. They stress the universality of problems and lessen the feelings of guilt about not being able to solve one's own difficulties.

THE CONS

The critics of call-in radio point out that such programs set up expectations for instant cures and for active therapists who give advice. Thus, when listeners go into therapy, they have negative responses to the style of the average psychotherapist. Material may be presented which is too explicit for listeners, who may become upset. Or listeners may hear a symptom described, and, feeling that it resembles their own, take drastic actions which may be harmful. Callers may be disappointed if they do not get on programs after waiting a long time and are frequently left with their original problem unresolved plus the frustration of the call. Critics of radio psychology often object to particular hosts, pointing out a lack of professional qualifications or misrepresentation of credentials; they complain that there are insufficient disclaimers explaining that radio psychology is not psychotherapy. In addition, they point out that diagnosis and treatment are offered without sufficient data, that hosts frequently criticize other therapists as well as whole schools of psychotherapy, that hosts do not keep current with literature or are not sensitive to the needs of minority groups, and frequently make statements which are offensive to other professions.

Some of these arguments are true about some of those doing radio psychology; quality differs from person to person and even from one call to another. Critics do not take into account that many program hosts are not trained to work in media, and that increased experience, peer consultation, and training can modify or eliminate these unacceptable aspects of performance. Of course, this raises the uncomfortable ethical issue of limiting activities to an idividual's areas of competence. Even more difficult to address are arguments about time limitation inherent in the medium, which necessitates responding to minimal information with advice that in many instances, sounds simplistic and superficial; or the need to cut callers short even when more attention is needed; or problems of confidentiality, especially in rural areas, where voices or life circumstances can be recognized.

ETHICS AND THE FUTURE OF RADIO PSYCHOLOGY

Is radio psychology an area in which clinicians should become involved at all? Advice given through the media was prohibited for psychologists until the change in the APA Ethics Code in 1981. The code now reads, "Individual diagnostic and therapeutic services are provided only in the context of a professional relationship. When personal advice is given by means of public lectures or demonstrations, newspaper or magazine articles, radio or television programs, mail or similar media, the psychologist utilizes the most current relevant data and exercises the highest level of professional judgment" (Principle 4k). Just what constitutes "professional judgment," or how one keeps informed on the "most current relevant data" for all of the topics which surface during radio programs is yet to be spelled out. Even if capability existed for retrieval of the latest research on every problem, say, through computer terminals available to each call-in host, there is still a question about the usefulness of such information, since frequently research problems differ markedly from action problems (Kerlinger, 1977).

Of further concern is the lack of data on the effects of radio call-in programs upon the listeners or callers. To date, there has been little published research done in this area. Recently, the Markle Foundation has granted funds to the author and Patricia Keith-Spiegel, former chair of APA's Committee on Scientific and Professional Ethics and Conduct, to carry out several studies which are in various stages of completion. When we know more, we will be in a better position to evaluate the pros and cons of radio call-in programs. Meanwhile, we do know that being the host of a radio call-in program is not for everyone. It demands high verbal ability, quick response rate, the skill to translate psychological concepts into everyday language, an absence of unnecessary equivocation, a flare for directness, and above all, the ability to project caring and warmth. It also requires the ability to assist listeners and callers in dealing with problems themselves where possible, or in seeking assistance where necessary. In previous years, it also demanded an ability to operate in isolation and without the wholehearted support and recognition of a professional organization. This has changed since the establishment of the Association for Media Psychology.

THE ASSOCIATION FOR MEDIA PSYCHOLOGY

The Association for Media Psychology began as an interest group which grew out of a 1981 symposium on radio call-in programs chaired by the author, during which many of the program hosts talked about their feelings of alienation, isolation and lack of peer support. AMP was founded in February, 1982, with the following purposes:

1. To unite and provide a common meeting ground for those engaged in, or interested in, the use of media as they relate to mental health and human behavior;

2. To assist the mental health sciences and professions to disseminate information through the media;

3. To stimulate research on the potential contribution of the mental health sciences and professions to the media and through the media to the public;

4. To assist in effecting behavior change through the media for those individuals seeking to improve their quality of life, physically, emotionally and environmentally;

5. To improve the quality of the use of media by the mental health professions through establishment of standards of competence, professional ethics, and guidelines, as well as through skill building, peer review, and consultation.

Since its founding, AMP has grown rapidly and has broadened its focus from radio to include motion pictures, television, and print. Guidelines for media usage are in preparation, and seminars and workshops are planned for national, regional, and state conventions to train mental health professionals who would like to become involved with media. For the interested reader, more information on this organization can be obtained by writing to AMP, 228 Santa Monica Boulevard #3, Santa Monica, CA 90402.

PREPARATION FOR MEDIA PARTICIPATION

Mental health professionals are accustomed to "hanging out a shingle" and waiting for clients or patients. It is difficult for clinicians to recognize that media generally do not seek professionals out, except to act as unpaid experts. Even the choice of a particular expert has been haphazard, usually through recommendation of a friend who sees a psychologist. If one wishes to work in media, opportunities must be created, and training must have been completed beforehand in order to utilize opportunities.

It is unfortunate that in most instances our clinical training has not included instruction in media. Some professional organizations are beginning to offer continuing education workshops on media usage which allow members to obtain "hands-on" experience with cameras, tapes, and other materials, as well as on-camera practice. Many cable companies are offering free or low-cost seminars to individuals who might be sources of future programming material, and they are frequently eager to include mental health professionals. A phone call to the local cable station can usually elicit information about availability of such classes, which fill up rapidly and frequently require enrollment several months ahead of time. Community colleges and extension division courses in writing, programming, and producing for radio or television or the popular press are generally available and often provide excellent preparation, even though not specifically designed for mental health professionals.

More and more psychology departments are purchasing tape equipment for teaching interviewing skills, supervising sessions, providing case consultation, and so forth. There were workshops on Video Research at the 1981 and 1982 American Psychological Association conventions.

After you have learned about writing, cameras, production, and public speaking, how do you use your new abilities? You can prepare samples of your work and send them directly to a number of the program directors of either television, radio, or press or, if you live on the East or West Coast in a large urban center, you can hire an agent.

AGENTS, CHOICE AND USE

Agents have been described as "engineers who link creators and businessmen together with golden chains." If mental health professionals desire to be creators, serious thought should be given to working through an agent. If you live in a small community and can meet with program directors, you will, of course, work without an agent; but access to people responsible for "buying talent" in an urban metropolis is more easily obtained by an agent. Wherever you live, you are considered "talent." A mental health professional is considered a "performer" just like anyone else who appears on media, and the number of people who listen or watch your program or read your books or articles will determine your success. An agent obtains opportunities for you to show your work, advises you as to the way it should be shown, and negotiates the circumstances under which it will be shown. The pay, benefits, perks and problems such as make-up, transportation, dressing rooms, hours, vacation, and so on, all must be negotiated, and that is what an agent will do for you. One of the major problems is obtaining a reputable agent, since there are only about 800 licensed agents in the entire United States, and most of them are on either coast. Also, most agents will not handle more than one or two mental health professionals at any time, since there could be a conflict of interest. It is frequently difficult for mental health professionals to talk in terms of bargaining, wages, working conditions, or other issues, because of their nonbusiness orientation. Realistic approaches to the entertainment industry are emphasized by agents, who point out the basic tenets of business: If they don't pay you, they don't value you; in business, nothing is ever given away; and someone is making money on your services and you deserve a share.

SOME BASIC CONCERNS

Whether you are planning to work in print or the electronic media, you will be dealing with industry. If you write for the popular press, you must tailor your message toward book sales; if you host a talk radio program, you will have to be concerned about the Arbitron Reports; if you are on air or provide material for television, you face severe time and content restrictions. Whatever mass medium you choose, you face loss of control over your material (to some degree) and even over your style. Changes may be required in your message, your looks, your approach, and even, at times, your values. The twin sirens of stardom and profit may beckon you, with the potential to undermine your ethical stance and your professional dedication. The antidotes are difficult to find. Private funding for independent production or self-publishing, and increased use of public radio and cable or educational television are viable alternatives to working with the entertainment industries, which must rely on numbers. Audience appeal is their criterion of success. The broadest possible transmission of information about psychology is through the mass media. The choice of depth versus breadth remains with the mental health professions.

CONCLUSION

Professionalization of media use by mental health practitioners has begun with the establishment of the Association for Media Psychology, the promulgation of guidelines for media usage, and the acquisition of skills. Ability, preparation, and practice are necessary for the beginning media professional. Many important questions remain unanswered about ethical issues and the effects of media psychology on readers, listeners, viewers, and participants. The future of media psychology will depend not only on outcome studies of media's effectiveness in the prevention of mental and emotional disorders, but on the response from the public about the usefulness of mental health information provided by mental health professionals through the media.

> Jacqueline C. Bouhoutsos, Ph.D., is currently in private practice as a clinical psychologist in Santa Monica, California. She is Founder/President of the Association for Media Psychology and Clinical Professor of Psychology at the University of California at Los Angeles. Dr. Bouhoutsos may be contacted at the Association for Media Psychology, 228 Santa Monica Boulevard, Suite #3, Santa Monica, CA 90401.

RESOURCES

American Psychological Association. COMMUNICATING WITH THE PUBLIC VIA THE MEDIA ABOUT PSYCHOLOGY. Washington, DC: Author, 1979.

American Psychological Association. ETHICAL STANDARDS OF PSYCHOLOGISTS. Washington, DC: Author, 1981.

American Psychological Association. MEDIA GUIDE. Washington, DC: Public Information Office, APA, 1980.

American Psychiatric Association. Guidelines for psychiatrists working with the communications media. AMERICAN JOURNAL OF PSYCHIATRY, 1977, **134**, 609-611.

Joslyn-Scherer, M. S. COMMUNICATION IN THE HUMAN SERVICES. Beverly Hills, CA: Sage Publications, 1980.

Keith-Spiegel, P. & Koocher, G. ETHICS IN PSYCHOLOGY (Tentative title). Reading, MA: Addison-Wesley, in press.

Kerlinger, F. N. The influence of research on educational practice. EDUCATIONAL RESEARCHER, 1977, **6**, 5-12.

Larson, C. Media psychology's new roles and new responsibilities. APA MONITOR, 1981, **12**, pp. 3; 9; 12.

McAlister, A., Puska, P., Koskela, K., Pallonen, U., & Maccoby, N. Mass communication and community organization for public health education. AMERICAN PSYCHOLOGIST, 1980, **35**, 375-379.

McCall, R. & Stocking, S. Between scientists and the public: Communicating psychological research through the mass media. AMERICAN PSYCHOLOGIST, 1982, **37**, 985-995.

Miller, G. A. Psychology as a means of promoting human welfare. AMERICAN PSYCHOLOGIST, 1969, **24**, 1063-1075.

National Institute of Mental Health. TELEVISION AND BEHAVIOR: TEN YEARS OF SCIENTIFIC PROGRESS AND IMPLICATIONS FOR THE EIGHTIES, 1982, **1**, 1-94.

Rosen, G. M. Guidelines for the review of do-it-yourself treatment books. CONTEMPORARY PSYCHOLOGY, 1981, **26**, 189-191.

Schwebell, A. I. Radio psychologists: A community psychology/psycho-educational model. JOURNAL OF COMMUNITY PSYCHOLOGY, 1982, **10**, 181-184.

Turkat, D. CABLE TELEVISION IN PSYCHOLOGY: FUTURISTIC CONSIDERATIONS. Paper presented at the American Psychological Association Convention, Washington, D.C., August, 1982.

NEW ROLES IN CONSULTATION
WITH POLICE

W. Parke Fitzhugh

My goal in preparing this contribution is to offer readers an introduction to consultation with police. The observations discussed are based on over a decade of work, primarily with a large metropolitan police department. My functions during that time have been varied and the discussion which follows will focus only on certain aspects of consultation. It is my hope that readers will come away with a valuable perspective on police issues and needs as well as a foundation upon which to build consultation in this area.

As pointed out by Miller (1982), it is important to be familiar with factors which can influence the consultation process when working with almost any group. This may be especially so when working with the police (Mann, 1973). Primary factors which affect consultation effectiveness with police agencies include the police culture and the type of expectations that individuals in a police agency have for the consultant.

CULTURAL CONSIDERATIONS

Although there are some variations, norms are fairly consistent among police agencies. Police value dominance, suspiciousness, and aggressiveness. While individual values may range from conservative to liberal, the predominant outlook tends to be conservative. Discipline is emphasized by police managers in order to keep police aggressiveness within reasonable bounds. Police management styles tend to be autocratic. The emphasis on discipline and autocratic management results in criticism or punishment far outweighing rewards for performance by officers. Communication may go down the chain of command from higher ranking to lower ranking individuals with some effectiveness, but communication from lower ranks up to higher ranks tends to be limited and ineffectual. Lower ranking personnel are also likely to complain of poor supervision, excessive paperwork, lack of proper equipment, and favoritism based on personality rather than performance. While police may also complain about the ineffectual criminal justice system, especially the courts, as well as the type of people with whom they come in frequent contact, the majority of their complaints are likely to be directed at the agency for which they work. Eisenberg (1975) provides a thorough summary of the factors affecting lower ranking police personnel.

Mid-management personnel (lieutenants, captains) may have a different set of job pressures. They often describe themselves as caught in the middle between upper management and lower management, having to enforce regulations for lower management personnel including ones with which they may not agree. Mid-management personnel also may bear the brunt of complaints from the officer and sergeant level but feel powerless to act on the complaints if they are directed at policies of upper police management or the governmental body for which they work.

Upper level management (majors, colonels, chiefs) are faced with the challenge of responding to political pressures, budgetary demands, and maintaining disciplinary and administrative control of the organization.

Police organizations generally are not readily open to change, although there may be individuals who very much want to introduce and see change occur within the organization. Change has been occurring with some regularity in police organizations since the late 1960's, particularly because of external pressures such as riots, pressures from minority groups for more equitable treatment, and federal money from the Law Enforcement Assistance Administration which was used as seed money to induce new programs. More recently pressure for the development of psychological service programs in police agencies has developed in part by incidents involving violence by officers who had a history of instability. Also, through federal and local dollars, police have been much more involved in education and training in the last decade and have become considerably more aware of the potential use of psychological expertise in crisis intervention, hostage negotiation, and dealing with patterns of deviant behavior.

The factors I have noted reflect some of the challenges to be faced in consulting with police agencies. Additionally, police are likely to want specific techniques and answers to their everyday problems, rather than being interested in theoretical explanations of behavior or conceptual strategies. Police value survival, both on the street and within the organization. They tend to respond most readily to information or approaches which they feel provides immediate assistance for their own survival. Police also tend to be suspicious of "outsiders," believing that only those experienced in police work can understand what the police officer faces. Police experience with professionals in social service agencies has also led to skepticism about the motives and commitment to service by professionals. Police often find social service agencies closed when police most need help in dealing with disturbed or destitute individuals.

With this background it should be apparent that police may be skeptical of the commitment of a consultant, unless they believe the consultant is available at times other than the usual 9 to 5 weekday work hours. A study by Brown, Burkhart, King, and Solomon (1977) shows the response of police officers to a survey in which role expectations from mental health specialists working with police were rank ordered by police and by psychologists. Highest ranked expectations of police, in addition to being taught human relations skills, included having the consultant always be on call for consultation and available to provide assistance in crisis intervention, as well as presenting the police officers' viewpoint to the community.

Keeping these factors in mind, it is important for a potential police consultant to consider the amount of time available and the scheduled time commitment that can be made, as well as the nature of activities in which he or she has, or can, develop consultation skills.

DETERMINING AREAS OF CONSULTATION

There are numerous areas of behavioral science application within police work in addition to the traditional ones of selection (Spielberger, 1979), crisis intervention (Bard & Berkowitz, 1967), and counseling. Such areas include recruit and in-service training programs, including the design and the actual execution of training, management consultation, and consultation in investigations of various types. Specific suggestions for various interventions will be listed later in this chapter.

The first issue, of course, may be gaining entry into the police agency. If a police agency has not requested specific services, the consultant might approach the agency offering services in which he or she feels most qualified. As Miller (1982) has indicated, listening is an important first step in the consultation process, and this is especially useful in approaching consultation with police agencies. A listening approach allows the consultant to gradually become familiar with not only individuals, but some of the culture and the jargon of the police world, and it can reduce the perception of the consultant as an "outsider."

If a professional approaches the police agency seeking consultation opportunities, contacting either the head of the agency or the training bureau, if the agency has one, may be the best entry point. It is even more useful if he or she can establish contact beforehand with an individual or individuals who can provide information about the organization, its philosophy, its politics, and possible areas most subject to consultation needs. If the consultation hours are to be limited to certain times, it is best to provide services which will fit those hours readily, such as training or management consultation. If a contract is made to provide emergency counseling services for police officers or to assist in crisis intervention, the likelihood of the consultant being called at other than normal working hours increases. With small departments (25 to 50 people), such calls may not be frequent. With larger departments, however, such calls can occur very often.

CONTRACTUAL CONSIDERATIONS

Table 1 contains a summary of the contract I have used. In addition to specifying the duties for which the consultant is held responsible, an important part of the contract is the indemnification and hold-harmless section which protects the consultant from being sued personally and also obligates the agency to provide the defense of the consultant against civil suits. If it is possible that he or she may do work on an extra-hours emergency basis with the department, the contract should include an "upset clause" which provides compensation for any extra hours that are required. Consultants may wish to consult an attorney regarding the details of any contract before signing.

It is important that the consultant report to the head of the agency, rather than be shunted down to a lower ranking entity such as a Personnel Bureau. Reporting at the top of the chain of command gives the consultant a much better channel for identifying problems. It also lets other members of the organization know that the consultant does not have a number of people who would appear to have authority over him or her, and that the consultant does not have to struggle to get information up the ineffectual communication network.

**TABLE 1:   SUMMARY OF CONTRACT OF DR. PARKE FITZHUGH
             FOR CONSULTING SERVICES WITH METRO-DADE POLICE**

RESPONSIBILITIES OF DR. FITZHUGH

Dr. Fitzhugh is hereby awarded an exclusive right and contract to furnish, and Dr. Fitzhugh shall furnish, psychological consultation to the Dade County Public Safety Department (hereinafter the "Public Safety Department"), according to the following particulars:

1. Consult with the Director of the Public Safety Department concerning behavioral science applications in organizational management. Applications may include recommendations concerning: communications flow between the various divisions and between those divisions and the Office of the Directors, and communications flow throughout the Department; approaches which assist in effective communications in staff meetings; approaches which may assist in facilitating job motivation and performance of departmental employees; factors which affect morale; psychological dynamics affecting organizational functioning and effectiveness; and psychological aspects of personnel selection.

2. Consult with the Director of the Public Safety Department or his subordinates concerning the psychological stability of police personnel whose performance is suggestive of instability. Such consultation may include recommendations as to whether the concerned individual should be relieved of police authority, including badge and gun, and subsequent recommendations concerning the readiness of the individual to resume full police duties.

3. Consult with the Director of the Public Safety Department or his subordinates concerning training programs in: stress management and reduction, crisis intervention, hostage negotiations, dealing with emotionally disturbed individuals, interview techniques, supervisory counseling, and behavioral science applications in management.

4. Provide training in programs outlined in 3 above.

5. Consult with the Director of the Public Safety Department or his subordinates concerning officers who appear to have a pattern of unnecessary conflict with the public.

6. Consult with investigatory personnel concerning psychological aspects of investigations including but not limited to sexual battery, homicide, arson, and individuals making threats against public figures.

7. Provide short term counseling and crisis intervention for Public Safety Department personnel for issues which affect job performance.

8. Provide consultation for situations involving hostages or barricaded subjects.

9. Provide consultation to and/or concerning police involved in shooting or other traumatic incidents involving death and/or violence.

10. Provide professional staff supervision for the Public Safety Department police officer serving as Assistant for Psychological Services and Training.

11. Periodically visit Public Safety Department facilities for consultation.

12. Provide office space for counseling, crisis intervention, and other consultation requirements for the Public Safety Department.

13. Serve in the delivery of these services for a maximum of 23 hours total per week for 47 weeks per year.

INDEMNIFICATION AND HOLD HARMLESS

The County agrees to indemnify and hold Dr. Fitzhugh harmless from any and all claims, liability, losses and causes of action which may arise out of the rendering of services contained herein, unless the result of an act or acts conducted in bad faith or with malicious purpose or in a manner exhibiting wanton and willful disregard of human rights, safety, or property. The County shall pay all claims and losses in connection herewith, unless excepted as detailed above, and will undertake the defense of Dr. Fitzhugh against all civil suits which may arise out of any acts or events occurring pursuant to the provisions of this contract, and pay all costs and judgments which may issue therefrom.

CANCELLATION OR TERMINATION

The county shall have the right to terminate this contract, in whole or in part as relates to one of the departments involved, after a minimum 30 calendar days written notice to Dr. Fitzhugh.

Dr Fitzhugh shall have the right to terminate this contract, in whole or in part as relates to one of the departments involved, after a minimum 30 calendar days written notice to the County by certified mail or other appropriate receipt.

A summary of the time distribution by type of duties in my experience working with a police agency of about 2500 employees is found in Table 2. The summary includes activities of an assistant for psychological services who is a police experienced individual at the master's level in psychology. We have found that a cost effective approach to presentation of psychological services for police works well with the master's level individual who is available on 24-hour call for police emergencies such as shootings, hostage situations, and barricaded persons. Additionally, the master's level person's credibility among qualified police personnel as an experienced officer has assisted significantly in the development of a positive attitude among police toward the psychological service program. Such a program also takes some of the pressure off the consultant in terms of handling emergency situations on a 24-hour a day basis. I find this a very important consideration as police emergencies seem more likely to occur during evening and weekend hours. A master's level assistant with police experience and authority can also work in active police enforcement situations in which it would not be appropriate for a civilian to be present.

TABLE 2: DISTRIBUTION OF TIME OF CONSULTANT AND ASSISTANT
BY TYPE OF ACTIVITY FOR A POLICE DEPARTMENT OF 2,500 PEOPLE

Area of Consultation	Consultant (Ph.D.) Hours Per Month	Assistant (M.A.) Hours Per Month
Organizational development	4	4
Employee performance problems	7	10
Personal development problems	1	4
Evaluation of emotional stability	2	0
Personality factors in investigations	1	3
Hypnosis	4	0
Suitability of employee for specific job	1	0
Callouts for hostage and barricaded subject negotiations	0	16
Training program design	3	15
Recruit performance	0	4
Stress Management Seminars	6	16
Hostage Negotiation Training	8	20
Training in behavioral science applications to management	1	8
Spouse and family groups	1	1
Brief counseling in death, injury, and shooting situations	2	25
Long term counseling in death, injury, and shooting situations	2	0
Counseling in personal crisis and stress management	19	15
Human relations problems: conflict with supervisors, subordinates, peers, public	13	15
Public relations contacts with the media	2	1
Public speaking engagements	1	3
Attendance at seminars	0	4
Administrative duties for department: reports, answering letters	0	16
Supervision of assistant	14	0

AREAS OF INTERVENTION

SELECTION

Spielberger (1979) gives an excellent overview of issues in psychological assessment for selection purposes in police work. This section will give a brief review of issues in the area.

An important concern is whether psychological screening of police applicants, even if it were highly reliable, is of critical importance in increasing the likelihood of appropriate and effective police behavior. In my view there are many other factors besides the entry level personality characteristics of an officer that determine police behavior. The nature of the organization in which the officer works, the experience which that individual has on the job, the amount of stress in his or her off-duty life, the type of training he or she receives, and, most importantly, his or her day-to-day supervision will be critical in performance. Therefore, effective application of psychological principles with the goal of assisting and producing more effective police work should be directed at many areas in addition to selection, which has been the traditional utilization of psychologists. It is important, however, to utilize a screening process as it is not unusual for individuals with personality disorders to apply for police work, and there is little likelihood that the sophisticated disorder will be recognized in recruit training or in field assignments until he or she is involved in gross police misconduct. Among the types of personality patterns to be screened out are individuals with any of the following characteristics: a tendency to be very passive or very aggressive, especially in conflict situations; a need for very high levels of excitement; neurotic behavior patterns; over control of anger and hostility; highly authoritarian patterns of behavior; poor self-concept; psychotic behaviors.

The "screening out" approach may be more realistic to attempt than "screening in," or predicting levels of police performance. Even attempts to use a screening out approach can be fraught with difficulties, as certain testing procedures may be subject to court challenge, especially in the area of ethnic bias. A complicating problem is that guidelines established by the Equal Employment Opportunity Commission in 1970 and those established in 1976 by the Federal Executive Agency appear to be in conflict as noted by Baer (1979), since the FEA guidelines seem to shift emphasis more to merit considerations than equal opportunity considerations.

A major problem in establishing the effectiveness of screening in procedures, which attempt to differentiate between levels of effectiveness in police performance, is that of establishing valid criteria which can be objectively measured. This tends to be especially difficult in police systems, as supervisors have a propensity to give most employees satisfactory or average ratings unless they are at extremes of performance. The development of behaviorally anchored rating systems is an important area in criteria establishment and can be a useful area for psychological consultation.

An important issue concerning criteria is their transportability from department to department. A study by Baer and Oppenheim (1979) indicated there were differences in specific job activities for patrol officers in five different cities, and for state troopers in five states. Thus, caution should be applied in assuming that job criteria established in one police locale will be totally suitable in another locale.

Even the apparently less complicated objective of screening out unsuitable personnel becomes difficult when establishing which instruments might best be used. The Minnesota Multiphasic Personality Inventory (MMPI) is controversial because of its emphasis on psychopathology, and there are conflicting opinions concerning its possible racial bias. The California Psychological Inventory (CPI) has been well researched in this area and has scales whose supposed area of measurement relate to police behavior (Spielberger, 1979); however, it is not likely to be as sensitive to psychopathology as the MMPI. The Sixteen Personality Factor Questionnaire (16 PF) might also be considered as an adjunct to the MMPI or CPI in terms of examining consistency between patterns on the respective tests. Axelberd (1982) has found that the MMPI and 16 PF complement each other well in assessing applicants based on his experience with over 3,000 police applicants. Fabricatore, Azen, Schoentgen, and Snibbe (1978) found the 16 PF had small but significant correlations with police performance based on superior performance criteria rather than "screen out" performance.

An alternative approach to psychological testing in screening now being developed is the Assessment Center. Filer (1979) outlines the approach in which multiple assessment techniques are used, including job simulation exercises. Trained observers provide judgments about behavior based on specially developed assessment simulations. To date, the assessment center approach seems to offer promise, although it takes time to get established and for assessors to be trained. The assessment center approach may have particular utility in selection for promotional positions within police work as it offers a chance for the development of valid criteria for supervisory positions.

Currently, individual psychological assessment for selecting applicants or promotional candidates is very much limited by the lack of adequate job performance criteria for the positions. The content of psychological evaluations provided for police agencies should be carefully considered by consultants in this area. Reports should be written with the understanding that they may be public record and that the individual about whom it is written, as well as the media, may ultimately have access to the report. The police department to which it is sent should also make a commitment to the limited distribution of the evaluation and responsibility for file maintenance. The psychologist may provide a description of an individual's behavior patterns, but should not take responsibility for determining whether the individual should be hired. The department should be responsible for working out its own standards and criteria for applicants and should assume final responsibility for decision making.

RECRUIT TRAINING IN STRESS MANAGEMENT

A popular area of training for recruits is stress management. The consultant in this area will probably face the dilemma of being requested to design and execute a thorough stress management program while being offered insufficient time and follow-through to support the initial training. Police recruits receive training in a number of areas which they see as critical to their survival and as likely to be more exciting than stress management training. Those areas would include felony stops, criminal law enforcement, firearms, search and seizure, and self-defense training. Consequently, if the techniques and values advanced in stress management training are not consistently reinforced through the training period, the likelihood of their retention begins to decrease significantly.

A critical factor in training effectiveness is the philosophy and demeanor of the training staff who, in their day-to-day contacts with the recruits, can either support the training or effectively undermine it. For this reason it is important to work with training staff to insure as much as possible their support for stress management programs, as well as their participation in reinforcing the concepts of stress management when recruits are involved in other training procedures. For example, a supportive and knowledgeable staff will be able to reinforce stress management principles during felony stop training, crisis intervention training, moot courtroom training, self-defense training, and on the firearms range. That participation is often best fostered by training the trainers, then involving them in program design and in-team teaching efforts. I have found that once police trainers understand the concepts and feel confident in explaining and using them, they can become excellent instructors and are powerful in terms of shaping the attitudes of police recruits.

The content of stress management training should be very explicit in its application to police recruit training and subsequent performance. Effectiveness of training is usually heightened when the content is directed towards specifics of how the police recruit can protect himself or herself. I have found a series of films by Harper & Row, including INTERNALIZING PROBLEMS, EXTERNALIZING PROBLEMS, and DEATH AWARENESS, to be excellent tools in relating stress management directly to police work. Also it is very useful to bring into the classroom a police officer who has experienced and mastered high stress situations such as having been in a serious shooting situation, or an officer who has been shot and survived. Especially helpful is the officer who can openly talk of his or her feelings, the importance of dealing with them, and the effects of the experience on family members.

The inclusion of family members in a session designed for the effects of police stress on family interaction is a useful adjunct to recruit training. In addition to giving the trainee and his or her family an opportunity to learn stress mastery techniques as they affect marital and family relationships, it also seems to increase the likelihood that the trainee and family members will appropriately seek professional help later in response to psychological stress. A particularly important part of stress mastery training for police recruits is providing them with information on how they may seek professional help and how they may be protected by privileged communication and need not reveal any assistance they seek.

Stress mastery techniques for specific groups such as minorities and women in police work might also be considered as part of police recruit training. Glaser and Saxe (1982), for example, report a program which is designed to help women cope with the conflicting demands they find others make upon them or they make upon themselves to be both feminine and aggressively masculine in the police role.

Murray and Grace (1982) outline a basic approach for a stress management workshop. Martin (1982) summarizes the stress inoculation approach, and Novaco (1977) presents an anger management procedure for training law enforcement officers. Territo and Vetter (1981) have edited a text which provides an excellent overview of stress related issues in police work. The content of that text can provide a good familiarization for the consultant concerning the difficulties which are likely to be encountered by police recruits in their future work.

Other areas of training useful for police recruits include nonverbal communication, crisis intervention strategies, specifics of how to deal with mentally disturbed individuals and relaxation techniques. The latter have been particularly useful for many recruits during firearms training in overcoming anxiety and muscle spasms which can significantly impair the individual's ability to control the weapon.

IN-SERVICE TRAINING

Strategies of in-service training may be similar to those applied in recruit training as outlined previously. Stress mastery courses for the experienced officer should cover stress identification, stress prevention, and methods of recovering from stress. Axelberd and Valle (1981) outline a 40 hour in-service stress mastery program covering psychological, physiological, and nutritional components.

Hostage Negotiation. A major area of police interest in psychological principles is in hostage negotiations. Bolz and Hershey (1979) give examples of the type of hostage situations which can occur. Many departments have special weapons teams used for the tactical aspect of such situations, but fewer departments have well trained police negotiators.

My philosophy has been to have the negotiation process confined to police personnel with the consultant functioning as a trainer and/or on-the-scene consultant. There are several advantages to this approach. Most importantly, the police officer is likely to be aware of legal and procedural matters with which the consultant may be unfamiliar. I have found also that police officers become much more committed to the learning process when they know that they will be the ones responsible for implementation of the training.

A model which I have found successful for hostage negotiation training begins with a 40-hour course. The first 16 hours involve presenting guidelines for negotiation situations and basic behavior observation and listening exercises, with the last 24 hours of the course involving simulations of hostage situations of increasing complexity and difficulty. The simulations include audio and video tape recording and replay, with the simulations stopped about every 15 minutes for review of the process to that point. Field simulations are conducted during night hours and bad weather in order to simulate as closely as possible the types of incidents that are likely to occur. Police endorsement of the program increases proportionately to the realism and challenge involved in the training. It is also important for training to occur on a regular basis so that police negotiators can maintain skill levels, confidence, and field support for the program. The Metro-Dade Police Department with which I consult has three four-person teams of negotiators who are scheduled for 16 hours of training per month.

Hostage negotiation training principles apply not only to hostage situations, but to incidents in which individuals barricade themselves in stores or residences. Such incidents may occur in the case of individuals undergoing emotional crisis or those involved in criminal activity who are surrounded by police. Generally, negotiation strategies involve the use of time and effective listening approaches to reduce the level of tension and excitement involved with the situation as well as to induce rapport between the negotiator and the person involved. I do not think it is appropriate to make specific strategies publicly available. If you are interested in more specific information, please contact me directly.

In starting a negotiation training program, it is important to get the endorsement of the department concerning the philosophy and implementation of that program. The principle of moving slowly rather than using force quickly is not in keeping with traditional police enforcement tactics. Since much of the training may emphasize dealing with individual emotions in a highly sensitive manner, even if those individuals are involved in criminal behavior, it may appear to be in conflict with other police enforcement approaches. Although police practices are gradually changing, there remains a tendency to favor action over words and patience. I have found that one of the most important factors in gaining support for the negotiation approach is the reduced risk to police safety when negotiations rather than tactical assaults can be utilized. Indirect benefit of a negotiation program is that the officers involved may become a cadre of instructors in behavioral science approaches, and they may also become highly credible sources of referral to psychological services for those individuals needing help.

Other In-Service Training. Other areas of opportunity for psychological consultation in in-service training programs are patterns and factors in deviant and criminal behavior, dynamics of group psychology as they relate to crowd and riot situations, principles of effective interviewing, the application of behavioral science principles to supervision and management, and factors in stress and decision making. In the latter area, I have found research by Janis and Mann (1977) to be very useful. Decision making in stress situations is very relevant to day-to-day police functioning, as they typically face circumstances in which any decision that is made appears to be associated with some risk. I have used a training program which involves simulation of high stress decision situations along with a requirement that the participants analyze the process which affected their decisions.

Another area that merits attention is police work with informants. Ironically, in spite of traditional police suspiciousness, some officers may be readily manipulated by sociopathic informants because a combination of the stress of the situation and relative naivete about the sociopath results in vulnerability on the officer's part.

COUNSELING AND CRISIS INTERVENTION FOR POLICE PERSONNEL

When establishing counseling services with a police agency, it is important to have clear guidelines as to the extent of services and length of therapy that will be provided. Providing long term therapy can quickly fill up all of a consultant's time since the job stress and marital and family problems can result in a significant number of individuals seeking professional help, especially if the agency covers all the cost of that help. A model I have found to be successful is to provide short term crisis intervention and problem solving counseling which is typically limited to a maximum of 6 hours. Those needing longer term assistance are referred to community agencies or individual practitioners. The model for each agency will be affected by the budget limitations of that agency.

Vehlow and Kropp (1982) summarize principles in developing employee assistance programs. Their strategies may also apply for designing consultant services with a police agency.

Referrals for Counseling or Evaluation. A most important area in establishing availability of counseling services for police is the outline of procedures which provide reassurance that counseling contacts are confidential and cannot be used against the officer. If an officer is to be directed to a psychological evaluation, which is often within the authority of a head of a police agency, the individuals in the organization who have such authority should be clearly specified. Such individuals should be of high rank, and guidelines should call for a consultation with the consultant before referral to determine if it is, in fact, appropriate. Since reports from resultant evaluations are usually public record, as with entry level screening reports, they should be carefully worded. I have found it best for a psychologist other than the individual who does the day-to-day counseling to conduct such evaluations. Both consultant and officer could be placed in a compromised position if the individual were directed to report for psychological evaluation to the same professional who had already done counseling on a confidential basis.

Police supervisors are becoming more likely to refer subordinates for counseling or evaluation, since it has become evident that they can be in a position of vicarious civil liability if they recognized an emotional problem and failed to take action. In my experience, when officers are presented with a choice of reporting to counseling voluntarily so that there is privileged communication, versus being ordered for evaluation with no privileged communication, they consistently choose the former. Also, as a psychological service program gains credibility, voluntary self-referrals increase significantly, and there are fewer instances of individuals being ordered for evaluation. The most notable exception to this principle lies in the area of alcohol abuse.

A significant percentage of counseling is likely to be related to marital and family problems. A typical police pattern is to carry over from job to family relationships patterns of dominance, suspiciousness, cynicism, and covering of emotions. Families can experience intense anxiety about the physical welfare of the officer, and the officer may be caught between the demands of the family to leave the job and his or her attraction to the excitement and rewards of the position. Officers may also become over-protective of their families, based on regular exposure to violence and alcohol and drug abuse. In many police agencies the divorce rate is high, which serves to worry officers' families and, in some cases, seems to create expectations of the inevitability of broken marriages.

A consultant can also be very helpful in crisis situations such as those involving the death or injury of a police officer. Assisting both family members and police co-workers, who function much as a family, can assist in reducing the potential for long term maladaptive reactions to the experience.

Post Traumatic Situations. Another constructive area for consultant intervention involves work with post shooting and traumatic incident reactions. Police who are involved in shootings, especially those in which the officer kills someone or in which another officer is shot, are often negatively affected by the experience. Shooting experiences can be highly personal to the officers involved and can result in feelings of helplessness and vulnerability, poorly directed anger, concerns with "what if," and guilt. The guilt reaction may be very powerful if the officers somehow feel they did not handle themselves as they "should have." This is especially common in situations in which one police officer survives a shooting without injury, while one or more other officers are shot. In my experience, if the affected officer has a high need for control or is a perfectionist, the subsequent negative reaction seems to be more pronounced.

Frequent reactions to shootings include sensory distortion in which time seems to slow down in the memory of the incident, flashbacks to the incident, temporary sleep disturbance, and trying to act as though "nothing really happened," including not discussing the situation with spouse or family "so as not to upset them." If the officer is unsuccessful in resolving initial doubts or conflicts over the incident, more serious long term reactions including psychosomatic illnesses, serious marital and family conflict, overaggressiveness and risk taking, or depression may occur.

Early intervention helps reduce the likelihood of severe or sustained post traumatic reactions. An effective approach is one in which the officer is contacted immediately after the shooting for debriefing concerning psychological reactions. The debriefing centers on what some of the typical reactions might be, how normal those reactions can be, indicating that the officer is "not losing his or her mind," and what mastery approaches would be useful. Emphasis is placed on the officer's being able to verbalize and accept the feelings typical of such experiences and to share those feelings with family members. If the officer has been involved in a fatal shooting, the debriefing must not interfere with homicide investigators' gathering of information. Consultants involved in this type of work should be fully informed about privileged communication statutes which may apply in their state and discuss implications with interviewees before proceeding.

For such a program to be effective, it should receive the formal sanction of the police department. The Metro-Date Police Department has supported this kind of program through an administrative order, and the majority of police officers have reacted very favorably. Working with the department in the establishment of the program can also reduce the probability of supervisors and peers treating the officer involved in the shooting as if he or she were a hero, which can often put the officer in more of a quandary as to how to react. Provisions for the involved officer to have one or more days off after the shooting are also appropriate.

Other police activities, such as work at a major disaster or accident scene, have potential for creating post traumatic stress. Wagner (1980) outlines a debriefing program for police who handle an airline disaster, which also has the potential for producing post traumatic reactions.

MANAGEMENT CONSULTATION

The principles of organization development which are outlined elsewhere in this volume (Goodstein & Cooke, 1983) will help develop effectiveness in most police organizations. This can, however, be a most difficult area to implement due to the cultural norms outlined at the beginning of this chapter. Preserving the **status quo** rather than becoming involved in risk taking and exploring possible organization problems happens to be the favorite style of many managers. Nevertheless, more individuals in leadership positions are being exposed to progressive management ideas in college courses and are becoming interested in exploring ways to improve organizational effectiveness.

It is best to work cautiously and gradually with organization change or development programs. Before any program is instituted, the risk involved should be considered, especially factors which could result in the program being stopped abruptly or gradually losing its emphasis. Any program which results in management feeling uncomfortable or appears to underline serious problems in their units is likely to have great difficulty in succeeding. The exception to this guideline would occur in the case of such a program being implemented under a strong leader who leaves no alternative to subordinates but to explore management effectiveness, and who also makes a point of rewarding such efforts. There should be a strong commitment to regular follow-through on any program. This is particularly important in police agencies which must respond regularly to crisis, a process which can consistently disrupt scheduled activities. A useful approach in management consultation involves the use of a team building format. I have found the Team Building Survey developed by McGregor (1967) to be valuable for this purpose. Another resource to which interested readers my wish to refer is **IMPROVING WORK GROUPS: A PRACTICAL MANUAL FOR TEAM BUILDING** by Francis and Young (1979).

An area of functioning that is often in need of improvement in police agencies is conflict management. In keeping with cultural norms noted previously, conflict is often handled by either avoidance or the use of power plays to overwhelm those in opposition. I have found that self-assessment tools such as the Conflict Management Survey and the Power Motivation Inventory by Teleometrics (see Resource section) are useful in helping managers look at their leadership styles. Use of the surveys also provides a conceptual basis and useful behavioral labels for subsequent analysis of group process. For individuals who are not threatened by self-assessment, I have found the California Psychological Inventory to be very useful in helping managers examine their styles.

OTHER AREAS OF CONSULTATION

Other areas which may provide consultation opportunities are reflected in the Table 2 which describes my activities. Of those areas, the application of hypnosis for victims and witnesses merits particular consideration. Although Reiser (1980) reports success in the use of hypnosis, including teaching police investigators hypnotic techniques, acceptance of testimony gathered under hypnosis is not accepted in all courts. Incorrect information elicited under hypnosis was critical in Arizona and Minnesota courts ruling testimony developed under hypnosis is inadmissible (Bodine & Levine, 1980). As reported by Loftus and Loftus (1980), hypnotic memory is not necessarily accurate, and the type of questions asked of the subject under hypnosis may influence that subject's reported memories. Additionally, if a subject's memory reports are altered under hypnosis by leading questions, that process may alter subsequent memory based reports (Turkington, 1982). Such factors emphasize the importance of the hypnotist asking only general and nonleading questions.

Recording the session can be useful in responding to any subsequent challenges concerning the proper handling of the process.

CONSULTATION AREAS AND ETHICAL CONSIDERATIONS

The range of consultation possibilities covered above suggests the many issues or dilemmas a police agency consultant may face, including confidentiality, responsibility to the client, representation of competence level, conflicts of interest, and other general ethical issues (e.g., it is important not to overstate one's qualifications in areas such as personnel selection or forensic hypnosis). The consultant's responsibility to the client should include the education of the client concerning the skills, limitations, and ethical principles of the consultant. Mann (1980) provides an in depth review of such issues to be faced by psychologists in police agencies. In my experience, a basic guideline for consultants is to make only those commitments to individuals or to an agency that can be met within the constraints of ethical principles, the consultant's skill level, and time availability.

W. Parke Fitzhugh, Ph.D., is currently in private practice in Miami, Florida. He holds a doctorate in clinical psychology and is Consulting Psychologist to the Metro-Dade Fire and Police Departments. His primary interests are in the areas of organizational dynamics, stress management, hypnosis, and family therapy. Dr. Fitzhugh may be contacted at 2400 South Dixie Highway, Suite 202, Miami, FL 33133.

RESOURCES

Axelberd, M. PERSONAL COMMUNICATION, July 7, 1982.

Axelberd, M. & Valle, J. Stress control program for police officers of the City of Miami Police Department. In L. Territo & H. J. Vetter (Eds.), STRESS AND POLICE PERSONNEL. Boston: Allyn & Bacon, 1981.

Baer, M. E. Impact of civil rights legislation and court actions on personnel procedures and practices. In C. Spielberger (Ed.), POLICE SELECTION AND EVALUATION. New York: Praeger Publishers, 1979.

Baer, M. E. & Oppenheim, A. B. Job analysis in police selection research. In C. Speilberger (Ed.), POLICE SELECTION AND EVALUATION. New York: Praeger Publishers, 1979.

Bard, M. & Berkowitz, B. Training police as specialists in family crisis intervention: A community psychology action project. COMMUNITY MENTAL HEALTH JOURNAL, 1967, 3, 315-317.

Bodine, L. & Levine, D. Hypnosis runs into court wall. THE NATIONAL LAW JOURNAL, June 2, 1980, 1-2.

Bolz, F. A. & Hershey, E. HOSTAGE COP. New York: Harper and Row, 1979.

Brown, S., Burkhart, B. R., King, G. D., & Solomon, R. Roles and expectations for mental health professionals in law enforcement agencies. AMERICAN JOURNAL OF COMMUNITY PSYCHOLOGY, 1977, 5, 207-215.

Eisenberg, T. Labor management relations and psychological stress: View from the bottom. THE POLICE CHIEF, 1975, pp. 54-58.

Fabricatore, J., Azen, S., Schoentgen, S., & Snibbe, H. Predicting performance of police officers using the Sixteen Personality Factor Questionnaire. AMERICAN JOURNAL OF COMMUNITY PSYCHOLOGY, 1978, *6*, 63-69.

Filer, R. J. The assessment center method in the selection of law enforcement officers. In C. D. Spielberger (Ed.), POLICE SELECTION AND EVALUATION. New York: Praeger, 1979.

Francis, D. & Young, D. IMPROVING WORK GROUPS: A PRACTICAL MANUAL FOR TEAM BUILDING. San Diego: University Associates, 1979.

Glaser, D. F. & Saxe, S. Psychological preparation of female police recruits. PERSONNEL, January 1982, pp. 5-7.

Goodstein, L. & Cooke, P. The concepts and techniques of organizational development: An introduction. In P. A. Keller & L. G. Ritt (Eds.), INNOVATIONS IN CLINICAL PRACTICE: A SOURCE BOOK (Vol. 2). Sarasota, FL: Professional Resource Exchange, 1983.

Harper & Row. OFFICER STRESS AWARENESS SERIES. Harper & Row, 10 East 53 Street, New York, NY 10022. (Film)

Janis, I. L. & Mann, L. DECISION MAKING: A PSYCHOLOGICAL ANALYSIS OF CONFLICT, CHOICE, AND COMMITMENT. New York: The Free Press, 1977.

Kroes, W. H. & Hurrell, J. J., Jr. (Eds.). JOB STRESS AND THE POLICE OFFICER: IDENTIFYING STRESS REDUCTION TECHNIQUES. Washington, DC: U. S. Department of Health, Education, and Welfare, 1975.

Kroes, W. H., Hurrell, J. J., Jr., & Margolis, B. Job stress in police administrators. In L. Territo & H. J. Vetter (Eds.), STRESS AND POLICE PERSONNEL. Boston: Allyn & Bacon, 1981.

Kroes, W. H., Margolis, B. L., & Hurrell, J. J., Jr. Job stress in policemen. In L. Territo & H. J. Vetter (Eds.), STRESS AND POLICE PERSONNEL. Boston: Allyn & Bacon, 1981.

Loftus, E. F. & Loftus, G. R. On the permanence of stored information in the human brain. AMERICAN PSYCHOLOGIST, 1980, *35*, 409-420.

Mann, P. A. Ethical issues for psychologists in police agencies. In J. Monahan (Ed.), WHO IS THE CLIENT? Washington, DC: American Psychological Association, 1980.

Mann, P. A. PSYCHOLOGICAL CONSULTATION WITH A POLICE DEPARTMENT. Springfield, IL: Charles C. Thomas, 1973.

Martin, R. A. Primer on stress inoculation. In P. A. Keller & L. G. Ritt (Eds.), INNOVATIONS IN CLINICAL PRACTICE: A SOURCE BOOK (Vol. 1). Sarasota, FL: Professional Resource Exchange, 1982.

McGregor, D. THE PROFESSIONAL MANAGER. New York: McGraw-Hill, 1967.

Miller, F. T. Consultation: A practical approach. In P. A. Keller & L. G. Ritt (Eds.), INNOVATIONS IN CLINICAL PRACTICE: A SOURCE BOOK (Vol. 1). Sarasota, FL: Professional Resource Exchange, 1982.

Murray, J. D. & Grace, J. E. How to develop a stress management workshop. In P. A. Keller & L. G. Ritt (Eds.), INNOVATIONS IN CLINICAL PRACTICE: A SOURCE BOOK (Vol. 1). Sarasota, FL: Professional Resource Exchange, 1982.

Novaco, R. A. A stress inoculation approach to anger management in the training of law enforcement officers. AMERICAN JOURNAL OF COMMUNITY PSYCHOLOGY, 1977, *5*, 327-346.

POLICE STRESS: A SELECTED BIBLIOGRAPHY. National Criminal Justice Reference Service, Department F, Box 6000, Rockville, MN 20850.

Reiser, M. THE HANDBOOK OF INVESTIGATIVE HYPNOSIS. Los Angeles, CA: Lehi Publishing Co., 1980.

Reiser, M. POLICE PSYCHOLOGY, COLLECTED PAPERS. Los Angeles, CA: Lehi Publishing Co., 1982.

Sarason, I. G., Johnson, J. H., Berberich, J. P., & Siegel, J. M. Helping police officers to cope with stress: A cognitive-behavioral approach. AMERICAN JOURNAL OF COMMUNITY PSYCHOLOGY, 1979, **7**, 593-603.

Spielberger, C. D. (Ed.). POLICE SELECTION AND EVALUATION: ISSUES AND TECHNIQUES. New York: Praeger Publishers, 1979.

Teleometrics International, 1755 Woodstead Court, The Woodlands, TX 77380. Source for the Conflict Management Survey and the Power Motivation Inventory.

Territo, L. & Vetter, H. J. (Eds.). STRESS AND POLICE PERSONNEL. Boston: Allyn & Bacon, 1981.

Turkington, C. Hypnotic memory is not always accurate. APA MONITOR, March 1982, 46-47.

Vehlow, C. M. & Kropp, C. L. Developing employee assistance programs. In P. A. Keller & L. G. Ritt (Eds.), INNOVATIONS IN CLINICAL PRACTICE: A SOURCE BOOK (Vol. 1). Sarasota, FL: Professional Resource Exchange, 1982.

Wagner, M. Airline disaster: A stress debrief program for police. POLICE STRESS, 1980, **1**(4), 16-19.

INTRODUCTION TO SECTION V: SELECTED TOPICS

In the SELECTED TOPICS SECTION we have included several useful articles dealing with clinical practice as well as a selection of useful handouts the reader can copy for use with clients and patients. This section is designed as a sort of potpourri to allow for contributions which may not fit neatly into one of our other categories but should be of interest to our readers. As with the other sections in this volume, the contributions included here have a practical emphasis.

In the first article, Smith provides an introduction to roles for clinicians in assessment and treatment of traumatic injury cases. As more mental health clinicians develop linkages with medical and rehabilitation settings, this topic grows in importance. The material covered is not of the type typically included in clinical training.

Ewing discusses a number of ethical issues frequently encountered in clinical practice. As a student of the law, as well as a clinician, the author is in a unique position to comment on the issues discussed.

One of the requests commonly received by clinicians in recent years relates to the assessment of claimants for Social Security benefits. In his contribution, Anderson offers many practical suggestions on the preparation of reports for this purpose. The article identifies areas where oversights on the clinician's part could interfere with client's claim.

In an unusual contribution, Russell presents a wide range of structured group exercises which might be of interest to experienced as well as novice group leaders. The author emphasizes appropriate application of the exercises, and a context for each exercise is suggested.

Three client handouts are included in this section. Lacks, Stolz, and Levine have constructed an excellent beginning guide to psychotherapy which should find wide use in clinical practice. Murray's handout on coping with loss and grief should be of value to clients struggling with these issues. The final handout is a brief introduction to psychological testing which would be appropriate to give clients prior to an assessment session.

SELECTED TOPICS

ROLES FOR CLINICIANS IN ASSESSMENT AND TREATMENT OF TRAUMATIC INJURY CASES

Harold H. Smith, Jr.

Every year, 3.5 million individuals are injured in automobile accidents, resulting in 250,000 people being hospitalized and 3,000 crippled for life (Wall Street Journal, 1982). The National Safety Council estimates that at least 2 million are injured in industrial accidents and an additional 2 million are injured in home accidents. The consequences of closed head injury, chronic pain, and incapacitating psychological reactions to injury (as reflected in the number of lawsuits, loss of employment or inefficient work performance, sick pay benefits, and medical and psychological treatment costs) are staggering.

Clinicians, particularly clinical psychologists, but also psychiatrists and psychiatric social workers, have the opportunity to make significant contributions to the assessment of traumatically injured individuals and to their treatment and rehabilitation. Detailed assessment can provide valuable information regarding an individual's psychological adjustment to injury, various correlates of chronic pain, relative assets and limitations relating to higher level cognitive skills, motor and sensory-perceptual abilities which are valuable for treatment considerations, as well as information to give the patient's family, and for the development of opinions in expert witness testimony. Indeed, Beals and Hickman (1972) have reported that the predictions by psychologists regarding the return to work of back-injured patients are more accurate than those by physicians.

Knowledge of the mechanics of traumatic injury is important for understanding the effects produced. Rapid acceleration of the body, which may result when a vehicle is struck from the rear, or rapid deceleration, which may result when a vehicle collides with a stationary object or another moving vehicle, or an injury received in a fall, produce different primary effects. Primary effects are those that are mechanical and occur at the time of impact; secondary effects may be due to ischemic or anoxic lesions, edema, alterations in cerebral blood flow, or intracranial hematoma (von Zomeren, 1981). Primary effects of rapid acceleration may include concussion and whiplash injury, while rapid deceleration may cause concussion and more severe closed head injury, but perhaps no "whiplash."

A blow to the head may result in concussion and closed head injury, with or without contusion or compression. Concussion, the diagnosis of which does not require transitory loss of consciousness, has generalized cerebral effects but usually does not produce gross lesions, although there is ample evidence of microscopic changes (Courville, 1953; Stritch, 1969). Holbourn (1943) has outlined a mechanicophysical model of brain damage from **closed head injury** which describes laceration of the brain and tearing of blood vessels due to shear-strains that develop as a result of the brain sliding in its dural compartment. Where the brain is confined, such as the frontal and middle fossae of the skull, damage occurs most frequently. Pudenz and Shelden (1946) used high speed cinematography to record the effects of cranial trauma on the underlying brain as viewed through a transparent lucite calvarium that replaced the convex portion of a monkey's skull. Using subconcussive blows to freely movable monkey heads, they were able to explain subdural hematoma as being due to cerebral rotation. The velocity required to produce such lesions was about 20 miles per hour.

A variety of symptoms may occur as a result of closed head injury and, collectively, these are referred to as **post concussive syndrome.** Frequently, headache, nervousness or psychic symptoms, dizziness, vision disturbance, fatigue, and tinnitus are experienced. A more serious closed head injury may result in a variety of memory deficits, including retrograde and/or post traumatic amnesia; residual memory deficits affecting a larger time span frequently occur and may be related to temporal lobe and hippocampal damage as well as diffuse damage (Whitty & Zangwill, 1977). Subtle memory deficits are easily missed upon clinical evaluation but are clearly demonstrated during psychometric examination. Impairment in the learning and retention of new verbal information occurs despite seemingly adequate short-term memory, such as that measured by digits recall.

Visuospacial memory deficits may also occur, especially with injury to the right cerebral hemisphere in right-handed individuals. Some individuals become disoriented when they cannot find their automobiles in a parking lot, or cannot remember the most efficient route of travel from one place to another.

The higher integrative functions of the brain, intelligence and cognition, are also affected by traumatic head injury. The patient may show evidence of perplexity or distrust of his or her own judgments and continue to solve problems according to old learned habits when new problem solving strategies are necessary.

Rapid acceleration also results in "whiplash," or **acute flexion-extension injury** of the neck. The term "railway spine" identified this type of injury that occurred to passengers involved in railway collisions in the 1800's (Trimble, 1981). Gorman (1979) has noted that of the 16 million automobile accidents yearly, 7 million are rear end collisions, and that about 1.75 million of these cause significant injuries. As a result of these injuries, which can be incurred at speeds as slow as 10 miles per hour, victims may experience spinal concussion, acute myelopathy with paraplegia, and brachial neuropathy if they have a tight fit of the spinal cord, injury to the auditory and vestibular structures, visual difficulties, including maculopathy and impaired visual acuity, cervical muscle sprain, and fractures or dislocations of cervical vertebrae. Sometimes brain damage occurs without direct impact to the head (Ommaya, Faas, & Yarnell, 1968). The post traumatic "whiplash" symptoms frequently are chronic and include poor concentration, insomnia, restlessness, subjective vertigo, high levels of neuromuscular tension, headaches, nausea, vomiting, sweating, palpitation, lacrimation, tinnitus, nuchal pain, and mood changes (Gay & Abbott, 1953; Ishii, 1969). Litigation does not appear to be a significant factor contributing to these symptoms (MacNab, 1974; Toglia, 1976).

The **post accident anxiety syndrome** (Modlin, 1967), similar to the post traumatic stress disorder, occurs in about 35% of trauma patients referred for psychiatric examination. Symptoms include chronic free floating anxiety, muscular tension, startle reaction and irritability, subjective memory deficits due to impaired concentration, repetitive nightmares, sexual inhibitions and social withdrawal. While some cases of post traumatic neurosis are clearly nonorganic in origin, it is evident that many individuals who seem to have post traumatic neurotic symptoms may also experience significant post concussive and/or cervical syndrome interaction effects.

ASSESSMENT

Multiple approaches to the assessment of patients' complaints provide a wealth of information that allows a formulation of their problems, provides baselines from which to demonstrate therapeutic change, and gives data that are pertinent in personal injury litigation proceedings. Regular use of such data is also expected to improve clinical acumen and improve therapeutic efforts.

Symptom monitoring by pain patients may include behavioral charting of activity levels (time spent sitting, standing, walking, reclining), times and amounts of medications or other treatments used, and results achieved (Fordyce, 1976). Such monitoring forces the patient to be aware of what his or her behavior is and that changes do occur. Being able to see even slight changes gives hope and increases motivation to alter behavior patterns.

Biofeedback instruments may be used to assess physical-physiological functioning through measures of temperature, muscle activity level, and skin conductance. Visual or auditory feedback gives concrete evidence of a patient's distress and provides an avenue for learning self-control of a variety of behaviors such as posturing, muscle tensing or bracing, and elevated levels of autonomic reactivity.

Psychological difficulties after trauma frequently are as disabling as the physical injury (Mann & Gold, 1966), and perhaps more so when visible evidence of injury is absent. Frequently, chronic pain is the complaint. An understanding of the psychosocial factors which contribute to chronic pain can be obtained through the use of a structured interview, such as The Psychosocial Pain Inventory (Heaton, Lehman, & Getto, 1980), or an objective questionnaire such as the Millon Behavioral Health Inventory (1979), which provides information regarding coping styles and likely response to medical treatment for chronic pain.

A detailed clinical interview is critical for eliciting information that may lead to differential diagnosis, and a Structured Clinical Interview (Burdock & Hardesty, 1968) may provide guidelines. Judgmental ratings may be made using the Brief Psychiatric Rating Scale (Levin & Grossman, 1978; Overall & Gorham, 1962), which is reproduced in this volume. Standardized instruments, such as the Minnesota Multiphasic Personality Inventory (Dikman & Reitan, 1977; Shaffer, Nussbaum, & Little, 1972) and the Sixteen Personality Factor Test

(Cattell, Eber, & Tatsuoka, 1970) clearly reflect evidence of emotional distress among traumatically injured persons. There appear to be differences in symptoms developed, depending upon whether the patient had "actively" or "passively" risked trauma (Sathananthan, Gershon, & Lenn, 1975).

Unconscious individuals may have their behaviors monitored by the Levels of Cognitive Functioning Scale (Hagen, Malkmus, & Burdett, 1979) which measures eight levels of functioning with descriptions of general, cognitive, and language behaviors at each level. The Glasgow Coma Scale (Teasdale & Jennett, 1974) similarly measures three components of wakefulness (eye opening, motor response, and verbal response). These scales provide a quantitative assessment of the severity of the injury received and have some prognostic validity.

Kurt Goldstein (1952) succinctly described the effects of brain damage on the personality, noting changes not only in abstract capacity, attention and memory, and emotional responses, but also in pleasure and joy, witticism, and friendship and love. More recently, Levin, Benton, and Grossman (1982) have reviewed the neurobehavioral consequences of closed head injury and have summarized well the present knowledge of the subject.

How to assess these neurobehavioral deficits is a matter of professional orientation. Russell (1979) has noted that adequate assessment of brain damage requires more than the Wechsler Adult Intelligence Scale. It has been shown that inexperienced clinicians, for example, make better interpretations of cerebral dysfunction using the Halstead Reitan Neuropsychological Battery (HRNB) as compared to some traditional techniques (Goldstein, Deysach, & Kleinknecht, 1973). The HRNB also predicts brain damage at a higher hit rate than EEG, x-ray, brain scan, and neurological examination (Filskov & Goldstein, 1974), and with a similar accuracy to that of computer axial tomography (Tsushima & Wedding, 1979). The results of neuropsychological evaluation should be interpreted cautiously in cases that involve personal injury litigation. Heaton, Smith, Lehman, and Vogt (1978) have shown that normal individuals may malinger "deficits" without detection.

Competence in neuropsychological assessment requires more than "workshop" training (Satz & Fletcher, 1981) but, with practice and supervision, clinicians are able to systematically assess head injured patients' cognitive abilities, overall level of intellectual functioning, verbal and communicative skills, remote and short term functions, and their social and economic competence. Such information is of immense importance for treatment and personal injury litigation proceedings.

TREATMENT

The psychotherapeutic and rehabilitative treatment of traumatically injured patients is a challenging task. Traumatically injured patients seek psychological assistance, usually after maladaptive coping behaviors have become fixed. Many have little understanding of the nature of their injuries, the treatment which they have had or are currently receiving, or the prognosis for their condition. A significant number anticipate "recover" to mean their "before injury" state of functioning. Patients may resume employment only to find that they cannot perform their tasks as efficiently as prior to the accident. Some patients are hesitant to seek psychological assistance, knowing full well that their pain and other symptoms are not "in their heads." Many patients are relieved, however, to find that a clinical psychologist or psychiatrist will listen to their complaints, and they find solace in learning that their symptoms actually are real and are shared by others similarly injured.

The treatment or psychotherapy that is provided may be multifaceted. Educating patients about their injuries and involving patients' families in treatment is often necessary (Lezak, 1978b). The victims' sudden exposure to the possibility of their deaths is quite disruptive to ego functioning, and frequently somatic defenses emerge. If not treated, psychological damage tends to become worse (Leopold & Dillon, 1963). Psychotherapy that substitutes "active recall and working through of the painful memories of the helplessness and separation for counterphobic behavior, passive reproduction of the experience in dreams, and magical ways of living out and re-enacting the trauma" (Titchener & Kapp, 1976, p. 299) is quite effective, as is the hypnotic affect bridge (Watkins, 1971), especially if combined with a variety of stress management procedures.

Deep relaxation through hypnosis or biofeedback training creates another bridge between physiological and psychological affect responses and allows the individual to re-establish a feeling of self-confidence and security as ego strengthening suggestions are given. Daily practice of these self-help techniques increases self-confidence that the patient can assume responsibility for his or her well being.

Individuals who experience chronic pain are often possessed. For many, the pain is with them constantly, unremittingly. It eats with them, sleeps with them, accompanies them everywhere, and frequently gives them an overlay of dejection, concern, and preoccupation that clinically and psychometrically resembles psychogenic pain. The reduction in mobility, social isolation (withdrawal from friends due to pain, loss of social contact because of unemployment), and iatrogenic effects of medication contribute to the development of neurotic symptoms. Many patients would gladly pay their litigation awards or workers' compensation receipts and more to be their "old selves," while others long for a visible sign of their injuries, noting that they could handle their lives better had they lost a limb or could display a scar.

Those with physical disfigurement, however, have similar neurotic adjustment patterns. Certainly the meaning of an injury varies from person to person. Those with burn scars (Andreasen & Norris, 1972; Andreasen, Norris, & Hartford, 1971) suffer the tactless curiosity and hostility from others and must undergo a progressive desensitization to their new selves, overcome the "why me" syndrome, learn new mastery and control of their lives, and, at times, dissociate themselves from their pain.

Despite the general similarities among trauma patients, numerous individual differences remain. Some individuals, especially those who experience post traumatic stress disorder, may show near remission of symptoms with brief treatment. Some regress significantly, resuming childhood habits such as thumbsucking. A few individuals may become acutely psychotic because of the stressors they experience, but most individuals who experience psychiatric symptoms manifest neurotic disturbances. Depression, usually related to anger and a sense of loss, frequently results in death wishes and suicidal ideation, and occasional suicide attempts.

In summary, the psychologist and psychiatrist face a challenge in assessing and treating the various consequences of a traumatic injury. Knowledge of the psychological consequences of closed head injury, flexion-extension neck injury, and chronic pain contribute to the understanding of the complaints and adjustment difficulties which these patients have. Supportive psychotherapy combined with re-educative strategies that include stress management procedures have proven effective in alleviating much of the distress experienced in post traumatic stress disorder. Hypnosis and biofeedback training may be effective in altering perceptions of pain. The head injured individual experiences a broad range of psychological difficulties, some of which may be unalterable. Nonetheless, the psychologist or psychiatrist can make significant contributions to the overall rehabilitation of the head injured patient.

Harold H. Smith, Jr., Ph.D., is currently in private practice as a clinical and forensic psychologist in Largo, Florida. He holds a Diplomate in clinical psychology, American Board of Professional Psychology and a Diplomate in forensic psychology, American Board of Forensic Psychology. He has particular interest in the areas of forensic and neuropsychology, as well as stress management. Dr. Smith may be contacted at 12775 Seminole Boulevard, Suite G, Largo, FL 33544.

RESOURCES

PUBLICATIONS

Andreason, N. J. C. & Norris, A. S. Long term adjustment and adaptation mechanisms in severely burned adults. JOURNAL OF NERVOUS AND MENTAL DISEASE, 1972, **154**, 352-362.

Andreason, N. J. C., Norris, A. S., & Hartford, C. E. Incidence of long term psychiatric complications in severely burned adults. ANNALS OF SURGERY, 1971, **174**, 785-793.

Beals, R. K. & Hickman, N. W. Industrial injuries of the back and extremities. JOURNAL OF BONE AND JOINT SURGERY, 1972, **54A**, 1593-1611.

Burdock, E. I. & Hardesty, A. S. STRUCTURED CLINICAL INTERVIEW MANUAL. New York: Springer, 1968.

Cattell, R. B., Eber, N. W., & Tatsuoka, M. M. HANDBOOK FOR THE SIXTEEN PERSONALITY FACTOR QUESTIONNAIRE (16PF). Champaign, IL: Institute for Personality and Ability Testing, 1970.

Courville, C. B. COMMOTIO CEREBRI. CEREBRAL CONCUSSION AND THE POST CONCUSSION SYNDROME IN THEIR MEDICAL AND LEGAL ASPECTS. San Francisco: Lucas, 1953.

Death on the road. WALL STREET JOURNAL, April 14, 1982, pp. 1; 24.

Dikman, S. & Reitan, R. M. Emotional sequelae of head injury. ANNALS OF NEUROLOGY, 1977, **2**, 492-494.

Filskov, S. B. & Goldstein, S. G. Diagnostic validity of the Halstead-Reitan Neuropsychological Battery. JOURNAL OF CONSULTING AND CLINICAL PSYCHOLOGY, 1974, **42**, 382-388.

Fordyce, W. E. BEHAVIORAL METHODS FOR CHRONIC PAIN AND ILLNESS. St. Louis: C. V. Mosby, 1976.

Fordyce, W. E. Use of the MMPI in the assessment of chronic pain. In J. Butcher, G. Dahlstrom, M. Gynther, & W. Schofield (Eds.), CLINICAL NOTES ON THE MMPI. Nutley, NJ: Hoffmann-LaRoche, Inc., 1979.

Gay, J. R. & Abbott, K. H. Common whiplash injuries of the neck. JOURNAL OF THE AMERICAN MEDICAL ASSOCIATION, 1953, **152,** 1698-1704.

Goldstein, K. The effect of brain damage on the personality. PSYCHIATRY, 1952, **15,** 245-259.

Goldstein, S. G., Deysach, R. E., & Kleinknecht, R. A. Effect of experience and amount of information on identification of cerebral impairment. JOURNAL OF CONSULTING AND CLINICAL PSYCHOLOGY, 1973, **41,** 30-34.

Gorman, W. F. "Whiplash": Fictive or factual? BULLETIN OF THE AMERICAN ACADEMY OF PSYCHIATRY AND LAW, 1979, **7,** 245-248.

Gronwall, D. M. A. & Sampson, H. THE PSYCHOLOGICAL EFFECTS OF CONCUSSION. New Zealand: Auckland University Press, 1974.

Hagen, C., Malkmus, D., & Burdett, C., 1979. Intervention strategies for language disorders secondary to head trauma. Cited by Hagen, C. Language disorders secondary to closed head injury: Diagnosis and treatment. TOPICS IN LANGUAGE DISORDERS, 1981, **1,** 73-87.

Heaton, R. K., Lehman, R. A. W., & Getto, C. J. PSYCHOSOIAL PAIN INVENTORY. Psychological Assessment Resources, Inc., 1980.

Heaton, R. K., Smith, H. H., Jr., Lehman, R. A. W., & Vogt, A. J. Prospects for faking believable deficits on neuropsychological testing. JOURNAL OF CONSULTING AND CLINICAL PSYCHOLOGY, 1978, **46,** 892-900.

Holbourn, A. H. S. Mechanics of head injuries. LANCET, 1943, **2,** 438-441.

Ishii, S. Significance of soft tissue neck injuries in the post traumatic syndrome. In A. E. Walker, W. F. Caveness, & M Critchley (Eds.), THE LATE EFFECTS OF HEAD INJURY. Springfield: Thomas, 1969.

Leopold, R. L. & Dillon, H. Psycho-anatomy of a disaster: A long term study of post traumatic neuroses in survivors of a marine explosion. AMERICAN JOURNAL OF PSYCHIATRY, 1963, **119,** 913-921.

Levin, H. S., Benton, A. L., & Grossman, R. G. NEUROBEHAVIORAL CONSEQUENCES OF CLOSED HEAD INJURY. New York: Oxford University Press, 1982.

Levin, H. S. & Grossman, R. G. Behavioral sequelae of closed head injury. ARCHIVES OF NEUROLOGY, 1978, **35,** 720-727.

Levin, H. S., O'Donnell, V. M., & Grossman, R. G. The Galveston Orientation and Amnesia Test. A practical scale to assess cognition after head injury. JOURNAL OF NERVOUS AND MENTAL DISEASE, 1979, **167,** 675-684.

Lezak, M. D. Subtle sequelae of brain damage. Perplexity, distractibility, and fatigue. AMERICAN JOURNAL OF PHYSICAL MEDICINE, 1978, **57,** 9-15. (a)

Lezak, M. D. Living with the characterologically altered brain injured patient. JOURNAL OF CLINICAL PSYCHIATRY, 1978, **39,** 592-598. (b)

MacNab, I. The whiplash syndrome. CLINICAL NEUROSURGERY, 1974, **20,** 232-240.

Mann, A. M. & Gold, E. M. Psychological sequelae of accident injury: A medico-legal quagmire. CANADIAN MEDICAL ASSOCIATION JOURNAL, 1966, **95,** 1359-1363.

MILLON BEHAVIORAL HEALTH INVENTORY. NCS Interpretive Scoring Systems, 1979.

Modlin, H. C. The post-accident and anxiety syndrome: Psychosocial aspects. AMERICAN JOURNAL OF PSYCHIATRY, 1967, **123,** 1008-1012.

Ommaya, A. K., Faas, F., & Yarnall, P. Whiplash injury and brain damage. JOURNAL OF THE AMERICAN MEDICAL ASSOCIATION, 1968, **204,** 285.

Overall, J. E. & Gorham, D. R. The brief psychiatric rating scale. PSYCHOLOGICAL REPORTS, 1962, **10**, 799-812.

Pudenz, R. H. & Shelden, C. H. The lucite calvarium - method for direct observation of the brain. JOURNAL OF NEUROSURGERY, 1946, **3**, 487-505.

Russell, E. W. Three patterns of brain damage on the WAIS. JOURNAL OF CLINICAL PSYCHOLOGY, 1979, **35**, 611-620.

Sathananthan, G. L., Gershon, S., & Lenn, E. Psychological profiles and effects in acute trauma: A pilot study. DISORDERS OF THE NERVOUS SYSTEM, 1975, **36**, 17-19.

Satz, P. & Fletcher, J. M. Emergent trends in neuropsychology: An overview. JOURNAL OF CONSULTING AND CLINICAL PSYCHOLOGY, 1981, **49**, 851-865.

Shaffer, J., Nussbaum, & Little, J. MMPI profiles of disability insurance claimants. AMERICAN JOURNAL OF PSYCHIATRY, 1972, **129**, 403.

Stritch, S. J. The pathology of brain damage due to blunt head injuries. In A. E. Walker, W. F. Caveness, & M. Critchley (Eds.), THE LATE EFFECTS OF HEAD INJURY. Springfield: Thomas, 1969.

Teasdale, G. & Jennett, B. Assessment of coma and impaired consciousness. A practical scale. LANCET, 1974, **2**, 81-84.

Titchener, J. L. & Kapp, F. T. Family and character change at Buffalo Creek. AMERICAN JOURNAL OF PSYCHIATRY, 1976, **133**, 295-299.

Toglia, J. U. Acute flexion-extension injury of the neck. NEUROLOGY, 1976, **26**, 808-814.

Trimble, M. R. POST-TRAUMATIC NEUROSIS. New York: Wiley, 1981.

Tsushima, W. T. & Wedding, D. A comparison of the Halstead-Reitan Neuropsychological Battery and computerized tomography in the identification of brain disorder. JOURNAL OF NERVOUS AND MENTAL DISEASE, 1979, **167**, 704-707.

von Zomeren, A. H. REACTION TIME AND ATTENTION AFTER CLOSED HEAD INJURY. Lisse: Swets & Zeitlinger, 1981.

Watkins, J. G. The affect bridge: A hypnoanalytic technique. INTERNATIONAL JOURNAL OF CLINICAL AND EXPERIMENTAL HYPNOSIS, 1971, **19**, 21-27.

Whitty, C. W. M. & Zangwill, O. L. AMNESIA. CLINICAL, PSYCHOLOGICAL, AND MEDICOLEGAL ASPECTS (2nd ed.). Boston: Butterworths, 1977.

ORGANIZATIONS

American Pain Society, Inc., 340 Kingsland Street, Nutley, NJ 07110.

International Neuropsychological Society, c/o Kenneth Adams, Division of Neuropsychology, K-11, Henry Ford Hospital, Detroit, MI 48202.

National Head Injury Foundation, 280 Singletary Lane, Framingham, MA 01701.

ETHICAL ISSUES IN CLINICAL PRACTICE

Charles P. Ewing

Like most organized professions, psychology, psychiatry, social work, and the other mental health disciplines have formal ethical codes to which their members are expected to adhere. In some respects these codes provide categorical rules of conduct. For example, the ethical canons of both psychology and psychiatry explicitly prohibit the clinician from engaging in sexual relations with a client. For the most part, however, such codes are written in rather general terms which often offer little in the way of concrete ethical guidance to the practitioner. Furthermore, no such code, however comprehensive, can be expected to illuminate all of the ethical dilemmas faced by the busy clinician. In many instances, ethical questions can and must be answered not by resort to any formal code but rather by a thoughtful consideration of the ethical traditions and enduring values of the practitioner's profession.

This chapter will examine several of the more common ethical issues faced by the mental health practitioner, many of which are covered only partially, if at all, by the formal professional codes of ethics. I should note from the outset that I do not profess to have "the answers" and that much of what follows has been informed primarily by my own experience as a clinician and student of the law and by my personal beliefs regarding the ethical traditions of my profession. The ethical issues to be considered are those related to: (a) confidentiality; (b) informed consent; (c) the client's "right to know"; (d) conflicts of interest; and (e) relations among professionals.

CONFIDENTIALITY

Confidentiality between client and therapist is obviously a vital element in successful psychotherapy and every psychotherapist, regardless of discipline, has a clear ethical responsibility to respect and safeguard client confidences. If psychotherapy took place in a social vacuum, it would be relatively easy to lay down a categorical rule regarding confidentiality. The rule would be simply this: Reveal nothing a client tells you unless the client requests otherwise.

Clearly, however, psychotherapy is not an entirely isolated or completely insulated enterprise. What goes on in the psychotherapist's office often has significant implications which extend well beyond the therapist-client dyad. As a result, society, through its various institutions including the law, has chosen to place certain restrictions on psychotherapist-client confidentiality. Thus, active psychotherapists are constantly confronted with demands for the release of what would otherwise be considered strictly confidential information about their clients.

The obvious problem for the psychotherapist is how to deal with the tension which inevitably arises between ethical duty and social-legal responsibility. In other words, how does he or she respond in a way which both meets the ethical duty to maintain confidentiality and complies with legitimate requests or demands for client information. In some cases, this conflict may be readily resolved by securing the client's informed consent to release the information. In other situations, however, the therapist may feel compelled to release confidential information regardless of client consent.

Situations of the former sort include those involving requests for information made by insurers, employers, schools, public agencies, health care professionals, and other institutions with which the client is voluntarily associated. In such cases, it is often apparently advantageous to the client to have certain confidential information released and most clients will readily consent. These situations are routinely handled by having clients sign standard pre-printed consent forms provided by the clinician or by the institution seeking the information. (See **INNOVATIONS IN CLINICAL PRACTICE: A SOURCE BOOK**, Vol. 1, pp. 219-221, for examples of various release forms.)

In most cases of this sort, such routine procedure poses no problem for client or therapist. However, clinicians who regularly handle requests for release of information in this fashion often run the risk of failing to adequately discharge their ethical responsibilities to the client. At the very least, securing **informed** consent to release confidential information requires careful discussion between client and therapist. In every case, the therapist should call the client's attention to any possible adverse consequences of releasing the information and require the client to specify exactly what information he or she is willing to have released. Under no circumstances should the therapist accept a "blank check" authorization from the client to release information. Furthermore, even after securing the client's informed consent, if the clinician has any doubt as to the client's willingness to have specific information (e.g., a diagnosis or clinical report) released, that information should first be provided to the client (this is discussed in detail further on in this chapter).

In what might be called nonvoluntary disclosure situations (those in which release of confidential information is mandated by law), a different approach is required. For example, virtually every state requires psychotherapists to report any reasonable evidence of child abuse. Some jurisdictions now also require psychotherapists to warn any third parties against whom clients have made threats of physical harm. In some instances, a psychotherapist may have a legal duty to disclose suicidal threats in an effort to prevent self-destructive behavior. Since the law regarding disclosure in these and other such situations varies from state to state, clinicians must make it a point to learn the legal requirements of the jurisdiction in which they are practicing. State and local professional associations and state licensing boards can be good sources of information for such requirements.

The clinician's awareness of legal requirements is necessary but not sufficient in dealing with nonvoluntary disclosure situations. Not all threats are serious and not all suspicions are fully warranted. Often clinicians must rely upon their own best judgment in determining whether the relevant legal standard is applicable to a given situation.

My advice to the clinician faced with such a determination stems from both ethical and legal considerations. In case of doubt, the clinician should first discuss the threat or suspicion at length with the client. If doubt remains, the clinician should seek the advice and counsel of other experienced therapists. In some instances, professional legal advice might also be sought. Failing all else, any error should be made on the side of safety. Ethically and legally, the therapist should inform the client of the legal requirement and seek the client's consent to report or warn, but ultimately make the necessary report or warning regardless of consent.

Clinicians who follow this course of action will not only discharge their ethical obligations to their clients but will also likely be immune from legal action for breach of confidentiality as long as they have acted in "good faith." Good faith is a legal term of art, but extended discussion with the client followed by consultation with experienced colleagues and the exercise of sound clinical judgment should be sufficient to establish that a clinician has met this requirement.

One further caution regarding confidentiality: Do **not** assume that **confidential** information is necessarily **privileged** information (i.e., immune from forced disclosure by legal process). In most jurisdictions, physician-patient confidences are privileged to some extent and many states accord the same treatment to psychologist-client communications. However, very few states have a privilege for communications between clients and other therapists, such as social workers or marriage counselors. Moreover, even where such privilege exists, it may be subject to significant exceptions.

All clinicians should become aware of the nature and limits of the psychotherapist-client privilege, if any, in the states where they practice. In any event, clinicians would do well to treat all clinical records as though they were subject to subpoena. Unless it is relevant to the client's treatment, potentially damaging information regarding a client should be excluded from case files.

Finally, it should be noted that much of the potential for ethical dilemmas regarding the release of confidential information may be mitigated, if not avoided altogether, by informing every client of the limits of confidentiality at the very beginning of the client-therapist relationship. Clearly, calling the client's attention to all conceivable conflicts would be impractical and counterproductive to treatment, if not impossible. A good deal of time and trouble could be saved, however, by offering each client a written statement regarding confidentiality and its limits and making sure that he or she understands this information **before** there is an opportunity for any disclosure. (See INNOVATIONS IN CLINICAL PRACTICE: A SOURCE BOOK, Vol. 1, pp. 379-380, for a sample handout on confidentiality.)

INFORMED CONSENT TO TREATMENT

Informed consent to treatment is often taken for granted by psychotherapists, particularly those in noninstitutional practice. The client who voluntarily seeks psychotherapy is assumed to have consented, at least implicitly, to the type of treatment the clinician ordinarily provides. It is often taken as a given that the client understands and accepts the nature of psychotherapy and thus has exercised informed consent simply by entering into a therapeutic relationship with the psychotherapist.

For a relative handful of sophisticated clients, these assumptions may have some validity. Most clients, however, have little, if any, explicit understanding of what the various forms of psychotherapy entail. They come seeking generic "counseling" or "advice" and are often surprised to learn that there are numerous schools of psychotherapy with varying time, financial, and personal commitments. Moreover, many clients have been socialized to "follow the doctor's orders" and not question the judgment of highly trained professionals.

Clinicians who fail to offer clients at least a rudimentary understanding of the psychotherapeutic process from the very start of treatment not only disregard a fundamental ethical responsibility but may well unwittingly foster client misconceptions which interfere with successful psychotherapy (e.g., the all too prevalent belief that psychotherapy is something "done" by the clinician "to" the passive client).

At a minimum, clinicians should explain to all new clients something of their own theoretical orientation and the kinds of techniques they generally utilize **before** the clients make any commitment to treatment. Ideally, each clinician should also explain to some extent how his or her orientation and techniques differ from those of other psychotherapists. This is especially important in cases where clinicians employ hypnosis, relaxation techniques, behavior modification regimens, family or conjoint sessions, or any other "nontraditional" psychotherapeutic approaches. Clinicians should also explain their own professional backgrounds (including training and experience with the sorts of problems presented by the client) as well as the limitations of their practices. For example, nonmedical clinicians (especially those with doctorates) should indicate from the start that they are not physicians and do not diagnose physical ailments or prescribe medications.

Additionally, clinicians should provide all clients with an understanding of the sorts of time, financial, and personal commitments which may be required over the course of treatment. Early on, it is especially important to give the client at least a working estimate of the duration of treatment and the number of sessions that may be required. The clinician should, of course, emphasize that any such estimates are subject to modification depending upon the needs of the client.

Finally, clinicians should advise clients from the outset of their freedom to terminate treatment in the event that they feel unable to establish a suitable therapeutic relationship. This point seems particularly important since many clients seem to feel that once they have begun treatment, they are "stuck" with the clinician, for better or worse.

Providing clients with these kinds of information not only avoids many sources of future conflict which may hinder treatment, but also insures that clients have the knowledge necessary to make informed judgments as to whether or not to pursue a therapeutic relationship with a particular clinician. Providing such information also often enhances client-therapist rapport and helps establish that a clinician is a forthright, truthful, and caring individual in whom the client may trust.

THE CLIENT'S RIGHT TO KNOW

Closely related to issues of confidentiality and informed consent is what might be called the client's "right to know." Psychotherapists, like many physicians, often seem to feel that client access to clinical information, particularly diagnostic impressions and test results, should be strictly limited. The notion appears to be that what clients don't know can't hurt them while what they do know may.

The "right to know" issue comes into sharpest focus when a client, generally after treatment has been terminated, demands a copy of his or her clinical file. This issue, however, is present (or should be) in every case, regardless of whether or not the client raises it.

Most clients expect, and all clients deserve, a careful explanation of the clinician's perceptions of their problems and functioning. Such explanation need not necessarily include a diagnostic label. Indeed, diagnostic labels often hide more than they reveal, especially to the client who is ignorant of psychiatric nomenclature.

Clinicians should strive to explain to every client, in terms the client can understand, the diagnostic formulations which will guide treatment. Where such formulations are tentative and subject to change as treatment progresses, as most are, clinicians should say so. Clinicians should not, however, use the tentativeness of their formulations and impressions as an excuse for denying clients the sort of clinical feedback they deserve (and for which they are paying). Furthermore, diagnostic feedback should not be limited to the earliest stages of treatment. A conscientious clinician will provide such feedback regularly as treatment progresses and will offer the client at least some sort of diagnostic summary upon termination.

Following this approach will not only enable clinicians to meet their ethical obligation to deal openly and honestly with clients but should also enhance rapport and stimulate client interest and involvement in the therapeutic process. Furthermore, clinicians who adopt such an approach should find that few, if any, of their clients end up demanding access to clinical records.

Since, however, client demands for access to their records may occasionally arise despite the clinician's genuine efforts to keep the client informed throughout treatment, this issue is worth at least some further consideration. In some jurisdictions, individuals have a legal right to obtain copies of their medical records, and this right has sometimes been viewed as applying to psychotherapeutic records as well. Thus, this is another area in which it behooves clinicians to become aware of the law in the state where they practice.

Regardless of the law, however, a clinician should treat clinical records as though they will be subject to review by the client. Records should, of course, be accurate and sufficiently detailed to serve their intended clinical purpose. A clinician will do well, however, to avoid using perjoratives and recording observations which could prove detrimental to a client if eventually revealed. Any essential notes a clinician feels should not be seen by a client are best kept mentally or in some cryptic fashion in the clinician's personal diary. While notes kept in this fashion may still be subject to revelation under legal process, they need not be revealed upon routine demand by the client for access to his or her clinical records.

In my own practice, very few clients have demanded personal access to their records. Generally, clients have been content to have the records (or a summary of them) forwarded to another clinician. In those few cases in which clients have demanded to see their records, I have granted such access but only with the proviso that I be present to answer questions or explain certain aspects of the records. I have never had a client refuse to accept this condition. Overall, I have found that this approach minimizes misunderstandings and avoids the kinds of suspicions and hard feelings which seem to arise when clients are denied access to their records or are offered only "laundered" summaries.

CONFLICTS OF INTEREST

Conflicts of interest which arise in the psychotherapeutic relationship generally take one of three forms: (a) client-therapist conflicts; (b) client-third party conflicts; or (c) client-client conflicts. Therapists are bound by the ethical standards of their professions to act in the best interests of their clients. In discharging this ethical obligation, therapists must strive to avoid actions which might place their own interests or those of others above the interests of their clients.

Admittedly, the psychotherapeutic relationship is fraught with potential for conflicts of interest, and avoiding such conflicts is not always easy. Yet, by anticipating potential conflicts and dealing with them openly and honestly before they arise, psychotherapists generally can avoid most of the more serious conflicts of interest known to arise in the course of psychotherapy.

CLIENT-THERAPIST CONFLICTS

Client-therapist conflicts of interest are among both the easiest and the most difficult to avoid. Most of the potential conflicts between client and therapist may be avoided simply by limiting the client-therapist relationship to the provision of psychotherapy. Obviously, any time a therapist simultaneously relates to a client in an extra-therapeutic fashion (e.g., sex partner, employer, colleague, business partner, lender, borrower), the potential for conflict of interest and exploitation rises dramatically.

While conflicts of this sort are easy enough to avoid, other potential client-therapist conflicts of interest may not be so readily prevented. Perhaps the most difficult conflict to deal with arises when a client, in the midst of ongoing long-term psychotherapy, becomes unable to pay the therapist's fee. The client's best interest, of course, generally lies in continuing the psychotherapeutic relationship, but doing so may well threaten one of the therapist's most important interests - that of earning a living.

In these days of economic instability and high unemployment, therapists must anticipate the potential for this sort of conflict in almost every case they accept for treatment. Ultimately, in some cases, therapists must be prepared to forego their usual fees if they are to take seriously the ethical duty to serve their clients' best interests. Often, however, such a difficult situation can be avoided by carefully clarifying financial arrangements in advance of treatment.

Before either client or therapist commits to a lengthy (and generally expensive) course of treatment, the therapist should provide the client with a liberal estimate of the number of anticipated sessions and the cost per session, stressing the importance of timely payments, preferably made at the time of each session. Obviously such estimates must be made subject to revision, but they at least let the client know from the start what sort of financial commitment he or she is being asked to make.

Once the therapist has reviewed the financial aspects of treatment with the client, an effort should be made to determine whether the client can reasonably anticipate being able to meet the projected costs of treatment. Many clinicians find it difficult to confront such issues with clients, but I know from painful experience that failure to do so can sometimes lead to later embarrassment and frustration for both therapist and client.

Once the therapist has reviewed the client's ability to handle the projected costs of treatment, a decision should be made and "lived with." If the therapist feels that the client is a poor risk financially, this is the time to refer the client to a clinic or agency with a sliding fee scale. If the therapist believes that the client is capable of meeting the costs of treatment (personally or through insurance), the client may be accepted for treatment. Then if, by some later unforeseen circumstance, the client becomes unable to afford the therapist's fee, the therapist should endeavor to work out an alternative fee arrangement (e.g., temporarily lowering the fee, allowing the client to delay payment or, if need be, seeing the client free of charge) so that therapy may continue as needed.

Such a financial screening process may seem difficult, if not distasteful, to some. In the long run, however, it should help insure that therapists are able to discharge their ethical obligation to act in the client's best interest. Most busy clinicians can afford to make alternative financial arrangements with a few clients, if necessary, but few are able to continue long-term treatment with large numbers of clients under such circumstances.

Where a client is apparently able to pay for treatment, but repeatedly fails to do so and runs up a large outstanding balance, the situation is much different. Here the client's failure to make timely payments may, and often does, create a situation in which effective therapy is impeded and it may no longer be in the client's best interest to continue treatment with the frustrated therapist-creditor. In such cases, the therapist would seem ethically justified in terminating or suspending treatment unless the client is willing to make a sincere effort to rectify the situation.

CLIENT-THIRD PARTY CONFLICTS

Conflicts of this second sort have already been discussed to some extent in the section on confidentiality. There are, however, other sorts of client-third party conflicts of interest which may arise in the private psychotherapeutic setting. Several aspects of such potential conflicts are worth noting at least briefly.

Client-third party conflicts of interest seem most likely to occur when there is some doubt as to which party is the true client. Therapists in correctional and other criminal justice settings face such conflicts on a daily basis, but the problem is by no means unique to those practices. Psychotherapists in private practice are often sought out by employers, probation officers, parents, and other third parties who ask them to provide treatment for another individual, the so-called "identified client."

If the "identified client" is willing to be treated and no limiting conditions are attached by the third party who has retained (and may well be paying) the therapist, there may be no conflict of interest. More often than not, however, the third party seeks to impose certain constraints or conditions upon treatment, to make the "identified client's" continued enjoyment of some benefit (e.g., employment, school attendance, or probation status) contingent upon progress in treatment, or to otherwise interfere directly with the therapist-client relationship.

The therapist should be exceedingly wary in accepting cases initiated by third parties. Where such cases are accepted, the informed consent of the "identified client" takes on even greater than usual significance. Informed consent in all such cases must include a clear understanding and acceptance by the client of third party involvement in **any** aspect of the psychotherapeutic relationship.

Furthermore, in all such cases, therapists should make it unmistakably clear to all parties that the therapist's ethical and professional responsibility is to the "identified client." In doing so, therapists should also clearly indicate that this means any client-third party conflicts of interest which may arise in the course of treatment will be resolved in favor of the "identified client's" best interests.

Finally, as in any case, all matters of financial responsibility (including the "identified client's" ability to arrange payment for services in the event that the third party declines to continue payment) should be clarified prior to initiation of treatment.

CLIENT-CLIENT CONFLICTS

Conflicts of interest of this final sort arise in those cases where a therapist is simultaneously treating more than one client (e.g., marriage counseling, family therapy, and, to some extent, group therapy). The prevention and resolution of conflicts of this nature can be extremely complex and a thorough consideration of this topic is well beyond the scope of this brief discussion. However, since such problems are likely to be of significance to many therapists, a number of points warrant at least brief consideration.

First, as was emphasized earlier, therapists are ethically bound to act in the best interests of their clients. The problem which arises in multiple client situations is, of course, that what may be in one client's best interest may be detrimental to the interests of one or more other clients. Hoping to avoid such a dilemma, some marriage and family therapists take the position that the "client" to whom they owe their ethical obligation is "the relationship" or "the family" rather than any individual spouse or family member. In my experience, there is much to recommend this approach, but the therapist who adopts it should realize that ultimately it is nothing more than a metaphor for the difficult clinical task of delicately balancing competing needs and interests.

In any event, the therapist who chooses to approach the problem in this fashion should make such intent clear to all clients at the outset of treatment and obtain their unanimous informed consent. Furthermore, the therapist must strive constantly to clarify and obtain client consensus regarding therapeutic goals. Where such goals are ill-defined or contrary to the wishes of one or more of the clients, there simply is no collective "client" in whose best interest the therapist may purport to act.

Clearly, in obtaining such unanimous informed consent, the therapist will have to face squarely issues of confidentiality and privileged communication. Regarding confidentiality, there seems to be no universally accepted approach among marriage and family therapists. The couple or family is, of course, entitled to the same assurances and warnings as would be given to an individual client. But the group nature of marriage and family therapy requires even further discussion and clarification of the limits of confidentiality, particularly if the therapist anticipates one or more sessions with individual members of the group.

Some therapists attempt to deal with the confidentiality problems posed in these contexts by flatly refusing to keep "secrets" between or among family members. Anything revealed to the therapist by one client will be revealed to the other(s). Other therapists take the position that individual confidences are to be respected. Still others attempt to avoid the problem by refusing individual sessions. It should be noted, however, that this latter tactic often fails since clients who want to speak individually with the therapist generally find a way to do so. Whatever approach a therapist takes in this regard, it is essential that the policy be spelled out to the clients and accepted by them prior to commencement of treatment.

Regarding privileged communications, the marriage or family therapist must keep in mind that, to the extent there exists a client-therapist privilege (see discussion of confidentiality), that privilege may well not apply to statements made by one client in the presence of the other(s). At a minimum, the therapist should explain this legal uncertainty to clients in advance of treatment and be certain that they understand it. Additionally, the therapist may find it helpful, especially in marriage counseling, to secure the written agreement of the clients that none will call the therapist as witness in the event of intra-family litigation. Even where such written assurances are obtained, therapists should recognize that, in some instances, courts may refuse to enforce such agreements.

RELATIONS AMONG PROFESSIONALS

While most of the ethical concerns which arise in everyday clinical practice involve therapist-client relations, there is yet another set of such concerns worth at least brief consideration: those involving relations between and among therapists. Virtually every therapist interacts professionally with other therapists on a regular basis. Many of these professional interactions have significant implications for the well-being and proper ethical care of clients. Here I will discuss briefly one of the more common interprofessional conflicts and the ethical basis for its prevention and resolution.

The conflict I want to consider is one many therapists refer to colloquially as "client-snatching." Most therapists are familiar with the phenomenon, although some may know it by a less accusatory name.

Obviously, every client is free to choose his or her own therapist, and some clients make it a point to "shop around" for a therapist with whom they feel most comfortable. Most clinicians recognize this approach to selecting a therapist and some have encouraged it by offering initial consultations without charge. The therapist who sees and accepts for treatment a client who has been "shopping around" can hardly be accused of client-snatching. However, once a client is in treatment with a therapist and such treatment has not been formally terminated, another therapist who accepts that client for treatment, knowing of the already existing treatment relationship, might well be accused of unprofessional, if not unethical, conduct.

In my experience, such client-snatching (or whatever one chooses to call it) has occurred most often when a therapist with an ongoing relationship with a client has sent that client to another therapist for a consultation around a specific issue (the need for medication, for example). The client is seen by the consultant therapist who, for one reason or another, establishes an enduring psychotherapeutic relationship with the client which excludes the initial therapist. In some areas, such situations are so common that therapists begin to take a proprietary interest in their clients and are reluctant to seek consultations from other therapists, even when they are appropriate to sound professional care. For instance, I know of colleagues, nonmedical therapists, who have lost so many clients to psychiatric consultants (to whom the clients were sent for assessment of possible medication needs) that they have adopted a policy of flatly refusing to seek such consults for any of their clients. In fairness to psychiatry, I hasten to add that some of my psychologist colleagues have also been known to "snatch" clients referred to them for psychological testing.

Client-snatching, as I have outlined it here, not only tends to increase the rivalry among the professions (which I believe is largely rooted in economics) but, more importantly, holds the potential for much harm to the client. Client-snatching is often a prime example of the client-therapist conflict of interest resolved in favor of the therapist.

Client-snatching, of course, would not be a significant problem if all therapists behaved ethically. The therapist called in as a consultant, or contacted independently by the client of another therapist, would refuse to engage in extended psychotherapy with the client unless it was unmistakably in the client's best interest, and only after conferring with the client's current therapist. Since, however, some therapists consistently fail to achieve this ideal, it is worth noting some ways in which the problem of client-snatching might be obviated.

First, every nonmedical psychotherapist should establish an ongoing relationship with a trusted and capable psychiatric colleague, someone to whom the therapist may refer a client for medical consultation without fear that the psychiatrist will add the person to his or her own roster of psychotherapy clients. Where the psychotherapist and psychiatrist have such a relationship and understanding, the client's need for medication and medical monitoring generally can be handled without disrupting the ongoing therapist-client relationship. In some areas, it may be difficult to find a psychiatrist willing to function only as a consultant and to share in the overall treatment plan, but the search for such a practitioner will be well worthwhile, not only to the psychotherapist but to the clients. The same may be said, of course, of the search for a trusted and capable psychologist to whom the psychiatric therapist can turn for psychological testing of clients.

Second, therapists can protect their own interests and those of their clients by carefully clarifying in advance of referral the relationship the consultant therapist is to have to the client. Obviously such arrangements are not binding on the client, who may well decide to transfer to the consultant for psychotherapy, regardless of prior arrangements between the professionals. Advance arrangements of this sort do, however, help to set the expectations of the client and the professionals, thus lessening the chances of a professional tug of war with the client in the middle.

Conscientious therapists who follow one or, better yet, both of these approaches will do more than simply protect their own economic and professional interests. They will put themselves in the position of not having to balance their own needs against those of their clients every time an outside consultation is clinically indicated. In so doing, they can only advance the cause of ethical professional care, care which serves the client's best interests.

Charles P. Ewing, Ph.D. is a clinical and forensic psychologist who has been in private practice since 1978. He is currently a J.D. candidate (Class of 1983) at Harvard Law School. He may be contacted in care of The Professional Resource Exchange, Inc., 635 S. Orange Avenue, Suites 4-5, Sarasota, FL 33577.

RESOURCES

American Association for Marriage and Family Therapy. CODE OF PROFESSIONAL ETHICS & STANDARDS FOR PUBLIC INFORMATION AND ADVERTISING. Upland, CA: Author, 1979.

American Personnel and Guidance Association. ETHICAL STANDARDS (Rev. ed.). Washington, DC: Author, 1974.

American Psychiatric Association. THE PRINCIPLES OF MEDICAL ETHICS WITH ANNOTATIONS ESPECIALLY APPLICABLE TO PSYCHIATRY. Washington, DC: Author, 1981.

American Psychological Association. ETHICAL STANDARDS OF PSYCHOLOGISTS. Washington, DC: Author, 1981.

Everstine, L., Everstine, D. S., Heymann, G. M., True, R. H., Frey, D. H., Johnson, H. G., & Seiden, R. H. Privacy and confidentiality in psychotherapy. AMERICAN PSYCHOLOGIST, 1980, **35**, 828–840.

Grossman, M. Right to privacy vs. right to know. In W. E. Barton & C. J. Sanbord (Eds.), LAW AND THE MENTAL HEALTH PROFESSIONS: FRICTION AT THE INTERFACE. New York: International Universities Press, 1978.

Keller, P. A. & Ritt, L. G. INNOVATIONS IN CLINICAL PRACTICE: A SOURCE BOOK (Vol. 1). Sarasota, FL: Professional Resource Exchange, Inc., 1982.

National Association of Social Workers. CODE OF ETHICS. Silver Spring, MD: Author, 1980.

Smith, D. Unfinished business with informed consent procedures. AMERICAN PSYCHOLOGIST, 1981, **36**, 22-26.

Van Hoose, W. H. & Kottler, J. A. ETHICAL AND LEGAL ISSUES IN COUNSELING AND PSYCHOTHERAPY. San Francisco: Jossey-Bass, 1977.

155 EXERCISES: A STARTING POINT FOR LEADING STRUCTURED GROUPS

John M. Russell

This contribution offers, in summary form, a listing of structured exercises which I have found helpful in a variety of personal growth, therapy, and workshop groups. The instructions are presented in outline form and need to be augmented to appropriately introduce the exercises in an actual group. The exercises are organized in the following five categories:

1. Early Group - warm-ups, demonstrations, easing-in exercises;
2. Mid-Group - feedback, working through, "heavy" or target learning exercises;
3. Focal Exercises - narrow, specific, limited focus exercises;
4. Guided Imagery - test exercise and visualization-dependent exercises;
5. Closing Group - consolidating, transferring learning, saying goodbye exercises.

I have included a number of sources at the end of the contribution for those readers who wish to obtain other useful exercises.

Structured exercises are one way to guide a group into a limited territory or focus of learning. This delimiting often helps to reassure cautious members who may be afraid to enter into more open learning experiences where they fear that "anything" might happen. At the same time, the exercises are designed to be sufficiently open to preserve the member's freedom to learn by doing on their own and in their unique ways. This translates into a freedom to learn within leader-imposed limits. It might be described as escorting people into a large pasture bounded by fences and telling them to explore the potential riches of learning or reflection available within.

As is the case with any technical aids, there are a number of advantages and disadvantages to the introduction of structure into an ongoing group. Exercises must be creatively woven into the group fabric in order to encourage group exploration and development. In my experience, the people who have reacted negatively to exercises have been either highly creative, politically "freedom" conscious, or felt alienated and oppressed; these people have tended to prefer the freedom to create their own learning experience. These

Portions of this contribution have been adapted from an earlier article by the author which appeared in VOICES, Summer, 1971, and are reproduced here by permission.

individuals may have felt deadened, defeated, or diminished by earlier experiences with the imposition of unnecessary, apparently irrational, and unilaterally dictated rules and procedures. The leaders must learn to select exercises carefully and introduce them at appropriate moments, to time the exercises so that most individuals have sufficient time to reach a stopping point, to allow for creative and accepting processing to take place, to avoid mechanically using exercises when the leader is bored or unprepared, or running ego or "mind trips" as if the exercise has some presumed unilateral message for all members. When the leader maintains a discovery model of learning, introduces the exercises as a learning experiment, and is honestly accepting of each member's experience, then I think he or she can minimize the potential legitimate objections to the use of exercises.

Structured groups are one way for beginning leaders to develop their skills (Russell & Easton, 1979). Once a group leader is experienced and comfortable with a number of standard exercises, like the ones listed here, the next step is to invent exercises, metaphors, mirrors, and other tasks that are spontaneously created to assist the group's development or an individual member's learning process. Then structured exercises become a flexible, spontaneous group resource available to enhance creative moment-to-moment learning and personal growth.

Though it is not possible for me to cite all of the leaders who taught me how to use these exercises, I do want to thank the many individuals who contributed to the list. Since group techniques are often passed on from leader to leader, I am also indebted to the originators of each of these techniques. The summary format of this paper both allows and can encourage the reader to expand upon, improve, adapt, and revitalize these learning aids.

John M. Russell, Ph.D., is currently the Director of Behavioral Science in the family practice residency program of the Greenville Hospital System in addition to maintaining a part-time private practice. He was formerly Director of the Counseling Center and Associate Professor of Education at Northern Michigan University and Assistant Professor of Psychology at Purdue University. He has developed academic courses designed to train group leaders and now emphasizes group work in his private practice. Dr. Russell may be reached at the Center for Family Medicine, 701 Grove Road, Greenville, SC 29605.

STRUCTURED EXERCISES

I. EARLY GROUP EXERCISES

NAME OF EXERCISE	CONTENT FOCUS OR THEME	DIRECTIONS - INSTRUCTIONS (Summarized)
Previous Attempts	Starting Points	Briefly describe your previous attempts to alter the behaviors (weight loss, no smoking, procrastination, guilt, depression) you want to change."
Graffiti Button	Warm-ups	"Create a humorous slogan or saying on a button which relates to your expectations for this group experience."
Well Excuse Me	Rationalizations	"What excuse or rationalization will you use this time if your learning needs are not met?"
Ask Your Question	Agendas	Write down the one question you would like to be able to answer as a result of this group experience."
Hopes/Fears	Goals	"Write down your 'hopes' and your 'fears' for this group."
3 Famous People	Associations	"Write down the names of 3 famous people that you admire....What does this say about who you are?"
Expected/Real Profiles	Self-Image	"Before I distribute the results of your test, I want you to draw the profile you think will approximate your actual results."
Name	Self-Image	"Describe your reactions to your own first name."
3 Wishes	Ideals	"If you could have 3 wishes come true, what would your wishes be?"
Designs	Information Accuracy	In pairs - each person draws 4 geometrical shapes, then take turns directing others to try to duplicate their designs by giving one-line-at-a-time (not repeating) verbal directions only.

NAME OF EXERCISE	CONTENT FOCUS OR THEME	DIRECTIONS - INSTRUCTIONS (Summarized)
No Leader	Entry, Ambiguity	"Your leader(s) will be here in a few minutes. He/She/They would like you to introduce yourselves and begin to get to know each other."
Names Game	Ice Breaker (No silent members)	Go around the circle with first names (real or "Group" name). Then one person tries to say each person's name, the group helps when someone misses. Then another person tries until each member has given every other member's name.
Credentials Bag	Status	"Each person take a card, write down all the formal titles you have, all the academic degrees, all honors you have received...Now place the card in this bag. I will now throw away (or burn) the bag and you are not to refer to **anything** you have written during your group here." (Thus, we all start out equal, equally acceptable, equally vulnerable).
Expectations	Entry	"Let's go around the group and ask what each of us **expects** to **happen** in this group."
Descriptions	Entry	One person gives his/her first name, a personally descriptive verb and adverb both beginning with the first letter of the first name: John Jousts Joyously. Each person gives their own and then repeats all names and descriptions already given.
Deception	Introduction: "Trust yourself, not directions"	"Each of you has a name tag with different colors; your task is to find out what the different colors represent." (Random, Birth Order, Sun Signs, Age, and so on). Debrief.
First Impressions	Stereotypes	(Beginning of group) "Let's go around and verbalize our first reactions to one another; just say what your first impressions are."
Past	Background Sharing	Each, "In 5 min., tell us the experiences that made you who you are now. In the last minute describe a peak experience when you felt elated, 'up,' joyous."

NAME OF EXERCISE	CONTENT FOCUS OR THEME	DIRECTIONS - INSTRUCTIONS (Summarized)
Adjectives	Indirect Feedback	"Write down an adjective that best describes the person on your left. Use no names, put the piece of paper in the center." Each one is read, and group reacts to who **might** be represented by that trait.
Secrets	Indirect Disclosure	"Write down a secret that you have told few, if any, people. Use no names, place the folded paper in the center." Papers read and reacted to one at a time.
Milling	Making Contact (Loneliness)	"I want you to experience the room we are in. Move around and familiarize yourself with this room. Do not look at anyone's face...Now move around the room and begin to be aware of the people here. Now look into people's faces. Without talking, try to make contact with the people here."
Passing Objects	Spontaneity (Loosening up)	"Imagine this is a **square** object here in my hands. I want you to do something with the object and then pass it to someone else in the group. Do something with it and pass it on." (Then change shape to circular, cylindrical shapes.)
Dyads	Getting to Know Group Building	"Pick a person. Get to know that person....Now form into foursomes and get to know these people....Now get to know the people in the other foursomes." (Or pick a person you do not know or for some reason do not like and get to know him or her.)
Dichotomies	Labeling (want to be comfortable, yet move away from these labels as basic for inter-action)	"Imagine a deep crevice runs through the middle of the room from here to here. On this side of the room I want all the people who consider themselves to be _____ and on this side all those who think they are _____. Those who are on one side but would **like** to be on the other side, switch sides." (Talkers-listeners, introverts-extroverts, liberal-conservative, fighters-lovers, warm-cool, sharp-smooth, up-down, in-out, and so on.)

NAME OF EXERCISE	CONTENT FOCUS OR THEME	DIRECTIONS - INSTRUCTIONS (Summarized)
Humming	Label Feelings	"Close your eyes. Begin humming a single tone. Relax. Let your mind relax. If a tune comes to mind, hum that tune, and any other tune that happens to come out." Now how does that title or content relate to how you are feeling right now?
Animals	Entry	"If you had to be an animal (or a house, car, city, state, and so on), what kind of animal would you prefer to be? Why?" (Group's reaction to each.)
Pet Peeves	Practice in Negative Feedback	"Each of you write down your pet peeve - something that really irritates you about people - on a slip of paper, fold the paper and place it in the center; no names please." (Each slip is read and discussed.)
Lemons	Individual Differences (Lemons, like people, are very much alike, yet different at the same time. They look alike from afar, but are quite unique.)	"Take a lemon. Get to know your lemon. Introduce your lemon as worth knowing to someone else's lemon. Introduce your pair of lemons to another pair of lemons, then pass the lemons with your eyes closed and try to identify each lemon. Close your eyes, get into a circle and roll your lemon into the center; then find your lemon."
Lifting (Levitation)	Trust "Tripping"	One person lies on back, with eyes closed. Group reaches under and lifts. Begin swaying immediately after lifting, lift over head and still swaying lay him or her down on the floor.
Break In	Inclusion/Motivation (Anger)	Task for one person "talk yourself into the group" and ask for the group "to keep the person out until they assertively ask to join."
Blind Walk	Trust/Caring	Pairs. One person is blindfolded, other puts one hand on first's shoulder from behind. Task is to provide experiences (or show caring) for the blindfolded person. 10-15 or 20 minutes, then reverse. Talk about reactions.

NAME OF EXERCISE	CONTENT FOCUS OR THEME	DIRECTIONS - INSTRUCTIONS (Summarized)
Mirroring	Dominance-Submission	Pairs facing. "Imagine a glass pane separates you. Place your hands on the glass across, but not touching, from the other person's hands. Let them move as they will, but keep hands across from the other person's hands....Now one person dominate and the other person must follow the first person's movements....Now the other person reverse this and dominate, with the other person following or submitting." Talk about reactions.
Line Up	Dominance-Submission (Anger)	"I want you to form a line(s) against this wall. Now I want you to order yourself as follows: The most dominant person against the wall, then highly dominant people, then submissive people, and the most submissive at the end. If someone is where you think you should be, **do** something about it."
Show and Tell	Senses	"Bring in your favorite food, poem, flowers, music, and so forth and show that to the group." All react to the various Stimuli.
Permission	Noncoercion	"I want to make sure you understand that you have my permission **not** to do anything you do not want to do. Discuss this ground rule now and reach a concensus as to how this applies to this group."
Johari Window	Self-Awareness	After describing Johari grid (known to self/known to others - unknown to self/unknown to others), "draw your own sections with the size of each indicating your own estimate of how large are these areas in your life."
Health Paths	Assessment	In these 6 areas - social, emotional, physical, intellectual, spiritual, recreational - write down: 1. OK or not OK; 2. if you aren't OK, what is the cause, (3) what can you do to be OK in this area.
Brainstorming	Agendas	(Blackboard or newsprint) "Let's list all of the areas/questions you might want to cover" (or things that cause depression, and so on). "Just share anything you might want to cover."

II. MIDDLE GROUP EXERCISES

NAME OF EXERCISE	CONTENT FOCUS OR THEME	DIRECTIONS - INSTRUCTIONS (Summarized)
Associations	Projection	"If you had to be a _____, what would you choose to be?" (Vehicle, color, musical instrument, animal, season, song, house, garden, river, state, and such.)
Values Auction	Values	(1) Each person writes down their 5 most important values, (2) they are collated and the top 15 selected, (3) each person is given $10,000 "paper" money and 15 values auctioned off to the highest bidders.
Hot Potato	Conflict Styles	"Based on what's happened so far, typify each member's handling of conflict as either: placating, blaming, or super-reasonable."
Purr/Ouch	Interpersonal	"List the people you see each week on this dichotomy: Toxic-Nourishing (or energizers-deadeners)."
Scripts	Transactional	"Using all the magazines available, make a collage that represents the phases of your life and the T.A. scripts you have learned."
Splits	Polarity	"I want you to play out the two opposite parts of your polarity by role playing each side - one in this chair and, when talking for the other, move to this chair. Carry out a lively dialogue between these two parts of yourself."
Dear John	Health	"Write yourself a letter from your body about how it feels you are taking care of it and what suggestions it has for improving your health."
N.L.P.	Info Processing	Demonstrate neurolinguistic programming analysis of representational systems (visual, kinesthetic, auditory) with one member - then split into two's to practice (Bandler & Grinder, 1979).

NAME OF EXERCISE	CONTENT FOCUS OR THEME	DIRECTIONS - INSTRUCTIONS (Summarized)
Myths	Denial	"Finish the following sentences: 1. All of my life I have been waiting for someone to _____ 2. Sometimes, I think my whole life is based on proving that _____ 3. Never, ever, in this group, refer to me as a _____ 4. I have wasted a lot of energy denying that _____ 5. One myth that I have stubbornly held onto is _____."
Stroking	Values	"Write down a prescription for being really good to yourself - be specific."
Not Too Late	Values/Death	"Write down your answers: If you had 6 weeks to live, what would you do, what would you want said in your eulogy, what would you like to give away and to whom, what would you like inscribed on your tombstone?"
Too Busy	Time	"How much time are you spending 'earning' your answers to the previous exercise?" (Not Too Late)
Here and Now	Present Focus	"For the next hour we will only talk about what thoughts/feelings we are having **right now.**"
Life Line	Growth/Goals	"Draw a line across the length of your paper - starting at the left side, put your birth on the left and your death on the right - fill in your significant past events up to the present - and your 'hopes' for future events and getting old."
Tit-for-Tat	Interpersonal Payoffs	"Let's do an analysis of each person's interpersonal behavioral style and what the interpersonal 'payoff' is for that style. When they do X_____, what do they want in return from other people?"

NAME OF EXERCISE	CONTENT FOCUS OR THEME	DIRECTIONS - INSTRUCTIONS (Summarized)
Wheeling Dealing	Interpersonal, Style	"Using the interpersonal wheel on the blackboard (in order: dominance - anger - withdrawal - submission - nice person - socializer), based on your experience in this group, label yourself and each member by their **usual** or most chosen category."
P-A-C Person	Transactional Analysis	"Draw how large your current parent-adult-child circles are; then draw them how you would like them to be."
Body Talk	Body Feedback	"Examine the tension right now in your body; what is your body trying to tell you?"
Uppers/Downers	Loneliness	"List people you know from (1) the top of a page: people who make you feel great and leaving them is easy; (2) top middle: people you feel good with but have a hard time leaving them; (3) low middle: people you tolerate but are with only to avoid being alone; (4) bottom: people who make you feel lonely even when you are with them."
Strength Bombardment	Resources/Positive Feelings	Each person gives a list of his or her strengths. The group then adds to each list, giving only positive feedback.
Analogies	Feedback	Each member to each other member: "You remind me of a _____ because of _____." Example: Minister, because of "good guy" style.
Feedback	Feedback	One at a time (or in two's): "Look the other person in the eyes, touch him/her, and tell him/her what you think of him/her." (A potent exercise; may be repeated later in the group.)
Nonverbal Feedback	Feedback	"Now, without using words, give feedback to each group member."
Yell	Hostility, Release	The first person to sense hostility whispers a "code phrase" into the next person's ear; when the code reaches the first person, the group stands up and yells the code phrase.

Innovations In Clinical Practice: A Source Book

NAME OF EXERCISE	CONTENT FOCUS OR THEME	DIRECTIONS - INSTRUCTIONS (Summarized)
Creative	Expression, Projection	Assemble collages from magazines, paint pictures, make things out of clay individually to express past, present, or identity. This can also be done by the group to express molar group feelings. Alternately members can sing personal songs or create a dance, and so forth.
Who Are You	Uncovering	A stimulus question is asked **20** times, and the target person gives a different response each time. (Can be used as feedback, example: Joe is a person who _____) (10 times) I am a person who _____ .
Role Playing	Feedback/Uncovering	Direct two (or more) people to play out an interaction or situation that is problematic. Alter egos sit behind the principal players and voice the real-immediate reactions that the principal player may feel but are not socially approved. Roles may be **reversed**. Practice in constructive behaviors with group encouragement/suggestions so that member is successful or effective is the goal.
Coins	Giving-Taking (Imbalances)	"Take all the coins you have and give them to me. (Imbalances) How does that make you feel?" Give them back equal amounts of money. "Your first task is, one at a time, to give money to those you'd like to give it to. Look at how much you ended with, and remember who gave to you." Take the money and redistribute it evenly. "Now your task is to, one at a time, take money from those people you'd like to take from." Return money to members and **process.** "Now give each person a symbolic gift and take one from them." **Process.**
Fishbowl	Feedback	Inner circle completes task or interacts, outer circle members observe. Outer circle gives feedback on **process** of inner group. Reverse positions and repeat. (Observers can be used in this manner.)

NAME OF EXERCISE	CONTENT FOCUS OR THEME	DIRECTIONS - INSTRUCTIONS (Summarized)
Center of Group	Inclusion (Power)	"This paper represents the center of the group, place yourself according to how close you feel to the center and how close to various members in the group." Position yourself in relationship to both the center and to particular individuals. (Alternately, this exercise can be used as a group sociogram with one member placing all the other members in relation to center and each other.)
Penny-Nickel	Negotiation/ Competition	Split the group into two halves: Arrange 2 sets of four chairs facing each other; have each group select 3 people to sit together on one set of the chairs. "This group here has an infinite number of pennies. The task for this group is to buy nickels from that group. Only the people in the chairs can speak; if one of you in the outer group wants to speak you can come up and use the fourth chair, speak, and then return to the outer group."
Out Time	Processing Time	"Take time to look at what has happened and what you have been feeling. Go where you want, but do not talk to anyone."
III. FOCAL EXERCISES		
Dilemma	Negotiation/ Independence	When any unexpected problem presents itself or the schedule needs to be changed, describe the problem and assign the group the responsibility for resolving the problem. Process how the decision was made.
No Respect	Nonresponders/ Rejection	When a person is feeling that they are not being listened to, have that member carry on a conversation with another member who reads a paper and then turns back as the first member tries to talk to him or her.
What If	Catastrophizing	When a member becomes anxious ask, "What's the worst thing that can happen to you in this group right now?...How would you handle that if it did happen?"

NAME OF EXERCISE	CONTENT FOCUS OR THEME	DIRECTIONS - INSTRUCTIONS (Summarized)
Mom/Dad	Transference	"Write down how you feel about the leader and how you think the leader feels about you - in what ways are your comments similar to how you feel about one or both of your parents?"
Voice	Paralinguistic Cues	When one member's vocal cues are not congruent with his or her verbal cues, have members show the discrepant style by role playing. Have members repeat the same words with as many different uses of vocal cues as possible.
I Agree	No Conflict	When a member starts to argue, agree with everything he or she says. (Can then switch to disagreeing to contrast.)
FIRO	Group Process	"What group issues are most relevant for you now: inclusion, control, or affection?" (Schutz, 1966).
Ask Me	Silent Members	"Can you tell us why you have not spoken thus far? How can we help you to speak more comfortably?"
False Fronts	Facades	"List the facades/masks/false fronts that you hide behind...Why do you feel that you need them?"
I Object	Fighting	Have two conflicting members each select two "seconds" to help them prepare for a "fair" verbal fight. When both are ready, have them present their positions using a debate or courtroom metaphor.
Turning	Needs	To a discontented member: "Conduct a needs assessment on the group to see if the group is heading in the right direction or if we need to steer a different course."
Whined Downer	Complainers/ Regression	When group "griping" gets too heavy, have everyone complain in whiny voices and feel sorry for themselves. Then have everyone say positive things about the group and feel very good about themselves.
Anxiety Stomp	Anxiety, Substitution	When someone is anxious, have him/her put the "fear on the floor" and "stomp" it out in anger.

NAME OF EXERCISE	CONTENT FOCUS OR THEME	DIRECTIONS - INSTRUCTIONS (Summarized)
Changing Tapes	Thought Stoppage	When members can't free themselves of obsessive thoughts (e.g., food binging), have them imagine biting into a lemon to loosen their "obsession tape," then switch to a positive relaxation "fantasy tape."
Working	Vocational	"People can be placed in three vocational clusters; people people, things people, ideas/data people. Rank order these 3 for yourself."
Roles	Feedback	"If this were an Indian tribe and you were stepping down as chief - what roles in the tribe would you assign to the members here? Why?"
Living In	Values	"Design an ideal communal living arrangement."
Pair and Care	Affection	"Pick a person who you could have warm feelings for; choose or be chosen, you cannot refuse to be chosen. Show your feelings nonverbally."
Games	Interpersonal	"What do you expect me to do when you say (or do) _____?" Tie the **game** to expected reactions (and thus control) of others. Group games to watch for: Pied Piper, Saint, Wooden Leg, If It Weren't for You, Tease But Don't Touch, Sicky, You and Him or Her Fight, Spotlighter, Mr. Clean, Mr. Machismo, Superhelper, I Don't Care What You Think.
Waiting for Santa Claus (or the Easter Bunny or the Golden Egg)	Dependency	"Let's all imagine that we are children. It is Christmas and we have put our stockings over the fireplace and are waiting for Santa Claus to come. Everyone quiet, and let's all wait for him over here at the door." (Focus - **we** have to work for ourselves and not wait for others to nurture us.)
Unhooking	Manipulation	Once person is made aware of a major manipulation, have him/her evaluate the relationship, then say to manipulator, "You cannot push me around any more, I will not allow you to affect me, I am leaving your control now." Have the person turn and walk out of the room. Process **both** persons' feelings.

NAME OF EXERCISE	CONTENT FOCUS OR THEME	DIRECTIONS - INSTRUCTIONS (Summarized)
Tug-of-War	Dominance	Put dominant member (or 2) on one side and all others on the other end of an imaginary rope.
Elect and Do	Group Process	Form dyads, then quads (verbally and nonverbally), then eights. **Process.** Have each group elect a leader for a task to be announced later. **Process** how leader was chosen. Then announce a task to be completed cooperatively as a group. **Process** how group reached their goal. **Process** the whole group building exercise.
Today's Leader	Authority	To a member who attacks the leader, elect him or her leader for the day. (Look for behavior that the leader was being criticized for using.)
Goodbye	Separation	For someone unaccepting of a relationship's end (moving away, death) have him/her say goodbye to the "person" in an empty chair. "Say everything you wanted to say to _____, but didn't have a chance to."
Top Dog/Underdog	Learned Bias	Designate all blue eyed people as special and give them priority or special considerations. At the same time, punish and scapegoat the brown eyeds (less sensitive, less able, not as clean, and so on). Once bias is established in members' behavior, then **reverse** and reward the brown eyed members.
Produce or Else	Affection, Respect, Confusion, Authority	Play an authoritarian role where you demand that a passive aggressive (or other defense) member **produce** for you a tangible product. Play a conditional-withholding role and force a person to comply. For example, "be a good member, disclose, and I will then respond to you." (Remember, most people here want the **affection** of the authoritarian and yet feel they must lose their integrity (and produce) and **compete** for the affection being apparently withheld.)
Show Down	Feedback	Select a problem pair. Have them walk toward each other from opposite corners and "do what you feel like doing"; if they pass, have them approach again until they respond to each other.

NAME OF EXERCISE	CONTENT FOCUS OR THEME	DIRECTIONS - INSTRUCTIONS (Summarized)
Gossip	Problem Member	Put the member in corner with his or her back to the group. Discuss the person and then ask for his or her reactions.
Exclusion	Inclusion	Place the member who feels "out of it" in a corner and whisper about him or her inaudibly. Make the person come back to the group; or if the person does not come willingly, ask or carry him or her back to the group. (Processing is necessary; this exercise is designed to focus on feelings of alienation and difficulty breaking in.)
Gibberish	Communication	"Talk to each other in gibberish, try to communicate something and see if the other person can understand what you are saying" (focus on voice tone and gestures).
Remember	Feelings/Nonverbals	Arrange members in seated pairs. Explain, eyes closed, "Remember a time you felt very, very alone and without using words communicate this to your partner....then remember a time you felt very angry and communicate this nonverbally...a time you felt great joy and communicate this." **Process.**
Give Me	Manipulation/Guilt	Assess how a person has been manipulated (example, guilt) and use same tactics to have him or her give you (leader) a coin, ask for more, keep asking. Make the person borrow more; keep going until person sees and defeats the manipulation or gets so angry that he or she expresses it directly to you. Role play or practice behavior to overcome/avoid manipulations.
Lights Off	Voices/Communication	Turn the lights off; continue to talk. Focus is on listening to vocal cues only.
Hassling	Assertiveness	Set up a phone conversation (or situation) where a person has to be **assertive** in the face of authority or a strong person (such as a person who cuts in front of the person standing in a line waiting).

NAME OF EXERCISE	CONTENT FOCUS OR THEME	DIRECTIONS - INSTRUCTIONS (Summarized)
Upending Expectancies	Feedback	When a person unknowingly "asks" for, or his or her behavior pulls, a given response (example, sympathy), respond in an opposite manner. Then have the individual verbally ask for the response he or she has been forcing others to give. Assess: Is this really what the person wants from other people?
Taking	Taking	One person is placed in the center, eyes closed, no movement allowed. The rest of group **gives**; the person is **only** allowed to receive.
Cartoon	Group Process	"Write a cartoon (poem, fantasy) describing what is happening in this group (or class)."
Goal Setting	Accomplishment, Control	At the end of a session, a person states a believable, achievable, measurable, observable **goal** to be completed by the next session. Reports on attainment come at beginning of next group. (Focus on sense of personal control over environment.)

IV. GUIDED IMAGERY

These exercises should be done with eyes closed, instructions given, time in silence, and then debriefing. (Process these exercises very carefully - may have to have a member start over again to create a successful finish to an upsetting exercise.)

Test	Visualization Ability	"Close your eyes - imagine you are watching a bull fight in Mexico." Debrief after one minute - if they can visualize color, movement, detail, background - then guided fantasy will work OK - if images shift, are vague, can't hold whole picture together at same time, are slow to form - then will have to "talk" themselves through imagery exercises (may go slower and your verbiage may "bother" them) and exercises may have less impact.
Tug-of-War	Polarities	"Imagine each of your polarity extremes are at ends of a rope, involved in a tug-of-war. Imagine what they do and say, trying to dominate the other side."

NAME OF EXERCISE	CONTENT FOCUS OR THEME	DIRECTIONS - INSTRUCTIONS (Summarized)
Keep Away	Defenses	(To an angry member) "Imagine you have hidden yourself away from everyone by building a fortress with a moat surrounding it...people try to approach but you yell at them and refuse to let your drawbridge down to let them enter...you're safe and all alone."
Seeding	Growth	"Imagine you are a seed, placed in fertile soil and watered, you slowly grow into a full size plant."
Stay/Leave	Dependency/ Transitions	"Imagine you have been living in a very comfortable cell with all of the conveniences, books, food you have needed - then one day the jailer unlocks your cell and leaves without explanation - what do you do?"
Barriers	Frustrations	"You are on your life's journey when on the road in front of you is a huge barrier blocking your path - what do you do?"
Redreaming	Practicing Success	"Continue a troubling dream that you typically or recently have had - but in your fantasy make the dream have a successful or happy ending."
Learning Center	Supports	"Design your ideal learning center - pick your location and imagine yourself creating an optimal learning environment for yourself."
Ideal Image	Goals/Motives	"Picture how you would like to be after you reach your goals (or reasons) for coming to this group."
5 Years	Future Vocational	"Imagine yourself waking up 5 years from today on a weekday (or weekend day). Where are you, what kind of dwelling, are people there; you eat breakfast; what do you do in A.M. hours; during lunch, what do you talk about if with people or think about if alone; what do you do in P.M. hours; during dinner, who do you talk with and about what; how do you spend your evening hours; reflect on the day before you go to sleep."

NAME OF EXERCISE	CONTENT FOCUS OR THEME	DIRECTIONS - INSTRUCTIONS (Summarized)
Don't Forget	Aversive	"Imagine all of the bad implications of your previous problematic behavior – what are the worst things that happen to you when you continue to repeat that behavioral pattern" (example, being fat and not fitting into chairs, and so on) – "Remember these effects the next time you are about to use that behavioral style."
Cope Out	Coping	"Imagine the worst thing happening to you (in terms of failing) and imagine yourself creatively coping with your failure – make yourself handle the situation without catastrophizing."
Mini-Vacations	Relaxation	"Imagine you are in the most relaxing location in the world and doing the most pleasurable, relaxing thing you can do. Pretend you are there and, using all of your senses, get lost in the fantasy."
Slow Down	Relaxation	"Imagine: 1. You are a feather being blown up above the clouds on a beautiful day; you safely rise, circle, fall, and land softly in a warm meadow. 2. Walking on a country road on a dewy morning. 3. Lying in the grass, looking at clouds and trying to imagine what clouds/things the cloud shapes bring to mind. 4. Innertubing, blindfolded, down a lazy warm river until you are pulled out at a party location. 5. Lying in a hammock on a warm, breezy day in the shade of a tree."
Inner Space	Awareness, Awe	"Imagine being a miniature, remote control television camera – enter your body through your mouth – travel to the stomach – then to the intestines – you are absorbed by the blood – pass through the heart and lungs – flow in the blood out to muscles – to brain – leave the blood vessels and enter brain and explore eyes – ears – spinal cord – sexual parts – re-enter digestive tract at intestines and travel back out via the stomach and mouth – record sights and reactions."

NAME OF EXERCISE	CONTENT FOCUS OR THEME	DIRECTIONS - INSTRUCTIONS (Summarized)
Body Be	Awareness, Health	"Imagine you are looking at your body in a mirror as it looks now - then allow it to change in the ways that are both possible and that you would like it to be different."
Doorways	Significant Others/ Values	"Imagine a house,...this house holds all the different parts of your brain, enter; off the corridor each room has a different name on the door; enter the ones you want to; record your impressions in each room; finish up in the master computer room."
Reach Out	Grief	"Imagine a person you miss very much is across a ravine from you, build a bridge over to that person, cross the bridge and reach out and touch him/her, talk to him/her, imagine the comments he/she will make, then, when you are ready, say goodbye and cross the bridge again to the other side."
Quest	Learning/Wisdom	"Imagine you are a 12 year old Indian child living 200 years ago and you are ready to be sent on a vision quest to discover yourself and be assigned your adult name. The first night you are taken to a hill overlooking your village, you disrobe, are handed two warm buffalo robes and told to stay there without food or water for 24 hours....You are greeted warmly and then briefed: You are to travel to four lodges of symbolic learning; stay at each 3 days, learning from that place's perspective; you are given a symbolic gift, and then travel on to the next lodge." (Lodge of North is wisdom symbolized by the White Buffalo, Lodge of the East is knowledge of farsightedness symbolized by the Yellow Eagle, Lodge of South is up-close knowledge of innocence symbolized by the Green Mouse, Lodge of the West is introspective knowledge symbolized by the Black Bear.) "Make a shield of your gifts" - debriefing leads to a concensus symbolic name based on the preferred learning styles/symbols (Storm, 1972).

NAME OF EXERCISE	CONTENT FOCUS OR THEME	DIRECTIONS - INSTRUCTIONS (Summarized)
Sub Me's	Integration	"Imagine each aspect of your personality becomes a separate subpersonality seated at a large conference table – have them begin a lively conversation as to how they can work cooperatively together."
Gold Watch	Values	"Imagine a retirement luncheon is being held for you – what will the speaker say about you before he hands you a gold watch – how do you react?"
Eggshell	Protection	"Imagine a large circle of white light is hovering 3 feet above your head...now the light streams down through the top of your head, warms you, cleanses you, then exits out your stomach and surrounds you with a foot-wide sheet of gleaming white light...the light dissolves slowly, turning into a thin but strong Teflon-like eggshell that protects you from getting hurt."
Guru	Mentor	"Imagine you have traveled to a wilderness area, you walk into the densest section, and continue for half a day when you come upon a beautiful meadow – you see a house and you know a wise person is there waiting for you – you ask the person 3 questions which are answered, and you are given advice on how to live a better life – you exchange gifts and return."
Contact	Senses	"Imagine you have walked into the woods for an hour – you sit down at the edge of a clearing and without moving again for one hour you explore the area with your eyes closed using only sound and smell, the second hour you explore the area with only your eyes, the third hour you explore only your feelings about the area, and the fourth hour you combine the information from all of your senses."
I'll Be Fine	Trust/Relaxation	"Imagine that you do a dozen extremely pleasurable activities...now imagine taking those same feelings with you and holding onto them in the dentist's chair, operating table, or delivery room."

NAME OF EXERCISE	CONTENT FOCUS OR THEME	DIRECTIONS - INSTRUCTIONS (Summarized)
Keys	Discovery	"You discover a key hidden is some of your old childhood things, imagine finding a lock - opening the lock - the door opens - what do you find?"
No Thank You	Guilt/Scapegoating	"Imagine you are Mr./Ms. Clean who wears glowing white clothes and has never made a mistake in his or her whole life...now imagine someone coming up to you who seems to delight in making you feel guilty, inferior, worthless, or unlovable - imagine him/her accusing you or dumping all of the usual nonsense on you - but you remain super-reasonable, serene, unruffled, innocent, and puzzled. You declare your innocence and ask him/her why he/she needs to say those things to you - and ask if he/she is having trouble with those same statements. If he or she explodes into vicious anger, you maintain your serene innocence - if he/she reaches out or apologizes, you acknowledge it and hug - if he or she stays accusatory, you imagine him/her leaving you and being relieved."
Rescue	Nourishing	"Remember a time when you felt hurt and overwhelmed as a child. Now imagine yourself going back as a strong, capable adult and helping that hurt child in you to feel nourished and protected."
Left/Right	Balance	"Imagine entering the left hemisphere of your brain...you see a small opening which leads to the right brain - stretch open this small tube so you now enter the right brain...carry messages back and forth so you can act as the communication go-between for the two hemispheres."
Fingered	Blaming	"Imagine a finger pointed at you and an angry voice telling you something.
Relief	Pain	"Imagine entering your body and traveling to a hurt or stiff part of your right-now body - imagine stroking, gently stretching, and soaking that part in hot soothing oil so that the stiffness and pain is replaced by warm pleasant sensations."

NAME OF EXERCISE	CONTENT FOCUS OR THEME	DIRECTIONS - INSTRUCTIONS (Summarized)
Purging	Release	"Imagine all of the bad, hurt, angry feelings well up inside of your stomach and are squeezed up to your throat where they pass out through your left shoulder, down your left arm, and out through your fingers into a trash can. When all of the feelings have been drained, close the trash can, and put it into a bonfire – watching as the trash can and contents melt away."
Heal	Helping	"Imagine you were temporarily given healing power – you can touch each of the people you know just once to take away one problem they have."
Looking Up	Spiritual	"Imagine you have a spiritual center at the top of your brain – imagine opening the doors and entering this magical place in your brain."
Wise Person	Projection	"Close your eyes, imagine you see a wise person sitting in front of you, walk up and ask him or her a question and imagine his or her answer." (Can have person imagine a date on a calendar.) "How does all this relate to how you are feeling now" (or on the calendar date).

V. **CLOSING GROUP EXERCISES**

NAME OF EXERCISE	CONTENT FOCUS OR THEME	DIRECTIONS - INSTRUCTIONS (Summarized)
Contracting	Transfer	"Write out a contract as to how you plan to implement what you have learned here – be specific enough to assess later."
Next	New Goals	"What is the next learning experience for you to initiate based upon what you have learned here."
Good Luck	Support	"Give a symbolic gift to each member to help him or her after returning home. Also give a gift to the leader(s)."
How Now	Hopes/Fears (Repeated)	"Compared to your initial hopes/fears how are you feeling about this group experience?"

NAME OF EXERCISE	CONTENT FOCUS OR THEME	DIRECTIONS - INSTRUCTIONS (Summarized)
Tools	Resources	"What resources will you need to develop back home for your new learning to be successfully implemented and maintained."
Codes	Reminders	"Pick a 'code' word to remind you of each of the important elements you learned. Later use the word to remind yourself when you need to call upon that learning or when you feel yourself slipping into bad habits."
Goodbye	Letting Go	"Go around and say goodbye in your own ways to each group member."
Stumbling	Relapse	"Assume upon return home that after a while you find you have slipped into your old bad habits; anticipate how you will get yourself back on the 'right' track again."
Winding Down	Summarizing	"Let's talk about the group ending (mourning expected loss); let's try to pull together what we have done, what has happened to us here, and so forth."
Exit Triads	Re-Entry	"Form triads, think of going home now and anticipate your feelings when you go home and talk with people there."
Clinicing	Summarizing	Place an empty chair in front of the leader. Members can come and get summary feedback from (and give to) the leader.

RESOURCES

Bandler, R. & Grinder, J. FROGS INTO PRINCES. Moab, UT: Real People Press, 1979.

Clearinghouse for Structured Group Programs, Counseling Center, University of Rhode Island, Kingston, RI 02881. Outlines for a large number of complete workshops can be ordered; request their catalogue and order information.

Cooper, C. L. & Harrison, K. Designing and facilitating experimental group activities: Variables and issues. In J. W. Pfeiffer & J. E. Jones (Eds.), THE 1976 ANNUAL HANDBOOK FOR GROUP FACILITATORS. San Diego: University Associates, 1976.

Otto, H. A. FANTASY ENCOUNTER GAMES. Berkeley, CA: Nash Publishing, 1972.

Pfeiffer, J. W. & Jones, J. E. (Eds.). A HANDBOOK OF STRUCTURED EXPERIENCES FOR HUMAN RELATIONS TRAINING (Vols. 1-8); and THE ANNUAL HANDBOOK FOR GROUP FACILITATORS (1972-83). San Diego, CA: University Associates.

Russell, J. M. Personal growth through structured group exercises. VOICES, 1971, 28-36.

Russell, J. M. & Easton, J. Teaching the design, leadership, and evaluation of structured groups. PERSONNEL AND GUIDANCE JOURNAL, 1979, **57**, 426-29.

Schutz, W. C. THE INTERPERSONAL UNDERWORLD. Palo Alto, CA: Science and Behavior Books, Inc., 1966.

Stevens, J. O. AWARENESS: EXPLORING, EXPERIMENTING, EXPERIENCING. Lafayette, CA: Real People Press, 1971.

Storm, H. SEVEN ARROWS. New York: Ballantine Books, 1972.

University Associates, Inc., 8517 Production Avenue, P. O. Box 26240, San Diego, CA 92126. University Associates are publishers, trainers, and human resource consultants. Their publications contain a wide range of materials which would be of interest to group leaders.

HOW TO EVALUATE CLAIMANTS FOR SOCIAL SECURITY AND SSI BENEFITS *

Jack R. Anderson

The signs and symptoms of their illnesses prevent many mentally disabled Americans from establishing eligibility for the benefits to which they are entitled under the provisions of the Social Security and Supplemental Security Income disability programs. The purpose of this paper is to describe and recommend to the professional staff of public hospitals and mental health and retardation centers, where most of the mentally disabled are treated, some specific steps they can take to intervene on behalf of their patients in the adjudicative process for establishing eligibility for benefits.

By the end of 1980, a total of 550,000 mentally disabled individuals were receiving monthly checks from the Social Security and SSI disability programs for a total of some $2.25 billion for the year. These individuals make up about 11% of the total number of Social Security and SSI disability recipients. During 1980 an additional 65,500 new mental disability allowances were made (Atlanta Regional Office of Social Security, personal communication, 1981).

For the purposes of these programs, the mentally disabled include both the mentally ill and mentally retarded or, specifically, individuals with one of four diagnoses: organic brain syndromes, functional psychotic disorders, functional nonpsychotic disorders, or mental retardation.

ESTABLISHING ELIGIBILITY

Any individual who believes he or she is mentally disabled and entitled to benefits from either program may file, or have a representative file, an application with the local Social Security district office. The district office processes the application and forwards it to the appropriate state disability determination section. A team composed of a disability examiner, who has special knowledge of the evidentiary requirements of the disability program, and a physician then processes the application. These two work together in examining the medical evidence that may be submitted with the application, initiating requests for additional medical evidence when necessary, and scheduling consultative examinations when appropriate. The process of gathering medical evidence continues until the team members agree that the evidence is sufficient to prepare a disability determination.

Two definitions are of key importance in the processing of applications by the disability determination team; the first is that of "disability." Under Social Security law disability means "inability to engage in any substantial gainful activity by reason of any medically determinable physical or mental impairment which can be expected to result in death or has lasted or can be expected to last for a continuous period of not less than 12 months" (DHHS, 1980, p. 55586). The second definition is "a medically determinable impairment is one which has medically demonstrable anatomical, physiological, or psychological abnormalities. Such abnormalities are medically determinable if they manifest themselves as signs or laboratory findings apart from symptoms. Abnormalities which manifest themselves only as symptoms are not medically determinable" (DHHS, 1980, p. 55586). From this definition it can be seen that mental status findings for disability determination examinations must be much more detailed and must contain much more objective clinical data than are necessary for routine psychiatric examinations done for diagnostic and treatment purposes.

In adjudicating claims for chronic brain syndromes, functional psychotic disorders, and functional nonpsychotic disorders, the members of the team look for specific signs and symptoms listed in Social Security regulations (DHHS, 1980) and determine whether these signs and symptoms cause a "marked restriction in daily activities," "marked constriction of interests," "deterioration in personal habits," and "seriously impaired ability to relate to other people." If these determinations are all positive, the claimant's condition is said to **meet** the severity of the listings and an allowance is made, that is, the claimant is found eligible to receive benefits. If the claimant's condition or claimant's signs and symptoms are not included in the listings, the team may also make a finding that the severity of his or her condition **equals** the severity intended by the listings, in which case an allowance can also be made. If the claimant has more than one mental disability or has a combined mental and physical condition neither of which meets or equals the severity of the listings, it is possible that a combination of the conditions can be found to equal the severity of the listings, and an allowance can be made in these cases.

If the claimant's impairment is determined to be mental retardation, the team has to decide whether there is evidence of one of the following conditions: severe mental and social incapacity as evidenced by marked dependence upon others for personal needs such as bathing and dressing and inability to understand the spoken word, to avoid physical danger, to follow simple directions, and to read, write, and perform simple calculations; an IQ of 59 or less; or an IQ of 60 through 69 along with another mental or physical impairment that imposes additional significant work-related limitation of function (DHHS, 1980). If the claimant's mental retardation meets one of these three sets of criteria, then it is considered to meet the severity of the listings. As with the other mental conditions described, mental retardation that does not meet the severity of the listings may be combined with other mental or physical impairments and be found to equal the severity intended by the listings; thus an allowance can be made.

If the team determines that the claimant does not have a condition or combination of conditions that meets or equals the severity of the listings, the next determination that has to be made is whether the claimant can meet the mental demands of unskilled work. To do this, he or she must have the capacity to understand, remember, and carry out instructions; respond appropriately to supervision, co-workers, and customary work pressures; sustain work attendance for reasonable periods of time (40 hours a week); and exercise acceptable judgment concerning work functions. If the team finds evidence of a medically determinable mental impairment that would preclude the claimant from meeting any one of these mental demands of unskilled work, an allowance can be made on combined medical and vocational factors.

The processes described above constitute the initial adjudication level. Of the 65,500 new mental disability allowances made during 1980, a total of 45,600 (about one-third of the total applications) were approved at this level. Applicants whose claims are denied at the initial level are informed that they have the right to appeal to the same district branch for reconsideration. During reconsideration, applicants present any new medical evidence that supports their claim to a second adjudication team from the same disability determination service that denied their initial claim. During 1980, less than half of those denied at the initial level chose to appeal; only 15% of those who did appeal won approval at this level (SDIP, 1981).

Claimants who are denied at the reconsideration level are given another chance to appeal for a hearing before an administrative law judge of the bureau of hearings and appeals of the U. S. Department of Health and Human Services. In 1980, 65% of them chose to do so, and 58% of the appeals were allowed even though they had previously been denied at both the initial and reconsideration levels. Those who are denied at the hearing level are given two more chances to appeal: first to the standing HHS appeals council appointed by the Secretary of HHS and then to a U. S. district court. However, in 1980 only about 0.5% of the total allowances were made at these levels (SDIP, 1981).

RECOMMENDATIONS FOR ACTION

The two most important principles for mental health and mental retardation professionals to remember in assisting their clients in applying for benefits are persistence and documentation.

Persistence is necessary to keep the claim active. If the claim is not allowed at the initial level, the claimant should be assisted in preparing a request for reconsideration. This request must be submitted to the district office within 60 days of the claimant's receipt of the denial notice. At this point it is also advisable to consult a lawyer. Most legal aid services prefer that their clients enlist their assistance at this time. If public counsel is not available, or if the claimant prefers, private practice lawyers may be consulted. The law provides for payment of legal fees in an amount up to 25% of the award approved. If the claim is again denied at the reconsideration level, a request should immediately be made for an administrative law judge hearing. It is important to remember that, in 1980, 58% of the claims heard by a judge were allowed even though they had been previously denied twice.

Without the intervention of mental health professionals as advocates, many mentally disabled individuals drop their claims after denial at the initial or reconsideration levels. Some do so because they function at such a low level of intelligence that they simply do not understand their rights of appeal. Some are delusional and distrustful of the adjudication procedures. Others are too anergic to carry through the necessary actions of appealing. It is imperative that advocate assistance be provided to the level of the hearing before an administrative law judge.

There are a variety of reasons why so many denials at initial and reconsideration levels are reversed at the administrative law judge hearings. The sheer volume of claims to be processed precludes a deliberate and careful review of each claim at the initial and reconsideration phases. There are not enough psychiatrists willing to spend their time consulting with the state agencies to provide a professional review of each case. A large percentage of the decisions at the initial and reconsideration levels have to be made by the disability examiners without benefit of medical consultations. Moreover, the psychiatrists I have worked with in two state agencies have not agreed among themselves, with me, or I with them more than about 50% of the time on which claimants were so severely impaired as to be eligible for benefits. From what I have seen at the federal regional offices, I doubt that their interrater reliability is any better.

In fact, a report by the Comptroller General of the United States (CGUS, 1979) quotes a 1978 study showing that two federal reviewers disagreed in 44% of the cases they reviewed. The federal reviews of random samples of state agency decisions were intended to increase the accuracy of the state adjudicative decisions and ensure uniformity throughout the United States. Obviously, if they disagree 44% of the time, the goals of the federal review program will not be met, and determinations at the initial and reconsideration levels will depend as much upon the individual examiners and medical consultants who review the claims as upon the severity of the impairments.

The administrative law judge hearing also is the first level of adjudication at which the decision is made by a person trained in legal procedures. It is the first level at which the procedures are outside the jurisdiction of the disability determination program. It is the first level at which the claimant makes a personal appearance at the decision-making procedure, represented by legal counsel if he or she wishes.

Documentation is nearly as important as persistence. The treating mental health and retardation center or public hospital is in the best position to provide medical evidence to document the severity of the claimant's condition. The best time to submit evidence is just before the claimant submits his or her initial claim to the Social Security district office. If that is not feasible, it can be given to the claimant's attorney at the time the appeal is made for reconsideration or for the administrative law judge hearing.

The format for documentation is simple; there should be sections on history, mental status, daily activities, diagnosis and prognosis, and general remarks. The sections on mental status, daily activities, and general remarks can be tricky, though. For adjudicative purposes, the mental status section should contain a wealth of clinical data. The claimant's appearance and behavior should be described; information on flow of thought and conversation, affect and mood, mental content, sensorium and cognitive functioning, and insight and judgment should also be included.

Scores of standardized psychological tests may be included. Test protocols should be attached to reports. If an MMPI is administered, a copy of the profile is required. For the WAIS-R and WISC-R, verbal, performance, full scale, and all subtest scores must be included. For test results to have adjudicative value they must be supported by clinical signs and symptoms. Any discrepancies observed by an examiner between intelligence scores and the claimant's appearance, conversation, behavior, work history, or academic achievement should be discussed and if possible explained. Elevated validity scales on MMPI profiles may provide useful evidence of claimant's motivation even though the clinical scales cannot be taken at face value. Psychological data properly presented can be helpful both in establishing the diagnosis and in determining the degree of severity (Schaffer, 1981).

Sufficient detail should be provided to enable any reader at any level of adjudication to form an independent opinion of the severity of the claimant's condition. Examples should be given of symptoms such as illogical associations, abnormal affect or mood, or impairment of reality testing (delusions or hallucinations). If there is impairment of memory, or of the ability to calculate or to abstract, the recall assessment techniques, arithmetic problems, proverbs, or similarity items used to assess these capacities should be described. Opinions on the claimant's insight and judgment should be supported by clinical observations, and an opinion of the claimant's ability to manage his or her own funds should be included.

The section on daily activities is not usually found in psychiatric reports prepared for purposes other than disability determination. For this report, however, it is a must. By law, no decision is possible on a mental disability claim without an adequate description of the claimant's daily activities. This description should include how the claimant spends his or her time; how the claimant takes care of his or her personal needs, whether he or she is involved in taking care of other family members, or performing household tasks like cooking, shopping, or yard work. Recreational activities and hobbies should be noted. Most important, the description of daily activities should illustrate the claimant's ability to relate to others and the extent of his or her socialization.

Diagnosis should be according to **DSM-III**, and prognosis should indicate whether the condition is expected to remain severe, or has been severe for a period of 12 consecutive months from the estimated onset.

The general comments section provides an opportunity for caregivers to point out which of the claimant's symptoms can be expected to prevent him or her from meeting the mental demands of unskilled work. These remarks should be quite specific. For example, an organic brain syndrome may impair a claimant's memory to the point that he or she would not be able to understand, remember, or carry out instructions. A claimant's delusions or hallucinations may preclude his or her responding appropriately to supervisors, co-workers, and customary work pressures. If the preceding sections contain sufficient clinical detail, the general comments section can present conclusive medical evidence that the claimant is eligible for disability benefits.

Mental health and retardation professionals other than psychiatrists may be in a better position to prepare the documentation, since they have more personal contact with the claimant. However, the report should be signed by a psychiatrist so that it will have the maximum probative value.

SETTING PRIORITIES

I have had frequent opportunities to discuss the disability programs with staff members of state hospitals, Veterans Administration hospitals, and mental health and retardation centers. They usually agree that it would be desirable to provide assistance to claimants in establishing eligibility for disability payments, but they cannot spare the necessary time, money, materials, or manpower to do so. In my opinion, the disability payments are so important to the mentally disabled that the advocacy program described above should be given the highest priority in the operational budgets of all publicly funded mental health and retardation institutions and community-based centers.

There are hundreds of thousands of mentally disabled Americans who could be enjoying a higher degree of personal dignity, freedom, normalcy, and treatment in the least restrictive environment if only they were provided the necessary assistance to establish their eligibility for disability benefits. Mental health professionals, by following an advocacy program such as I describe, can help the mentally disabled achieve those goals.

Jack R. Anderson, M.D., is currently in private practice in Birmingham, Alabama, where he is also professor of clinical psychiatry at the University of Alabama Medical Center. Dr. Anderson is a retired U.S. Army psychiatrist and was Director of Public Institutions for Nebraska, with responsibilities for statewide programs in mental health, mental retardation, corrections, services for the blind, veterans' homes, and alcoholism. His interests include psychotherapy and forensic psychiatry. The author may be contacted at 2000 Old Bay Front Road, Mobile, AL 36615.

RESOURCES

Controls Over Medical Examinations Necessary for the Social Security Administration to Better Determine Disability. Washington, DC: Comptroller General of the United States, 1979.

U. S. Department of Health and Human Services. FEDERAL REGISTER (Vol. 45, No. 163:55585-55617). Washington, DC: U. S. Government Printing Office, 1980.

Shaffer, J. W. Using the MMPI to evaluate mental impairment in disability determination. In J. Butcher, G. Dahlstrom, M. Gynther, & W. Schofield (Eds.), CLINICAL NOTES ON THE MMPI (No. 8). Nutley, NJ: Roche Psychiatric Service Institute, 1981.

U. S. Department of Health and Human Services. SOCIAL SECURITY BULLETIN (Vol. 44, No. 3:2-48). Washington, DC: U. S. Government Printing Office, 1981.

Status of the Disability Insurance Program. Washington, DC: US House Committee on Ways and Means, March 16, 1981.

INTRODUCTION TO CLIENT HANDOUTS

Many practitioners have found that informational handouts and brochures are quite helpful in communicating with their clients. Well designed materials can provide clients with important information, prevent misunderstandings and facilitate treatment. Each **INNOVATIONS** volume includes a few carefully selected handouts which you may freely copy for use with your clients.

Lacks, Stolz, and Levine's guide to psychotherapy is the best client handout on this topic that we have reviewed. The authors pay careful attention to the wording of their contribution and provide clear and concise answers to many of the questions about therapy that are typically asked by clients. Patricia Lacks, Ph.D., is currently an Associate Professor of Psychology at Washington University, St. Louis, Missouri, and has research interests in psychological assessment and behavioral treatment of insomnia. Jeffrey L. Levine and Jennifer A. Stolz are currently completing requirements for doctoral degrees in clinical psychology at Washington University. All three authors may be contacted at the Department of Psychology, Washington University, Box 1125, St. Louis, MO 63130.

Murray's handout provides valuable information to clients who are struggling with loss and grief. The author is an experienced clinician and instructor in this area. His contribution should be of significant help to individuals who have personal questions and concerns about the topic. Dr. Murray has co-authored another contribution for this volume and biographical information on him may be found on page 286.

In the third handout, Keller offers information to clients who are scheduled for psychological testing. This contribution is designed to reduce pretest anxiety by briefly explaining testing procedures to clients who have never been through such a process and who might be apt to perceive testing as a mysterious and frightening prospect. Biographical information on Dr. Keller may be found on page 285.

A GUIDE TO PSYCHOTHERAPY

The decision to begin psychotherapy is one which may have important consequences for the rest of your life. Research has shown that when individuals enter this type of treatment with a good understanding of what they are about to undertake, the are likely to achieve more favorable results. This pamphlet contains information about the unique process of psychotherapy. It will provide you with a written record of the practices and responsibilities of the client and the therapist. Read it and then ask your therapist any remaining questions you may have. No pamphlet can hope to provide accurate information about all types of psychotherapy or all therapists. Use this pamphlet as the focus for a discussion with your therapist about his or her specific practices.

In the information which follows, the term therapist refers to either a licensed clinical or counseling psychologist, a certified social worker, or a professional counselor. The profession of psychiatry has not been included since its practice is complicated by the use of physical treatments such as the prescription of drugs. However, much of the information included in this pamphlet is applicable to psychotherapy as practiced by a psychiatrist.

DESCRIPTION OF PSYCHOTHERAPY

In psychotherapy, you and a trained mental health professional work out strategies for handling problems of daily living. Problems that can be effectively dealt with include:

--anxiety and fears	--interpersonal difficulties
--depression	--low self-esteem
--habit control	--guilt
(e.g., smoking, over-eating)	--alcoholism

In addition, therapy can lead to personal growth through clarification of your thoughts and feelings about yourself, others, and events in your life. If you are uncertain as to whether your current concerns would best be dealt with by this form of treatment, discuss this with your therapist during your first session.

The majority of the time you spend in therapy will consist of talking about the issues you have presented to your therapist. However, along with "talking therapy," other methods may be employed, such as relaxation and assertiveness training, hypnosis, and role playing. Furthermore, treatment can involve an individual, family, couple, or group, depending upon the nature of the problem. The specific form of your therapy will also depend upon the theoretical orientation and background of your therapist. Some therapists focus discussion on your childhood and the past while others will emphasize the present. For some, the essential goal is insight into the cause of problems, while others work for direct behavior changes using very specific techniques. You may wish to ask your therapist about his or her orientation at the start of therapy so that you will know what to expect during your treatment.

The length of treatment varies depending upon the therapist, the client, and the nature of the presenting problem but it typically will last at least 10 or 12 weeks for relatively specific or situational problems. If your problems are severe, affect many areas of your life, or have persisted for a long period of time, therapy can last up to a year or even several years. Usually, after several sessions, the therapist can give you some idea of the estimated length of treatment. Generally, sessions are scheduled for once a week and last 45-50 minutes, giving the therapist the remainder of the hour to make notes which will aid in planning further treatment and assessing progress.

THERAPIST RESPONSIBILITIES

The therapist will usually devote the first few sessions to assessing the types and extent of problems or concerns you have. This process requires him or her to ask detailed questions about your history, life situation, and present distress. After the therapist has identified the specific problem areas, the two of you will agree upon a therapy plan including goals, methods to accomplish these goals, and approximate length of time to achieve the goals. Periodically, there should be a joint assessment of progress which may include reformulation of the goals.

If you require some medical treatment such as medication, the therapist will refer you to a physician, usually a psychiatrist. Therapy ordinarily will continue at the same time that you are receiving the additional medical treatment. If, at any time, your therapist believes that he or she can no longer be of help to you, another appropriate professional will be suggested.

CLIENT RESPONSIBILITIES

As a client in psychotherapy you will also have certain responsibilities. It is important for you to attend all of your scheduled appointments on time. Unlike many other appointments you may have, psychotherapy will start promptly at the designated time. If you are late, you will not have the benefit of a full session.

Equally important are the responsibilities you have to be as active, open, and honest as possible with your therapist. Your most important responsibility, however, is to work toward the goals you and the therapist have agreed upon. Seeing a therapist for one hour per week will be of little benefit without additional effort outside the therapy office. This work can include thinking about the material covered in your sessions, making yourself aware of your behavior, or working on specific assignments made by your therapist. Examples of the latter might be keeping a log, reading a special book, or practicing a new skill.

FEES

Another client responsibility is the prompt payment of fees. Many therapists will discontinue the treatment if fees are chronically unpaid. Fees for psychotherapy vary depending upon locality, treatment setting, and type of helping professional. If you are unable to afford the fees of a private practitioner, many mental health clinics have a sliding scale so that fees can be adjusted somewhat according to family income or ability to pay. Therapists differ as to when they require the fee to be paid: following each session or after a monthly billing. Policies for payment of missed sessions also vary.

Some therapists will expect you to pay for a missed session unless you cancel at least 24 hours in advance; except, of course, if your absence is due to an accident or illness.

Part or all of your fee may be paid by health insurance. However, even if you have insurance coverage, you are still responsible for the treatment fee. Some therapists are willing to collect the fee directly from the insurance company, while others will want you to pay the fee directly to them and then be reimbursed by your insurance company. To determine if you are eligible for insurance benefits, read your contract and call the insurance company, since recent changes may have been made which are not included in your contract. In general, you will want to check on three key elements: Does your insurance cover mental health services, does it apply to outpatient care, and will your company reimburse for the helping professional you have consulted (e.g., psychologist, social worker, or other).

CONFIDENTIALITY

The codes of ethics for psychotherapists and the state laws regulating most kinds of therapists consider the personal information you discuss to be confidential. This means that the helping professional may not reveal any information about you to another person without your explicit permission. Records of your treatment will be kept in a locked file. There are some very special circumstances which are exceptions to this rule. The therapist may discuss your case with a supervisor or with other professionals clearly concerned with the case. If your fees are paid by a third party, such as an insurance company, certain details of your treatment (e.g., dates of treatment and diagnosis) must be revealed to obtain reimbursement. Many insurance companies now allow you to file claims directly with them so that this information will not be seen by your employer.

In a very small number of situations, therapists are legally required to disregard confidentiality. For example, if you reveal information that indicates a clear danger of injury to yourself or others (e.g., potential suicide or homicide), the therapist will need to contact appropriate authorities or family members. Also, all helping professionals are required by law to report any knowledge of the abuse or neglect of a child or an incompetent or disabled person.

Finally, with your permission, some therapists may make audiotapes of your treatment sessions for their own review or for supervision of their work. However, they will not disclose the contents of these tapes to others without your written consent.

EFFECTIVENESS AND RISKS OF TREATMENT

Psychotherapy is a time-consuming and expensive endeavor so you will want to know about its effectiveness. The success of your therapy depends on a large variety of factors including the nature of your problems, the effort you put into the process, the type and length of treatment, and the therapist's skill. Nevertheless, on the average, two-thirds of all clients show improvement during therapy.

At times this process will involve the stirring up of painful or uncomfortable thoughts and feelings. It may also lead indirectly to the loss of important relationships, such as when a client experiencing marital difficulties decides to seek a divorce. Nevertheless, the overall gains you achieve through therapy should generally outweigh these potential risks.

HANDLING DISSATISFACTION WITH TREATMENT

It is not unusual to feel angry and upset at times about what happens in therapy. Questions or concerns about the treatment you receive should first be raised with your therapist. Exploring your thoughts and feelings, even when they are negative, is an important part of the therapy process. If after discussing the issues with your therapist you are still not satisfied, you have several options. You may seek a second opinion concerning your treatment. Another approach would be to switch to a new therapist. Competent therapists recognize and accept that they will be able to serve the needs of some clients better than others.

If you believe your therapist's behavior is either unethical or does not adhere to professional standards, you again have several alternatives. If your therapist is employed by a mental health agency, you may bring the matter to the attention of the program director. Another option you may choose is to contact the appropriate state or national professional association or the state licensing or certification board.

ALTERNATIVE SOURCES OF HELP

You should be aware that other helping systems exist that may be used in conjunction with or in place of therapy. Before engaging in one of these activities, you should discuss the decision with your therapist to assure that it will be a useful option for you at this time. You may want to consider:

--Individual self help such as educational books, recreational activities, or changes in your living or job situation.
--Peer support groups such as Parents Without Partners, Alcoholics Anonymous, or Weight Watchers.
--Crisis intervention services including crisis hotlines, rape crisis centers, and shelters for battered women.
--Assistance from other kinds of agencies such as legal, vocational, or pastoral counseling.

OTHER SPECIFIC QUESTIONS YOU MAY WANT TO ASK YOUR THERAPIST

1. What are the therapist's qualifications to help you (e.g., training, credentials, experience)?
2. What is the therapist's treatment orientation or philosophy?
3. What are the therapist's values in areas that may have special pertinence to you (e.g.,homosexuality, divorce, religion, non-traditional life styles)?
4. Are you permitted to phone the therapist between sessions or at night?
5. What arrangements does the therapist have for emergencies or for when he or she is out of town?

This guide was prepared and is copyrighted, 1982, by Patricia Lacks, Ph.D., Jennifer Stolz, M.A., and Jeffrey L. Levine, M.A. Reprinted by permission of the authors.

COPING WITH LOSS AND GRIEF

Loss is a common experience in the normal course of life. As people change and grow throughout a lifetime, certain aspects of their lives are left behind and they may experience a sense of loss in the process. For example, a person becoming a parent for the first time, while delighted over the new role, may nevertheless feel a loss of carefree youth. A person moving on to a new job may have sad feelings about leaving the old one even though it is a good change. Many people, likewise, experience a sense of loss when a close friend relocates to a distant community.

The death of a loved one is a particularly painful loss and it can feel traumatic and overwhelming. Such a loss may not only be unexpected, but may cause a more intense grief over a longer period of time. Most losses engender some form of a grief reaction which is not only normal, but desirable, since grief can actually have a healing effect.

WHAT IS GRIEF?

Grief is the total process of reacting and responding to the losses in our lives. It can be viewed primarily as a psychological process, but one which affects all aspects of our lives. Grief is experienced emotionally but can also affect our physical health, ability to work, and relations with other people. Grief, however, is different from mourning. Mourning refers to the activities or practices associated with loss that are a result of society's expectations. While grief may be a universal process related to our basic biological and psychological needs, mourning practices, such as funeral rites and the public display of emotion, may vary among communities, churches, families, and even individuals within families.

WHY DO WE GRIEVE?

Grief seems to serve a useful healing function when it is allowed to operate normally. The outcome of the grief process should be the resolution of the hurt and the re-establishment of one's life. Grief allows a "working through" of all the feelings, thoughts, and decisions that a loss can generate.

Many people find that their emotions change frequently throughout the grief process. Shock, disbelief, anger, fear, and depression are generally experienced at different times during the course of grieving until eventually a feeling of hopefulness toward the future once again returns. These strong and often painful emotions of the grief process may be a necessary step toward a true resolution of the loss.

CAN GRIEF AFFECT HEALTH?

Bereaved people commonly experience sleep and eating habit disturbances, loss of energy, and emotional upset. In addition, there is evidence that major losses may make a person more susceptible to illness. Because of this, a bereaved person should try to avoid any additional stresses during the grief period. Counselors also advise the bereaved to be cautious about making sudden or premature decisions that could be regretted later on. A widow, for instance, should not rush to a decision about selling her house.

WHAT CAN HELP THE GRIEF PROCESS?

In coping with loss, it is important to accept the natural grief process. People frequently expect their sadness and feeling of loss to last a relatively short period of time when it is likely that grieving may continue (although less frequently or less intensely) for many months. Having someone who will listen to your story or with whom you are able to share feelings can be very helpful. A good listener is someone who can listen to you uncritically and encourage you to share whatever is on your mind. Grief emotions may not always seem pleasant or "proper" but they are real and should not be criticized.

Many people want to tell their "story" over and over again, sometimes with new details that sadden, anger, or even amuse them. By allowing these emotions (crying, laughing, trembling, making angry noises, or whatever) people seem to move more directly through the grief process and are able to function better between these periods. A friend, spouse, relative, or pastor who is a good listener can be an effective aide in this process. Some people also find it helpful to share their feelings with another who has encountered a similar loss. No two people have had the same experience but someone who has "been there" can be a powerful ally. Many communities and churches have organized support networks of people who want to help those who have had losses similar to their own. Such programs as Widow-to-Widow or the Candlelighters (for parents who have lost children) may be available in your community.

WHEN IS PROFESSIONAL HELP NEEDED?

Some people find they need extra help during a major loss and seek a professional counselor for any of the following reasons:

  - They feel stuck in the grief process and are becoming depressed.
  - They do not feel able to express their feelings.
  - They cannot find anyone in their daily lives who is able to be the listener they need.
  - This loss stirs up other, older losses, and has caused them to explore long-standing feelings or emotional concerns.
  - They need reassurance and support to trust the grief process and to believe they can work through a particular loss.

DOES THE GRIEF PROCESS EVER END?

In the midst of grieving for a loved one, it may seem that the grief process will go on indefinitely and that there will be no end to the painful feelings. No amount of grieving will ever change the facts of the loss or erase important memories. When the grief process is allowed to work, however, the intense hurt does subside and the bereaved person can again feel hope for the future. People generally are able to resolve the loss and reorganize their lives in such a way that they may emerge strengthened by the re-examination of their lives caused by the loss.

WHERE CAN I LEARN MORE ABOUT GRIEF?

In addition to consulting a counselor, pastor, or family physician, a few particularly helpful books are listed below. There are other good books and resource organizations that you may wish to consult. Your counselor or one of the other professionals mentioned should be able to help you assess your needs and find the resources you require.

THE BEREAVED PARENT by H. S. Schiff, New York, Penguin Books, 1978.

HELP FOR YOUR GRIEF by A. Freese, New York, Schocken Books, 1977.

LOSS: AND HOW TO COPE WITH IT by J. E. Bernstein, New York, Houghton Mifflin, 1977.

This information was prepared by J. Dennis Murray, Ph.D., Associate Professor of Psychology, Mansfield University, Mansfield, PA 16933.

ABOUT YOUR APPOINTMENT FOR PSYCHOLOGICAL TESTING

If someone asks you to take psychological tests, you should free to ask about the reasons for the testing and how the results will be used. When you meet with the psychologist for the first time, he or she will usually want to get to know you, answer your questions, and make sure you feel as comfortable as possible before the testing begins. Psychological tests are widely used and are given for numerous reasons. These include testing to find out more about your personality (including the ways you typically behave, cope with situations, and feel about different things), your skills or ability to do different tasks, or such things as your work or school interests, attitudes, and levels of achievement. In spite of what you may have heard, a psychologist cannot "read your mind". The usefulness of the testing will depend to a large extent on your willingness to be honest and cooperative.

Personality Tests may be administered many different ways. Psychologists select the tests to give to a particular person based on the questions they are attempting to answer. For example, you may complete some "objective tests". These usually ask you to indicate how words or statements about thoughts, feelings, and actions apply to you. Other personality tests may require you to draw something or do other tasks. You might also be asked to describe things that you see when you look at different kinds of pictures or drawings. Some of these tests may not make complete sense to you, but they have all been carefully designed to help psychologists better understand your personality. You will receive clear instructions with each test.

Ability Tests may be used to help predict areas of job or school success or your ability to cope with different situations. While these tests may sometimes give a specific IQ or intelligence score, experience and research have shown that other things (such as motivation, attitude, and how you feel about yourself) are just as important in predicting how you will behave in different situations. These tests may ask you to answer general questions, solve problems, or complete different kinds of puzzles. Your skill on these tasks can then be compared to others who have taken the tests. You should not feel bad if you find some of the tasks to be difficult for you. Most people find that some tasks are easier for them than others, because ability tests are almost always designed so you will reach a point when some of your answers will be wrong.

No preparation is required for psychological testing. Studying for the tests would be of no help. In fact, many of the tests do not have simple "right" and "wrong" answers. You should try to get a good night's sleep and avoid a heavy meal just before your appointment. If you feel ill or have any unusual discomfort, please let us know as soon as possible before the appointment. It is important for you to show up on time for your testing appointment(s) since the psychologist has probably reserved several hours for your use.

Your Testing Appointment(s) Are Scheduled for:

Day:_____ Date:_____ Time:_____ - _____

Day:_____ Date:_____ Time:_____ - _____

INFORMATION FOR CONTRIBUTORS

The editors of INNOVATIONS IN CLINICAL PRACTICE welcome the opportunity to review manuscripts which are consistent with the goals of the series as described in the preface. Manuscripts will be reviewed only with the understanding that they are not simultaneously under consideration elsewhere. While we will attempt to handle all manuscripts with care, it is important to note that we assume no responsibility for unsolicited manuscripts. Any obligations we make to contributors are specified by written contract, and we reserve the right to accept or reject manuscripts at our discretion. All manuscripts which are accepted are subject to editing.

MANUSCRIPT SUBMISSION

Interested contributors should submit an original and two copies of manuscripts addressed to: Senior Editor, INNOVATIONS IN CLINICAL PRACTICE, Professional Resource Exchange, Inc., P. O. Box 15560, Sarasota, Florida 33577. All manuscripts will be acknowledged and authors will be notified following review. Contributions not accepted for publication can be returned only if authors include a large, self-addressed envelope with sufficient postage.

MANUSCRIPT PREPARATION

Brief contributions are preferred, and unsolicited manuscripts should not exceed 20, double-spaced, typed pages. Each manuscript should begin with a title page which includes the names, addresses and telephone numbers of the author(s). The second page should have the title centered at the top but should not contain the names of the author(s). No abstract is required. Manuscripts should generally follow the style specified by the PUBLICATION MANUAL OF AMERICAN PSYCHOLOGICAL ASSOCIATION (1974). There is, however, an exception in that each article should include a "resource" instead of a "reference" section and "reference notes." The use of footnotes is discouraged. Contributors may refer to the contents of the present volume for a general sense of the style which should be followed. Three levels of headings may be used to facilitate the organization of contributions: (a) a centered main heading, (b) a flush side heading, and (c) an indented side heading. Manuscripts should be written in a concise, professional, but readable manner. For example, writing in the first person is quite acceptable. Sexist language should be avoided.

ASSESSMENT INSTRUMENTS AND FORMS

The INNOVATIONS volumes contain informal clinical assessment instruments and checklists. We do not usually publish formal psychological tests. Assessment instruments are designed to help the clinician be more thorough in collecting information. Contributors of assessment instruments should write for the special instructions which pertain to this type of material.

NOW AVAILABLE . . .

CONTINUING EDUCATION CREDITS

THROUGH HOME STUDY

INNOVATIONS IN CLINICAL PRACTICE: A SOURCE BOOK is now available for continuing education study in your home or office. This best-selling, comprehensive source of practical clinical information is complemented by an examination module which may be used to earn continuing education credits.

Credits may be obtained by successfully completing an examination based on those contributions in each volume which have been selected by the editorial advisory board. Each of the contributions explores a timely topic designed to enhance your clinical skills and provide the knowledge necessary for effective practice. After studying these selections, a multiple-choice examination is completed and returned to the Professional Resource Exchange for scoring. Upon passing the examination (80% of test items answered correctly), your credits will be recorded and you will receive a copy of your official transcript. If desired, your credits may also be entered in the American Psychological Association's Registry for Continuing Education (for a small additional fee payable to the Registry).

The continuing education module for Volume I of **INNOVATIONS IN CLINICAL PRACTICE** will be available in July 1983 and contains examination materials for 20 credits. The Volume II module will be available in September 1983 and will earn approximately 20 credits. The cost of each module (exclusive of the volume) is only $45.00.

The **INNOVATIONS IN CLINICAL PRACTICE** Continuing Education Program is one of the most efficient ways to stay current on new clinical techniques and obtain formal credit for your study. If your professional associations and state boards do not currently require formal CE activities, you may still wish to consider this program as an excellent means of receiving feedback on your professional development. This self-study program is...

Relevant – selections are packed with information pertinent to your practice.

Inexpensive – typically less than half the cost of obtaining credits through workshops and these expenses are still tax deductible as a professional expense.

Convenient – study at your own pace in the comfort of your home or office.

Useful – the volume will always be available as a practical reference and resource for day-to-day use in your professional practice.

Effective – as a means of staying up to date and obtaining feedback on your knowledge acquisition and professional development.

The Professional Resource Exchange is approved by the American Psychological Association to offer continuing education for psychologists. Approval is limited to organizations and does not necessarily imply endorsement of individual offerings.

ORDER FORM ON NEXT PAGE

CONTINUING EDUCATION

ORDER FORM

I want to order **INNOVATIONS IN CLINICAL PRACTICE: A SOURCE BOOK.** Please send me:

Deluxe Binder Editions ($44.95 per copy)........ ___Volume I ___Volume II ... $_____

Hardbound Editions ($39.95 per copy).......... ___Volume I ___Volume II ... $_____

Continuing Education Modules ($45 per module).. ___Volume I ___Volume II ... $_____
        *(See note at bottom of this form regarding the CE Program)

      Florida residents: please add sales tax (5%).......................$_____
      Shipping & Handling (Books = $2.50 per copy in US, $3.50 foreign,
            CE Modules = postpaid in US, $2.00 foreign)....$_____

TOTAL ORDER (ORDERS FROM INDIVIDUALS & PRIVATE INSTITUTIONS MUST BE PREPAID)..$_____

Check or money order enclosed (USA currency)__ Please charge my: Mastercard__ Visa__

Credit Card Number:_____ Expiration Date:_____

Telephone: (____) ____-_____ Profession:_____ Highest Degree:____

Have you previously ordered from the Professional Resource Exchange? Yes___ No___

SHIP TO.......... _____
  (please print)
             _____

             _____

             _____

Please make checks payable to the Professional Resource Exchange & mail your order to:

  Professional Resource Exchange / Post Office Box 15560 / Sarasota, FL 34277-1560

Phone Orders (MasterCard & Visa only), call (813) 366-7913 (weekdays: 10:00-5:00 EST)

We usually ship in-stock items within 48 hours. Items ordered prior to publication will be shipped within 15 days after publication. If shipment will be delayed 30 days over normal shipping time, you will be notified and a refund will be made if desired. Fifteen day return privilege if not satisfied. Availability and prices on all products are subject to change without notice.

* Volume I Module earns 20 CE Credits. Available July 1983. Volume II Module will earn approximately 20 CE Credits. Available September 1983. In order to participate in either CE program, you must purchase the Module and either purchase or have access to the corresponding **INNOVATIONS** volume.

                               Revised: April 1983